LOCAL PUBLIC HEALTH PRACTICE: *TRENDS & MODELS*

Glen P. Mays, PhD, MPH
C. Arden Miller, MD
Paul K. Halverson, DrPH, MHSA

APHA
AMERICAN PUBLIC HEALTH ASSOCIATION
800 I ST NW
WASHINGTON DC 20001-3710

American Public Health Association
800 I Street, NW
Washington, DC 20001-3710

Mohammad N. Akhter, MD, MPH
Executive Director

2 M 3/2000
Library of Congress Catalog Card Number 99-073689

ISBN: 0-87553-243-8

Printed and bound in the United States of America.
Cover Design: Kathy Keler
Book Design and Typesetting: Jean-Marie Navetta
Production Support: Susan Westrate
Set in: Palatino and Futura
Printing and Binding: Automated Graphics Systems, Inc.

Table of Contents

Table of Contents

Authors

Glen P. Mays, PhD, MPH
Department of Health Policy and Administration, and
Center for Public Health Practice
School of Public Health
The University of North Carolina at Chapel Hill

C. Arden Miller, MD
Department of Maternal and Child Health
School of Public Health
The University of North Carolina at Chapel Hill

Paul K. Halverson, DrPH, MHSA
Department of Health Policy and Administration
School of Public Health
The University of North Carolina at Chapel Hill, and
Public Health Practice Program Office
Centers for Disease Control and Prevention

Contributors

Nancy Rawding, MPH
Public Health Policy Consultant, and
Immediate Past Executive Director,
National Association of County and City Health Officials

Carol Brown, MS
Director of Data and Community Assessment
National Association of County and City Health Officials

Thomas A. Bruce, MD
Emeritus Professor of Medicine
University of Arkansas Medical Sciences, and
Program Consultant and Advisor
W. K. Kellogg Foundation

Steven Uranga McKane, DMD, MPH
Former President
The California Endowment

Foreword

William H. Foege, MD, MPH

This marvelous book invites awe at the ingenuity and energy of thousands of public health workers who labor quietly in thousands of local health departments. Over 40 years ago I started my public health career at the Seattle-King County Health Department. In subsequent years, employment at state, national, and global levels made it clear to me that while coordination and plans are needed at all levels, the work gets done at the local health department. Every immunization given, every water supply treated, every surveillance system deployed, every illness reported, and every early death prevented in the final analysis involves the local health department.

It is also clear that any intervention introduced at a state, national, or global level must be based on experience and evidence of success at a local level. Some successful local interventions are never replicated, some become the basis for national policy, and some, such as the introduction of child restraints in automobiles, move directly from a local area to a state and then to other states without ever involving a national program.

Finally, it is clear, if public health is to lead to social justice in health, it will happen local health department by local health department.

What is less clear is how that actually happens. This book provides a wealth of information, describing a vast spectrum of approaches and policies. It presents no single clear path to success, and the authors conclude that one of the few generalizations they can make is that local public health departments "Differ from each other and they differ from their past."

The changes faced by local health departments are overwhelming. The breadth of activities was once dominated by infectious disease problems. Infectious diseases continue to require involvement in immunization programs, sanitation, nosocomial control, food inspection, and outbreak response. However, added to those duties is the maintenance of a complex infrastructure, maternal and child health, attention to injuries, chronic diseases, environmental health problems, occupational health, and mental health. Knowledge has exploded, tools are increasingly complex, and political demands are daunting. Not the least of the political problems is the education of politicians regarding the scope of public health. The response of local health departments demonstrates evolution in action. Therefore, it is safe to predict that the local health departments not only differ from each other and from the past, but they certainly differ from their future.

As Mays, Miller, and Halverson show, the response to our public health burden is heartening. There is an attempt to define core functions and respond accordingly. Yet there is no "job description" accepted by all. No norm that defines the gold standard. Whatever the historic reasons for such variability, the creativity and parallel research by local public health workers provides a wealth of experience on ways to get the job done. That may be the unifying theme. Local public health workers are problem solvers.

One surprise is the degree of accommodation to changes in managed care. In one study profiled in this book, about half of the local health departments maintained relationships with managed care plans—and half of those departments formed contractual relationships with these plans. This finding demonstrates the agility of local health departments but also highlights a challenge. Public health needs to define positive health outcomes that are useful in expanding the current HEDIS report cards. This could be done by using

Disability Adjusted Life Years (DALYs) or a similar metric, in a way that clearly defines the desired health outcomes and therefore the prevention activities that could and should be provided by the market place. This, in turn, becomes the basis for determining which activities and infrastructure need to be the responsibility of local health departments that are appropriately focused on population based interventions.

The book is incredibly rich. It points out the spectrum and heterogeneity of local health departments, their budgets, staffing, services, involvement in personal health services, and their relationships with states. Given the array of approaches, are there some generic lessons that favor success? Two seem apparent.

One of the important lessons is found in the description of other agencies that contribute to public health. The lesson is that the health leader of the present and future is clearly the person who can organize and lead a coalition. Local health departments lack the resources to implement what is now known about public health and the generic problems of poverty, illiteracy, and fatalism. However, the health officer who can clearly define shared goals for the health department and other groups has the opportunity to mobilize communities, corporations, service clubs, schools, and churches. An invested community is one of the secrets of a successful local health department.

The other lesson is to accept the fact that public health is inextricably bound to politicians and the political process. The successful health officer has built relationships with politicians. Politicians interested in public health make a major difference in the success of local health departments. That suggests two solutions. Those of us in public health must, first, become much better at providing politicians with information that compels their interest, and second, we should encourage public health people to seek political office.

A final challenge, public health response is best when it responds to problems with optimal information. The education of politicians, community groups, and individuals is also based on having the best information possible. Knowledge is power. The fact that the authors are concerned about a decline in the assessment function of local health departments is disquieting. However, pointing that out as a problem is already a step toward a solution, a reason for optimism. Why? Because local public health workers are problem solvers!

William H. Foege, MD, MPH
Presidential Distinguished Professor
Department of International Health
The Rollins School of Public Health
Emory University
Atlanta, Georgia
January 1999

Preface

As originally conceived, this book was to serve as a sequel and update to the collection of local health department case studies written by C. Arden Miller and Merry-K. Moos almost two decades ago (*Local Health Departments: Fifteen Case Studies.* American Public Health Association, 1981). As one of the few available resources offering a detailed, comparative analysis of health department structure and operation, this earlier work was so well received that it has continued to be used long after its content grew outdated. Local health departments have proven extremely malleable, changing rapidly in response to shifts in community health needs, resources, and priorities. Such shifts have been particularly extreme during the decades of the 1980s and 1990s, including the following: new and resurgent diseases; economic fluctuation; changes in political leadership; alterations in public health funding streams; and changes in the organization and financing of health services. In light of these changes, we endeavored to conduct a new series of case studies that would examine the current practice of public health at the local level.

Several considerations led us to deviate somewhat from the approach used in the original book of case studies. First, there are now many new sources of information about local health departments that did not exist at the time the original book was written. The National Association of County and City Health Officials (NACCHO) has conducted periodic surveys of their membership since the late 1980s, creating a wealth of information about health department structure and function. A number of other research and demonstration initiatives in local public health practice have been conducted by government agencies, foundations, and universities—including our own. In addition to case study analysis, this book uses many of these new information sources to examine larger trends in local public health practice.

Second, this book devotes much more attention to the public health contributions made by organizations other than the local health department. Recent studies have suggested that these contributions play important roles in the overall effectiveness of the local public health system. Moreover, current marketplace and health policy trends—such as managed care growth and public health privatization initiatives—appear to create incentives and even imperatives for collaboration among public health and other community health organizations. In light of these trends, this book includes substantial material examining the public health contributions made by other community organizations. As a consequence, the book is more a study of public health practice than of strictly local health departments.

The book is organized in four parts. Part One contains a series of chapters examining major trends and policy issues relevant to local public health practice. Chapter 1 provides an introduction to major methods of defining local public health practice and describing its infrastructure. In Chapter 2, contributors Nancy Rawding and Carol Brown discuss national trends in local health department structure and function, using data from the NACCHO surveys. Chapters 3 and 4 use data from other recent surveys to examine local health department interaction with other community organizations, and to measure the public health contributions made by these other organizations. In Chapter 5, contributors Thomas Bruce and Steven Uranga McKane describe the findings from a W. K. Kellogg Foundation's Community-Based Public Health demonstration initiative, which was designed to facilitate community and university participation in local public health practice. Chapter 6 provides a comparative analysis of the efforts maintained by state health agencies for assessing the performance of local public health practice. As the last chapter in this Part One, Chapter 7 examines longitudinal trends in local health department organization and operation using a selection of fifteen health departments observed over almost two decades.

Part Two presents a series of eight case studies in local public health practice. Chapter 8 describes the case study methodology and selection criteria used for these studies. Chapters 9 through 16 present the individual case studies. Part Three concludes the book by identifying a set of durable trends and themes derived from the case studies and cross-cutting chapters that illuminate important issues in public health policy and management. Finally, Part Four contains appendices that may be of interest to local public health practitioners and policy-makers, including a performance assessment tool and a list of study participants.

This book is written for a wide audience in public health. Local public health practitioners at all levels of government may identify promising new interorganizational models, strategies, and trends from the material presented here. Managers of other health-related organizations such as hospitals, health centers, and managed care plans may gain valuable insight regarding ways to engage in public health activities within their communities. Students of public health and health administration may acquire an enhanced understanding of the mechanics of local public health practice. Finally, health researchers and policy-makers may gain new insight into the policy options and research issues that yet need to be addressed in public health practice. We hope that this book will add to the discussion about the evolving roles of public health in a changing health environment.

Glen P. Mays
C. Arden Miller
Paul K. Halverson

Acknowledgments

This book represents the culmination of several years' work in studying local public health practice, and many individuals and organizations have made important contributions to this work during this time. A grant from the W. K. Kellogg Foundation provided critical support for data collection, analysis, and manuscript preparation. Steven Uranga McKane, formerly of the Kellogg Foundation and The California Endowment, provided important assistance in the early conceptual design of the book. Funding for the initial data collection and case study analysis was provided through a cooperative agreement between the Centers for Disease Control and Prevention and the Association of Schools of Public Health. Thomas B. Richards, MD, formerly at CDC's Public Health Practice Program Office and now with the National Center for Chronic Disease Prevention and Health Promotion, provided invaluable guidance and support throughout this effort.

This book benefited greatly from the reviews and recommendations made by members of our advisory panel, including the following: Doris Barnette at the US Health Resources and Services Administration; Thomas Bruce, MD, at the W. K. Kellogg Foundation; Steven Uranga McKane, DMD, MPH, at The California Endowment; Thomas B. Richards, MD, at the Public Health Practice Program Office, Centers for Disease Control and Prevention; and the following faculty members in the School of Public Health at the University of North Carolina at Chapel Hill: Janice Dodds, PhD (Department of Nutrition, and Center for Public Health Practice); Richard House, EdD (Center for Distance Learning and Health Communications); Arnold Kaluzny, PhD (Department of Health Policy and Administration, and Public Health Leadership Program); and Rachel Stevens, EdD (Center for Public Health Practice, and Public Health Nursing Curriculum).

This book would not have been possible without the substantial contributions of time and the candid contributions of information by the many organizations examined herein. These organizations are listed in Appendix D and include local and state health departments, hospitals, managed care plans, community health centers, and an array of other community organizations. We are truly grateful for their assistance.

Finally, we would like to thank Leslie Alexander-Alkins for research and editorial assistance and Sherry Rhodes for help with manuscript preparation.

Part I:

Trends and Issues in Local Public Health Practice

Chapter 1

Public Health and Its Infrastructure

Modern society protects the safety and promotes the health of people in a myriad of ways. Most of these function so efficiently and unobtrusively that they are taken for granted and not often recognized for their many supportive and protective services. Water can be taken from almost any faucet and used with confidence either to quench a child's thirst or to wash the family car. A bottle of aspirin can be purchased from any retailer with assurance that the labeled dose is accurate and free of toxic adulterants. Almost any restaurant or fast food purveyor is presumed to offer food that is free of contaminants that might cause illness. Automobiles, elevators, schools, playgrounds, job sites, and public buildings are all used by most people without serious thought for possible hazards to health and safety. People swim in motel pools presuming them to be maintained for purity of the water. In the event of sudden illness or injury, we expect easy access to emergency rooms or urgent care centers that are staffed with qualified personnel offering diagnostic and treatment services that conform to high standards of professionalism. Patients and their families seldom question the reliability of hospital laboratories, blood banks, or medical record keeping. Parents send their children to school without expecting them to be exposed to measles or tuberculosis. Every minute of our lives we unwittingly depend on societal protections to assure health, quality of life, and longevity. As a consequence we are a healthier and longer-lived people than any generation in any place before us.

Not all of these protections work consistently. There are lapses. Isolated instances are known when public water supplies are rendered dangerous from contaminating parasites or industrial wastes. Aquifers are threatened by depletion and incursion of sewage or salt water. Some schools persist with asbestos ceiling tiles, and many homes continue to threaten the health of children with flaking lead paint or faulty heating systems. Not all job sites are carefully monitored for safety. Some populations of children are not adequately immunized, resulting in school-based outbreaks of measles. Personnel with fake or absent credentials sometimes are identified on hospital staffs. Mandated screening and treatment programs may fail to reach some populations with a demonstrated need for them. The many protective programs that are known to work effectively do not consistently reach all populations, especially those who are vulnerable for reason of socioeconomic or racial circumstance.

Protection of the Public's Health

Finding the causes for gaps and lapses in public health preventive and protective programs requires a look at the many entities, both public and private, that are responsible for implementing them. Many of the programs are undergirded by governmental standard setting and regulation. All levels of government are involved. The federal government is primarily responsible for programs that are involved with interstate commerce, such as safety of food, drugs, and appliances. State and local government are primarily responsible for safety of schools, water supplies, waste disposal, and housing. At local and state levels, officially designated public health agencies may share responsibility with environmental protection agencies to assure safety of air, water, and other environmental conditions. Multiple agencies are operative at every level of government in efforts to protect the public's health.

Governmental authority for public health is also extensively shared with private entities and professional groups. Licensure, accreditation, and standard setting for hospitals and health care professionals and providers are extensively regulated and implemented by nonprofit voluntary professional organizations. Their work is not as independent of governmental authority as may appear on the surface. The services rendered by licensed and accredited providers are extensively subsidized by governmental financing, often through public insurance programs such as Medicare and Medicaid. Eligibility for such financing is dependent on compliance with governmentally established standards and regulation.

In the domain of personal health care, private providers are paramount. Increasingly, they are organized into groups, many of which assume clinical and financial responsibility for the health care of defined populations through managed care plans. Such care is well established in the event of injury or illness. The extent that needs for preventive care, screening, and population-based health status assessments will be fulfilled by these plans is still uncertain. Early results suggest the probability of cost savings by the expansion of managed care plans, but the extent that this benefit derives from curtailment of legitimate and necessary care requires careful study. These matters are the subject of subsequent chapters.

In order for the complex array of society's protective and preventive health services to function well, certain essential or core functions must be assured. These include assessments of a population's health status, investigation of adverse health events such as injuries or disease outbreaks, and analysis of vital statistics data and reported diseases in order to identify trends. For standards and regulations to be meaningful, careful monitoring for compliance is essential if corrective measures are to be taken. Because resources are finite, priorities must be established and plans for improvements agreed upon. The effectiveness of all these efforts must be evaluated and entered into the dynamics of political process in order to assure and modify continuing support as necessary. The public must be informed and educated about behaviors that are detrimental and about supportive and protective community services that may not be readily visible but that are essential for maintaining a community's health. These essential public health services will be elaborated subsequently, but they are described in general terms here in order to emphasize the complex protective interactions of both private and public health care providers.

Tensions among all the public and private players in the provision of health care cannot be ignored. They must be recognized and freed of destructive influences that may jeopardize the public's good health. Some of the tensions are venerable, such as the suspicions with which private providers and public agencies sometimes regard each other. The private sector resists regulation, standard setting, and monitoring that may limit enterprise, cause delays, and appear to intrude into domains thought to be sufficiently protected by professional competence. Public agencies may, however, legitimately question the extent that profit seeking may be responsible for self-serving trade-offs with the potential for neglecting or exploiting the health of workers or vulnerable populations.

Disagreement with a long history centers around the extent to which public health agencies render personal health care that might also be provided in private offices or clinics. Early in this century, a federal program to help finance and improve neglected maternal and child health services in state and local public health clinics was abandoned under the charge that it represented unfair competition with private professional interests. Nevertheless, about 75% of local health departments provide personal health care for programs such as prenatal care, immunizations, diagnosis and treatment of sexually transmitted disease, tuberculosis control, family planning, screening for hypertension and diabetes, and similar services.[1] One view holds that these programs all should be left to private providers, as might be possible if everyone were enrolled in a managed care plan. Public health agencies could then devote themselves to a narrower role of community protection emphasizing health status assessments and environmental issues.

A rejoinder claims that the assurance function of public health requires that public agencies provide those services and reach those people that private markets fail to adequately address. Public health agencies in this context are regarded as the residual guarantor for essential services, whatever they may be. Not surprisingly, private providers have traditionally not rendered services in an equitable fashion when profits were not appealing. This was apparent even in the 18th century with the establishment of public hospitals and clinics in port cities to serve the medical needs of able seamen. Survival of the young republic depended on fostering a strong maritime trade. Assuring the health and vigor of seamen seemed a legitimate role for government in the absence of alternate providers. In the intervening years, the list of services and people requiring governmental support and protection has lengthened. The list includes health care for military personnel (and in emergencies, such as World War II, for their dependents); care of American Indians on reservations; and care of the poor or uninsured people, especially uninsured childbearing women and children unable to pay for care in private markets. Some conditions requiring a complicated mixture of expensive services over a prolonged period have not been attractive to profit-inspired providers with the result that extensive public service or financing systems have developed. These include programs to cope with mental illness and other chronically disabling conditions. Contagions that represent an epidemic threat to community health have tended to fall in the public domain, such as control of tuberculosis, leprosy, and sexually transmitted disease. Finally, medical care for some populations has come to represent a prerogative of privilege, such as medical care for high officers of federal government and care for military veterans in public hospitals and clinics.

Another challenge to personal health care as rendered in public health clinics is the charge that it represents poor care for poor people. This assertion is seriously cast in doubt by growing evidence that for some care the outcomes are better in public clinics than when comparable people are cared for in private offices and clinics.[2] This is true of pre- and postnatal care in public health department clinics. The advantage in those settings appears to be the combination of nonmedical supportive services, including nutritional supplementation and counseling, home visiting, and transportation and linkage to social services.

If all people had health insurance, or were enrolled as necessary in managed care plans at public expense, there is no question that the need for rendering personal health care in public clinics would be drastically altered. Best prospects would be for appropriate and universal care by private plans at the time of acute illness or injury. Doubts persist on the extent that such plans will routinely and universally provide preventive services such as immunizations and screenings for problems of hearing, vision, developmental delay, or chronic illness. In theory, such preventive programs are reasoned to be attractive because in the long run they will save money and reduce costs for more expensive care. But many managed care plans are not able to engage in long-range commitments to their enrollees. Contracts are written for a year or two at most. The average duration of a Medicaid client's enrollment in managed care is currently 9 months.[3] Managed care plans cannot be expected to invest in preventive programs that will lower costs only for their successor contractors.

Cost savings within the health care sector can reasonably result from protective and preventive services. For example, family planning costs less than the care and management of unwanted childbearing; immunization programs are less costly than coping with a measles epidemic. But additional substantial savings from preventive programs accrue to sectors outside of health care, such as the education and criminal justice systems. Children damaged by abuse and neglect or by measles encephalitis incur expensive costs in both these systems. The costs are not fully borne by managed care plans; therefore their prevention may not automatically be regarded as a profitable investment by market-driven plans.

The danger is that short-term cost savings may be obtained through neglect, i.e. failure to identify nonemergency chronic conditions requiring expensive care. No good evidence yet supports a claim that all managed care plans can or will provide the indicated specialty and supportive services for chronic illness, disabling conditions, or hard to reach vulnerable populations. The need for publicly provided supplementary services for some people and for some conditions will very likely persist.

Contracts written by the states to enroll Medicaid clients in managed care can, of course, specify the full extent of services that are obligated under the contract. Similarly, state and federal legislation can specify these service provisions for other managed care enrollees. Detailed specificity in contracts and in managed care regulations might assure that all indicated preventive services are rendered. A study by the George Washington University Health Policy Center revealed that among existing Medicaid contracts none specify the full range of services that are mandated by federal government as a part of the Early Periodic Screening Diagnosis and Treatment for children enrolled in Medicaid.[3] Most contracts fall back on phrasing that requires services "as appropriate." Recent rulings establish that in the absence of specifically detailed provisions in the contract the managed care plans are at liberty to determine what is appropriate. The states are not freed from the federal mandates. Fulfilling these mandates outside the managed care plans through work of the public health infrastructure may be necessary and possible provided the states have not given away all their health care money under terms of the faulty contracts.

In future years, Medicaid managed care contracts and managed care regulations may be tightened but probably at substantially increased cost. Whether managed care plans and the states can agree on a price for a full spectrum of preventive and supportive services for vulnerable populations is problematic. Many states may opt to contract for the predictable expense of care for the sick and injured and to provide directly the basic preventive services, many of which are of a nonmedical nature, through public clinics. Such duality of care is the pattern adopted by many other industrialized nations in order to assure full participation of all populations in basic preventive care.[4]

The need for continued personal health care in public health clinics seems assured. The need may even grow, as the nation appears to move farther from universal coverage for medical care. In this country, the number of uninsured people, especially children, is increasing and likely will increase even more as welfare revisions serve further to reduce Medicaid eligibility and benefits. Hospital ethics in this country probably will attend by means of cost shifting (increasingly difficult) to the acute care needs of these children and their families. Only public clinics convincingly show promise for attending to their well child care, preventive services, and nonmedical health care needs.

Defining Public Health

The patterns of health care in both public and private sectors are rapidly changing. Defining these patterns has attracted considerable careful thought. A decade ago the Institute of Medicine exercised leadership in these efforts by publishing a report on the condition of the nation's public health systems.[5] The analysis was not in every way flattering, giving emphasis to the many gaps and inconsistencies in the nation's public health services and agencies. These shortcomings led to the conclusion that public health was in disarray, a finding amply justified by many weaknesses identified in the report. The appearance of disarray is explained in part by the pernicious underfunding of public health services and agencies. For the past quarter century, money has been lavished on every sector of health care except for public health. In the dynamics of policy negotiation, the up-front needs of people and institutions coping with dread disease are much more obvious and compelling than backstage efforts to keep people healthy. Semblance of disarray is further promoted by the extensive local geopolitical discretion that characterizes public health effort. Organized public health programs come close to being considered a local option, taking a lesser priority than schools, prisons, and highways.

Having helped identify the need for improved public health services, the Institute of Medicine report made a major policy contribution by defining the public health mission in more precise and succinct terms than previously. The IOM formulations were reconfirmed in a report published in 1996.[6] The public health mission they describe is threefold: assessment, policy development, and assurance. A work group of public health leaders convened by the Centers for Disease Prevention and Control (CDC) elaborated these three core functions by linking them with a set of 10 public health practices as follows[7]:

Assessment is the regular systematic collection, assembly, analysis, and dissemination of information on the health of the community. Assessment practices are specifically the following:

1. Assess the health need of the community
2. Investigate the occurrence of health effects and health hazards of the community
3. Analyze the determinants of identified health needs.

Policy Development is the exercise of the responsibility to serve the public interest in the development of comprehensive public health policies by promoting the use of the scientific knowledge base in decision making. Policy development practices are specifically the following:

4. Advocate for public health, build constituencies and identify resources in the community
5. Set priorities among health needs
6. Develop plans and policies to address priority health needs.

Assurance is the assurance to constituents that services necessary to achieve agreed-on goals are provided by encouraging actions of others (public or private), requiring action through regulation, or by providing services directly. Assurance practices are specifically the following:

7. Manage resources and develop organizational structure
8. Implement programs
9. Evaluate programs and provide quality assurance
10. Inform and educate the public.

Under sponsorship by CDC, several groups of investigators used these definitions of public health practice to develop systems of surveillance in order to measure the adequacy of public health practice in local geopolitical jurisdictions.[8,9] Each of the 10 practices was linked to a set of measurable indicators for this purpose. The methods and results of these surveys will be subsequently reviewed.

As these efforts were in progress, major health policy deliberations were undertaken by the Clinton administration. An elaborate legislative proposal emerged featuring universal enrollment of everyone in managed care plans. Implicit in the proposal was the assumption that if everyone were enrolled in private plans that provided for the full range of personal health care, then the need for preventive and supportive personal health care from public providers would be greatly diminished and possibly not necessary at all. In the context of this thinking, the mission for public health was redefined. Seven essential public health services were proposed. They represented a constricted version of the public health mission, omitting any reference to the assurance function. The new formulation was defended by the office of the Assistant Secretary of the Department of Health and Human Services (DHHS) by claiming that in the negotiations for reform the assurance function was not well understood by all the interests represented, including the companies that would manage universal health insurance coverage. This assertion invited speculation that perhaps the assurance function was understood all to well by negotiators but was unacceptable to a vision of private hegemony over health care.

The administration's proposal for health care reform failed to pass Congress, but efforts by DHHS to redefine the public health mission continued. The list of 7 essential public health services was expanded to 8, and then for a time to 12.[10] The currently proposed list of 10 essential public health services restores the concept of an assurance function for public health among the following provisions:

- Monitor health status to identify and solve community health problems
- Diagnose and investigate health problems and health hazards in the community
- Inform, educate, and empower people about health issues
- Mobilize community partnerships and action to solve health problems
- Develop policies and plans that support individual and community health efforts
- Enforce laws and regulations that protect health and assure safety
- Link people to needed personal health services and assure the provision of health care when otherwise unavailable
- Assure a competent work force—public health and personal health care
- Evaluate effectiveness, accessibility, and quality of personal and population-based health services
- Research for new insights and innovative solutions to health problems.

This formulation of the public health mission has been reviewed and accepted by leading public health organizations and is being vigorously promoted by DHHS. As yet no measurable indicators have been attached to the services, although that effort is in progress. Until it is successfully completed, the descriptions for the 10 essential services are of limited value for measuring public health performance.

Another effort to define and describe core public health functions was initiated by the World Health Organization (WHO) in 1997, drawing on the knowledge and experiences of an international collection of public health experts.[11] By using a Delphi process with 145 public health administrators, educators, researchers, and practitioners, the WHO study identified and prioritized a list of 37 essential public health functions that fell within nine general categories:

- Prevention, surveillance, and control of communicable and noncommunicable diseases
- Monitoring the health situation (health status, determinants, risks, and interventions)
- Health promotion
- Occupational health
- Protecting the environment
- Public health legislation and regulations
- Public health management
- Specific public health services (school health, emergency services, and laboratory services) and
- Personal health care for vulnerable and high risk populations.

With straightforward modifications, the public health categorizations identified by CDC, DHHS, and WHO approximate each other, but it is likely that none of them represents the last word for defining the complex role of public health in modern society. A recent survey of state health commissioners revealed that many of them are attempting to measure public health performance in their local jurisdictions (see Chapter 6).[12] All of them appreciate the assistance that both of the above formulations have provided, but no state is using either formulation in an unaltered form. Although the means are still imperfect, the need to define the public health mission in measurable terms has become widely accepted; many constructive efforts are underway. Considering the great variability in public health structure and function in different states, it is not surprising that each state has found it necessary to develop methods responsive to their different local needs.

Measuring Performance

Proposals for measuring the adequacy of public health performance have been offered repeatedly in the United States for the past 70 years, since shortly after the establishment of local health departments became widespread. The conceptual bases for many of these proposals are reviewed elsewhere.[13] Even as the need for evaluating the adequacy of public health practice became well established, no consistent plan of evaluation was put into practice. Licensure of public health agencies and workers, based on some presumed national standard of performance, was often discussed but never implemented. Public health agencies justified their efforts largely through reports on encounter tallies such as the number of immunizations rendered, prenatal visitations, and septic tanks inspected. These reports seldom included population-based denominators or data on unmet need. The presumption was strong that if public health agencies increased their encounters each year, the population's health was well served and further support for the agency was justified.

New efforts to improve these circumstances by developing a surveillance system to measure local public health performance were initiated by CDC in 1991. Contracts were issued to several university-based schools of public health for this purpose. Turnock and Handler at the University of Illinois and Miller and colleagues at the University of North Carolina at Chapel Hill shared perspectives and developed similar proposals. This book features performance measures derived from the Miller approach for the reason that they center on assessment of the contribution to public health practice by all providers in a jurisdiction, both public and private, rather than limiting performance measure to the role of the local health department.

The organizing framework for the surveillance system consists of the three core functions formulated by the Institute of Medicine and linked to the 10 practices previously described (not to be confused with the 10 essential services of DHHS). A group of indicators was developed for each practice drawing on materials from many sources, including Objectives for the Nation for the Year 2000.[8] Eight to 10 indicators were selected for each practice, yielding a total of 84 indicators. Responses to the survey were obtained from local health department directors. Results yielded scores for the surveyed jurisdiction with regard to adequacy of performance for each practice, the proportional contribution to performance by the local health department, and the identification of other providers contributing to the coverage of each practice within the jurisdiction. Schematic representation of the results can be presented in graphic form as illustrated in **Figure 1**. Note that the top graph line for each public health jurisdiction illustrates the extent that it is served by all providers according to each of the 10 practices. The bottom graph

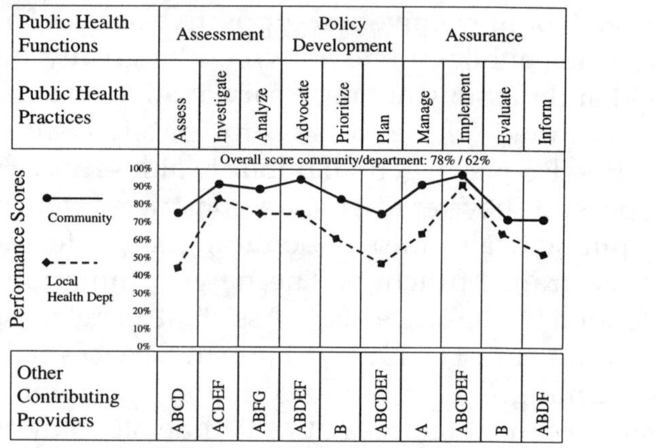

Other provider codes: A=state agencies; B=local agencies; C=nonprofit agencies; D=hospitals; E=community health centers; F=universities; G=other.

Source: Miller CA, Moore KS, Richards TB, Monk JD. A proposed method for assessing the performance of local public health functions and practices. Am J Public Health *1994:84(11):1743-1749.*

Figure 1. Public health performance profile for a sample community and local health department.

line illustrates the contribution to each of the practices by the local health department. The decimal notations in the line immediately under the graphs shows scores representing performance within the jurisdiction for each of the three core functions and the proportion of each function performed by the local health department. The alphabetical key at the bottom of the graphs gives an indication of providers other than the local health department that make contributions to each of the 10 practices. The survey protocol and scoring methods that yield these data are available in the appendix.

Although variation in levels of performance is great, on average across the country public health care is being performed at about 50% of a theoretical ideal level of practice, and on average about 25% of public health performance is rendered by organizations other than the local health department.[8]

A shortened version of the protocol (26 indicators) was tested in all local jurisdictions in six states and shown to correlate reliably with scores obtained from the longer protocol for overall public health performance, as well as for performance of each of the three core functions and for some of the 10 practices.[14] A subset of four indicators was shown to predict reliably the overall score.[15] The 26 indicators used for the abbreviated or screening survey follow. The four key overall indicators are shown in italics.

Assessment

1. In the past 3 years in your jurisdiction has there been a health needs assessment that included

using morbidity, mortality, and vital statistics data?

2. *In the past 3 years in your jurisdiction have there been age-specific surveys to assess participation in preventive and screening services?*
3. In the past 3 years in your jurisdiction has the population been surveyed for behavioral risk factors?
4. In the past year in your jurisdiction has there been timely investigation of any unusual adverse health event?
5. In the past 3 years in your jurisdiction has there been a review of hospital discharge data to determine age-specific leading causes of hospitalization?
6. In the past 3 years in your jurisdiction has there been a review of work-related morbidity and mortality?
7. In the past 3 years in your jurisdiction has there been an analysis of data on children two years of age who have been immunized with the basic series?
8. In the past 3 years in your jurisdiction has there been an analysis of health services needed by high-risk population groups?

Policy Development

9. In the past 3 years has there been a public review of the public health mission for your agency's jurisdiction?
10. In the past year, as a part of the job, have you and your senior staff embers regularly participated in meetings with other community health organizations?
11. In the past year in your jurisdiction has there been a formal attempt at informing elected officials about the potential public health impact of actions under their consideration?
12. In the past year in your jurisdiction have elected or other government officials been strong advocates for public health?
13. In the past 3 years in your jurisdiction have community health initiatives been prioritized on the basis of established problems and resources?
14. In the past 3 years has your health department published an explicit policy agenda for the department?
15. *In the past year has there been a formal attempt to inform candidates for elective office about health priorities for your jurisdiction?*
16. In the past year in your jurisdiction has a community health action plan, developed with shared input from local, regional, and state levels, been used?
17. *In the past year in your jurisdiction has a community health action plan, developed with public participation, been used?*
18. In the past 3 years has your health department entered into any written agreements with key health providers or funding sources to define service roles?

Assurance

19. In the past 3 years in your jurisdiction have local health codes been reviewed to assure they are up to date?
20. In the past 3 years in your jurisdiction have public health services been reviewed to assure they comply with applicable professional and regulatory standards?
21. In the past year in your jurisdiction has there been a program to assure environmental safety?
22. In the past year in your jurisdiction has there been a program to assure access to basic personal health services for those unable to afford them?
23. *In the past year in your jurisdiction has there been any evaluation of the effect that public health services have on community health?*
24. In the past year in your jurisdiction has there been any evaluation of the effect that budget changes for your health department would have on public health programs?
25. In the past year in your jurisdiction has there been a formal attempt at informing the public about health problems?
26. In the past year in your jurisdiction have reports on public health problems been provided to the local media?

The four key indicators in italics are of special interest. Scores on these items correlate closely with the overall performance score for the entire survey. Use of the four indicators independent of the others is of doubtful value, but they have important conceptual significance. They represent health status assessment, community-based planning, political action, and evaluation—a defensible foundation for all of public health practice.

In a later stage of analysis, the 26 indicators listed above were condensed and merged with similar indicators developed by Turnock and Handler.[13] The resulting 20 merged indicators are listed in the appendix. They show promise for standard setting in future surveys.[16]

Public Health Infrastructure

No one would claim that public health can be characterized fully by the work of local and state official public health agencies. Many other providers are appropriately and effectively involved. Conversely, no one would claim that public health practice requirements can be fulfilled without the official agencies. In major respects, their work undergirds all others.

This book is about local health departments, their work, their interactions with other organizations, both public and private at state and local levels, and their responsiveness to the current climate of rapid change in health care, emphasizing market-driven policies. Chapter 2 provides the most recent data available about the nation's approximately 3000 local health departments, drawing on information from the National Association of County and City Health Officials. Chapter 5, authored by individuals from the W. K. Kellogg Foundation, describes work with a group of local health departments constructively involved in demonstration projects featuring participatory action by community groups. Chapter 5 gives deserved emphasis to a concept of community different from the geopolitical orientation emphasized by other chapters. The demonstration projects feature community endeavor strengthened by a sociocultural approach to community action by users of public health services.

Other chapters describe findings from studies on local health departments that have been ongoing at The University of North Carolina at Chapel Hill School of Public Health for 20 years (Chapters 3, 4, and 7). Those studies include detailed case studies on a group of 15 departments identified in 1979 as exemplary in the performance of public health practice. Those departments continue to be studied over the intervening years. Findings are amplified by results from performance surveys of more than 300 other departments in 18 states. Detailed case studies are presented for a number of local jurisdictions (Chapters 9-16) in order to amplify findings and to provide models that may be of value to other jurisdictions coping with rapid change.

From these efforts, we demonstrate that public health as practiced at local levels in many communities, while by no means perfect, is dynamic, interactive with agencies involved with the latest trends in health care, and responsive to the changing circumstances of the demography and health status of populations within their jurisdictions. People who perceive that public health at local levels is bound by tradition will find no comfort in these presentations. Decision makers for public policy may well find evidence for favorable consideration of better support for the public health infrastructure in their own communities and across the nation as a whole.

References

1. National Association of County and City Health Officials. *1992-1993 National Profile of Local Health Departments*. Washington, DC: National Association of County and City Health Officials; 1995.
2. Buescher PA, Ward NI. A comparison of low birth weight among Medicaid patients of public health departments and other providers of prenatal care in North Carolina and Kentucky. *Public Health Rep*. 1992;107(1):54-59.
3. Rosenbaum S, Shin P, Smith BM, et al. *Negotiating the New Health System: A Nationwide Study of Medicaid Managed Care Contracts*. Washington, DC: Center for Health Policy Research, George Washington University; 1997.
4. Williams B, Miller CA. *Preventive Health Care for Young Children. Findings from a Ten-country Study and Directions for United States Policy*. Arlington, Va: National Center for Clinical Infant Programs; 1991.
5. Institute of Medicine. *The Future of Public Health*. Washington, DC: National Academy Press; 1988.
6. Institute of Medicine. *Healthy Communities. New Partnerships for the Future of Public Health*. Washington, DC: National Academic Press; 1996.
7. Dyal WW. *Public Health Infrastructure and Organizational Practice Definitions*. Atlanta, Ga: Atlanta Division of Public Health Systems, Public Health Practice Program Office, Centers for Disease Control; August 22, 1991.
8. Miller CA, Moore KS, Richards TB, McKaig CA. A proposed method for assessing public health functions and practices. *Am J Public Health*. 84(1):1743-1749.
9. Turnock BJ, Handler AS, Hall W, Potsie S, Nalluri R, Vaughn EH. Local health department effectiveness in addressing the core functions of public health. *Public Health Rep*. 1994;109(5):653-658.
10. Harrell, JA. The essential services of public health. Paper presented at the CDC Conference on Public Health Performance Measures. Atlanta, Ga: Centers for Disease Control and Prevention; June 1994.
11. Bettcher DW, Sapirie S, Goon EHT. Essential public health functions: results of the international Delphi study. *World Health Stat Q*. 1998;51(1):44-54.

12. Mays GP, Miller CA, Halverson PK. Assessing the performance of local public health systems: a survey of state health agency efforts. *J Public Health Manage Pract*. 1998;4(4):63-78.
13. Turnock BJ. *Public Health: What It Is and How It Works*. Gaithersburg, Md: Aspen Publishers; 1997.
14. Miller CA, Richards TB, Davis SM, et al. Validation of a Screening Survey to assess local public health performance. *J Public Health Manage Pract*. 1995;1(1):63-71.
15. Miller CA, Richards TB, Christenson GM, Kock GC. Creating and validating practical measures for assessing public health practice in local communities. *Am J Prev Med*. 1995;11(suppl 6):24-28.
16. Turnock, BJ, Handler, AS and Miller, CA. Core function related local public health practice effectiveness. *J Public Health Manage Pract*. 1998; 4(5):26-32.

Chapter 2

An Overview of the Nation's Health Departments

Contributed by Nancy Rawding and Carol Brown

The goal of this chapter is to provide an overview of the structure, functions, contributions, and challenges of local health departments nationwide. There are 2832 local health departments across the country, and they vary considerably with respect to services provided, size, budget, and many other characteristics (National Association of County and City Health Officials (NACCHO), unpublished data, April 1998). Along with these variabilities, there are important similarities in both mission and method for detecting disease and promoting health within communities.

Mission and Functions of Local Health Departments

The basic mission of local health departments nationwide is to protect and promote the health of the public. The specific services provided to fulfill this mission vary from state to state, within states, and over time. One significant change in the last 30 years has been a greater emphasis on local health departments as community leaders. In 1973, John Hanlon suggested that, "the official health agency might better concentrate upon its important and unique potential as community conscience and leader. Governmental agencies, such as local departments of health, are in the best possible position to sense the need for and to promote the establishment of social policy."[1] This point was further accentuated in 1979. The Model Standards for Community Preventative Health Services stated that public health must have "a governmental presence at the local level."[2] This concept, which became known as "AGPALL," provided a useful framework for the development of local health services and orientation to the community. Several other initiatives followed in the 1980s and 1990s that facilitated greater working relationships between the local health department and its community. The Institute of Medicine released its statement on public health, which described the mission of health departments in terms of three core functions[3] and later a federal workgroup delineated a set of 10 essential services for public health agencies.[4]

Historical Perspective

Local health departments (LHDs) have long played a major role in assuring and protecting the health of the nation's population. The first step in the formation of local health departments occurred in the late 18th and early 19th centuries when it became a trend to employ full-time persons to serve as the functional agents of local boards of health. City health departments were established before state health departments and well before county health departments. Health departments were established in Baltimore, Md (1798); Charleston, SC (1815); Philadelphia, Pa (1818); Providence, RI (1832); Chicago, Ill (1835); and Cambridge, Mass (1846). In 1866, New York City was the first to formally establish a central administration for health activities called the Metropolitan Board of Health.[5]

As the nation moved into the 20th century, many more public health departments were created, and these departments continued to refine their activities. In 1908, there were no county health departments, and by 1920, there were 131.[5] Gradually, American ambivalence about government interference gave way to a desire for the benefits that government intervention could provide to the public through sanitation, control of communicable disease, and other traditional public health activities.[5] By 1953, Joseph Mountin reported 1239 LHDs (963 county and 276 city units).[6] By the mid-1970s, 1980 local health departments were identified and their role in providing direct personal health services was documented.[7]

Since 1989 the National Association of County and City Health Officials (NACCHO) has conducted three separate studies of local health departments nationwide and has consistently found ~2900 health departments, though the precise number has varied a bit. In 1997, 2832 local health departments were identified by the following widely used definition of a local health department (NACCHO, unpublished data, April 1998): "an administrative or service unit of local or state government, concerned with health, and carrying some responsibility for the health of a jurisdiction smaller than a state."

Characteristics of Local Health Departments

Local health departments vary considerably with respect to their organization, specific services provided, the type and number of staff employed, and many other variables. These differences are primarily a function of the size and wealth of the community served, the organization within the state, state statutes, and availability of services from other providers.

The number of local health departments within each state can also vary tremendously and often has no direct relationship to the geographic or population size of the state. For example, California, one of the largest states in land size (nearly 156 thousand square miles) and also the most populous state with an estimated 30 million people in 1992, has 62 local health departments. This includes 58 county health departments and 4 city health departments. However, Massachusetts, one of the smaller states in land size (nearly 8000 square miles) and home in 1992 to an estimated 6 million people, has 325 local health departments/units. These are primarily city and town departments.

A question often voiced is why this number varies so greatly by state. The answer is complex and dependent, in part, on the history of state and local government and related culture. For example, it follows that the many townships developed in Massachusetts in the 1600s by the English incorporated many aspects of the English system, including a strong emphasis on town development and home rule. These towns were eventually incorporated and began to develop governmental services including health departments. Western states, largely organized some 200 years later, were more apt to organize local government functions around county political boundaries and in the context of expanded communication and transportation systems.

Relationship of Local Health Departments to State and Local Government

Today, local health departments are primarily entities of city, county, or town government. In some states, several counties with small populations have come together, or have been grouped together by the state, to form district health departments. Economies of scale have proved useful. In other states, county and city governments have not created local health departments; rather, the state health department has established offices throughout the state and provides services to the local level.

The majority of local health departments continues to be entities of county government. Nationwide, 61% are single county health departments, 10% are city-county jurisdictions, and 7% are multicounty health departments. Thus, a total of 78% are county related. Eight percent are entities of city government alone, such as New York City, Houston, Chicago, and Long Beach, and 10% are agencies of a town or township. Eleven percent of local health departments serve districts (NACCHO, unpublished data, April 1998).

Typically, local health departments derive authority from both state statutes and from their local government. The relationships between the state and local health departments vary from state to state, and even within states. The differences can be analyzed along lines of autonomy. In the majority of states, LHDs operate with some or considerable independence from state health departments. The local health department will develop its own budget, set priorities, and maintain its own staff and personnel systems. In other states, budget development, priority setting, and hiring and firing are conducted by the state health department. There may be little formal relationship with the local government unit. In other states, such as Florida, the local health departments are part of the state health department and also have a fiscal and reporting relationship to the county.

Advantages and disadvantages are found in each system. In highly centralized systems, health initiatives can be implemented statewide and can possibly make a very large and visible positive impact. Systems and procedures can also be developed once and then broadly implemented. These create opportunities for very efficient systems. However, local health departments with considerable autonomy may be better positioned to identify specific needs of the population and can tailor programs and policies to precisely what is needed in a specific community.

Regardless of the organizational structure within a state, close-working relationships between state and local departments will enhance the effectiveness of the public health system. Channels of communication between those in the state capital and those in local offices must be maintained to respond promptly to needs, to develop integrated systems useful to both levels, and to plan effectively for strategic development.

Relationships with Community and Local Boards of Health

Nationwide, there are 3186 local boards of health, and a recent study by the National Association of Local Board of Health provides interesting results. The following case definition was used in studying this group[8] "any officially constituted local body that establishes general public health policies for a local jurisdiction or that provides advice regarding the development of such policies to those responsible for policy development."

The boards of health comprises of a wide range of types of individuals including physicians, consumers, elected officials, other health providers, representatives of community organizations, and other government agencies. The individuals are overwhelmingly appointed to their positions, although in 29% the boards members are either exclusively elected or a mix of elected and appointed.[8]

As with local health departments, local boards of health exhibit different roles, responsibilities, and authorities. In the 1995-1996 study, 51% of the respondents indicated they perform a combination of advisory, governing, and policymaking functions. Eighty percent of responding boards indicated they have at least an advisory function. Seventy percent of respondents have responsibility for recommending public health policy, proposing, adopting, and enforcing public health regulations, and recommending budgets and priorities. Very few boards levy taxes or prepare grant requests.[8] Local boards of health play a very important role as a link with the community as a whole, advocate for the development of programs within the health department, and liaison to the state legislature. Because of their independent nature, boards of health often advocate in ways that are restricted for local health departments.

Furthermore, 85% of the responding boards indicated they are affiliated with a local health department.[8] According to the 1997 NACCHO study, 81% of LHDs nationwide report to local boards of health (NACCHO, unpublished data, April 1998). These results may represent an increase over the past decade. In 1989, 70% of responding health departments reported a board of health,[9] and in 1992-1993, 73% of local health departments, or ~2000, reported having such.[10] Although additional research is needed on the nature of these arrangements, several health departments have more than one board of health within their jurisdiction.

The boards of health tend to serve jurisdictions with smaller populations. Eighty-eight percent serve jurisdictions of less than 100,000 population, and 57% serve populations under 25,000.[8] None of the responding boards of health served jurisdictions of one million or more. According to a NACCHO study (1992-1993), boards of health in jurisdictions with populations of fewer than 100,000 tend to have greater statutory authority than those in jurisdictions with larger populations. The relationship between the size of the population and the presence or absence of a board of health was also observed in this study. Of health departments serving the smallest sized populations, 71% are governed by boards of health. Of those serving populations between 25,000 and 50,000, 80% are governed by boards of health. Of health departments serving populations over 500,000, 59% are governed by boards of health.[10]

The board of health study gathered data about areas of interest for additional training, information, or technical assistance for board members. Three out of four respondents noted the following areas: establishment of community health priorities, state and local health reform activities, community health assessment, and managed care and public health.[8] These same areas are high on the local health officials' agenda, as well.

Budget Expenditures and Sources of Funding

The NACCHO Profile series over the past 10 years has provided valuable information about the budget expenditures and financing of local health department services. Local health departments have relatively small budgets. Twelve percent report annual expenditures of under $100,000, and an additional 13% have annual expenditures between $100,000 and $249,999. This suggests that one out of four operate on less than $240,000 per year. Sixteen percent operate on budgets between $250,000 and $499,999, and 15% between $500,000 and $999,999. A large percentage, 44%, has budgets of over one million dollars. In fact, the mean expenditure for all health departments was $5,505,962, and the median total expenditure was $689,457 in 1997 (NACCHO, unpublished data, April 1998). (See **Figure 1**).

For health departments overall, 34% of their budgets come from local government (city/county/town

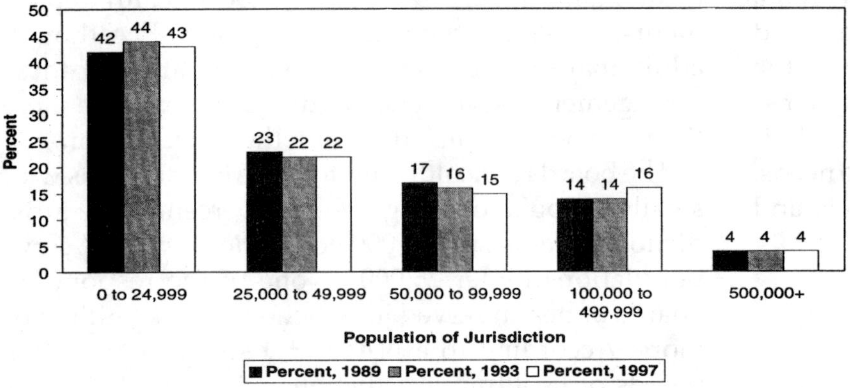

Figure 1. US local health departments, by population of jurisdiction served, 1989-1997 (n = 2,492).

funds). Forty percent is derived from the state health department, and this can include federal funds as well, such as infectious disease control dollars, maternal and child health block grants, etc. Seven percent of the funds results from services provided to patients covered by Medicaid and 3% from those covered by Medicare. This distribution is fairly consistent for health departments serving all population sizes.[10]

As part of a broader federal effort, case studies have recently been conducted regarding the feasibility of quantifying local public health expenditures according to the 10 essential public health services previously cited. Three case studies, conducted in Onondaga County, NY, North-East Tri-County Health Department, Wash, and Columbus, Ohio, demonstrated that expenditures could be described according to the 10 essential services without a major investment of time and resources. However, additional work is needed to compare information among agencies. Although pursuing this possibility would require great effort, having routine access to federal, state, and local public health expenditures by essential services would be useful for policy development and resource allocation decisions.

Findings of the case studies[11] suggest that for these three agencies, the highest percentage of total expenditures, 21.4% on average, were devoted to "assuring the provision of care when otherwise unavailable." The next 19.5% of expenditures were devoted to "informing, educating and empowering people about health issues." Next, 11.1% was spent on "enforcing laws and regulations that protect health and ensure safety."

Size of Local Health Departments

As previously stated, local health departments do vary considerably by size. Measures of this, in addition to expenditures as previously discussed, include population of jurisdiction served and staffing size.

Population of Jurisdiction Served

The 1997 NACCHO study of local health departments indicates that about two thirds of local health departments serve populations fewer than 50,000 (**Figure 2**). Only 3% serve populations between 500,000 and 1 million, with 1%, or 30, having populations greater than one million. The median population is 30,000, whereas the lowest reported population was 115 people, and the highest was 9,250,000 (NACCHO, unpublished data, April 1998). A consequence of this is that if a jurisdiction has a relatively small population, resources tend to be modest, and the health department may be challenged to accomplish a wide range of activities with limited resources.

Staffing Size and Type

In general, local health departments operate with relatively few staff members. Half of all health departments employ 20 or less and 25%, 8 or less (**Figure 3**). The number of staff members range from no staff to over 10,000. The average is 89 staff members.[10] As one would expect, the number of employees within a health department tends to increase as the population of the jurisdiction increases (**Table 1**). Whereas 44% of all health departments serving populations less than 25,000 employed four or fewer staff in 1992-1993, only 1% of health departments serving populations of 50,000 to 99,999 employed four or less. As Table 1 demonstrates, 98% of all health departments serving 500,000 or more people have a staff of one hundred or more.[10]

Services and Functions

Local health departments of all sizes provide numerous services to keep entire populations healthy. Exactly which services are provided is dependent on numerous factors: the needs of the community; the availability of services, such as primary care, by other providers; state statutes and the roles of other governmental agencies; the relative wealth of the community, and the historical origins of the department.

According to studies completed by NACCHO over the past 9 years and other studies before that time, local health departments have not and do not uniformly provide any one set of services nationwide. However, the

Table 1
US Local Health Department Staffing, by Population Size of Jurisdiction

	Population of Jurisdiction					
Number of Employees	0 to 24,999	25,000 to 49,999	50,000 to 99,999	100,000 to 499,999	500,000+	Overall total
0 to 4	37%	11%	2%	1%	0%	19%
5 to 9	24%	19%	5%	1%	0%	16%
10 to 24	24%	36%	22%	8%	0%	23%
25 to 99	10%	27%	56%	43%	2%	25%
100+	6%	7%	15%	48%	98%	18%

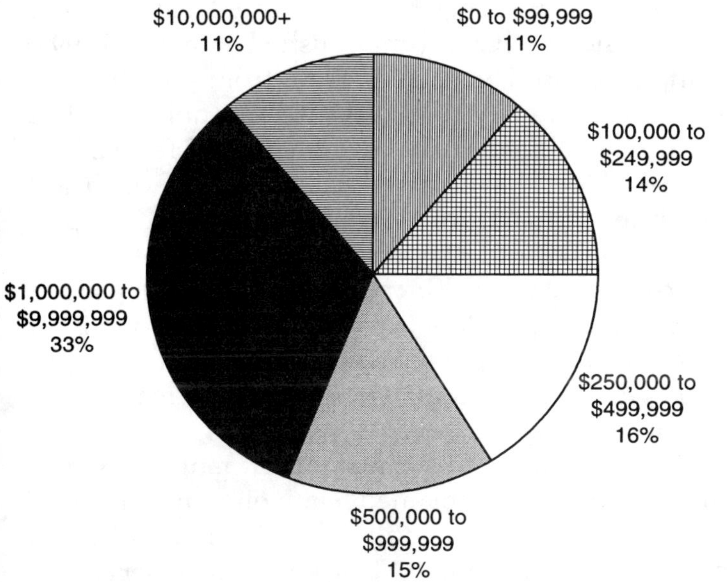

Figure 2. US local health departments: annual expenditures, 1997 (n = 2,492, unadjusted dollars).

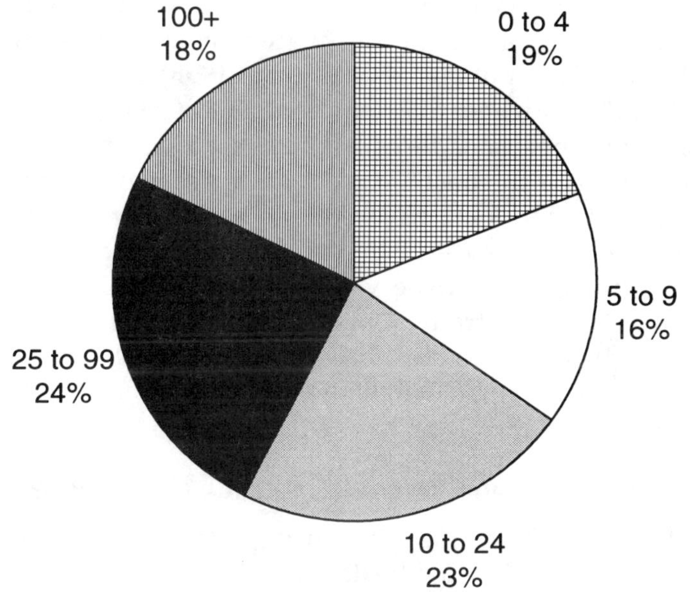

Figure 3. US local health departments, by number of full-time employees, 1997 (n = 2,492).

services that have historically been provided, or supported, at least in part, by the greatest number of local health departments concern the provision of immunization and other protections from communicable disease. In the most recent 1997 NACCHO local health department study, almost all respondents (93%) provided childhood immunization, and 92% provided adult immunizations. This is followed by communicable disease control services, provided by 91% of all local health departments (NACCHO, unpublished data, April 1998).

The following summarizes the types of services most commonly provided by health departments by selected types of essential services. Please note that in some cases comparisons are made between data from the 1992-1993 and the 1997 Profiles. These data are from two cross-sectional studies, and differences may be attributed to change over time as well as change in the sample population, sample size, and question wording. Further longitudinal analysis is needed and planned; however, preliminary analysis suggests that any changes noted are indeed due to more than differences in sample composition between the two studies.

Environmental Health

The practice of environmental public health focuses on the health interrelationships between people and their environment, promotes human health and well-being and fosters a safe and healthful environment. It involves the systematic development, promotion, and conduct of measures that modify or otherwise control those external factors in the indoor and outdoor environment that might cause illness, disability, discomfort, or death in humans. This includes health and safety factors and aesthetically desirable conditions in accordance with community demands and expectations.

Nearly all health departments provide some type of environmental service, and, in fact, this was the focus of many health departments when first established. In 1997, more than 8 out of 10 (84%) were involved in food monitoring and inspection. Lead screening and abatement followed in frequency (82%). The other three environmental health services provided by more than three quarters of the local health departments are inspecting restaurants (79%), monitoring sewage disposal systems (78%), and monitoring private drinking water systems (77%) (NACCHO, unpublished data, April 1998). The level of service has remained constant in several environmental health services. These include radiation control, at 22% in the most recent study, operation of sewage disposal systems at 78% , and monitoring of private drinking water systems at 77% (NACCHO, unpublished data, April 1998).

The data suggest that the provision of many environmental health services has increased or remained constant over the past 9 years. This is noteworthy because state and local governments have reorganized, and in some cases, the perception has been created that environmental health services have, in several cases, been split away from public health and that public health departments have become less involved. A review of the NACCHO data over the last 9 years challenges this perception.

Primary Care and Personal Health Care Services

The majority of local health departments provide some type of personal health care. In addition to the provision of childhood and adult immunizations already discussed, today many are involved today in the traditional areas of maternal and child health. Three out of four health departments are women, infants, children (WIC) providers, and 69% participate in the Early and Periodic Screening and Diagnostic Treatment (EPSDT) program for children (NACCHO, unpublished data, April 1998). These participation rates have remained fairly constant over the past 9 years (NACCHO, unpublished data, April 1998).

It is interesting to note, however, that the number of local health departments involved in the provision of, resource support, or contractual arrangement for well baby care and/or sick child care appears to have decreased. In 1989, 84% of all local health departments were active in these services, and in 1992-1993, 79% provided or contracted out for the provision of well child services.

Increases have been observed over the past 4 years in tobacco use control and prevention and personal health case management. In 1992-1993, 42% of local health departments directly provided tobacco use control programs, and an additional 3% contracted out for these activities.[10] In 1997, 68% reported activity in tobacco prevention (NACCHO, unpublished data, April 1998). These data correspond with the enormous increase in interest that has occurred regarding tobacco control during the past 6 years.

The data suggest that the provision of adult immunizations also increased during the past 5 years. The provision of pneumococcal vaccine increased from 48% in 1992-1993[10] to 62% in 1997 (NACCHO, unpublished data, April 1998). Hepatitis B immunizations changed from 77% to 89% in the same time period, and diphtheria and measles increased more moderately, from 77% to 83% and from 76% to 81%, respectively, according to National Association of County Health Departments[10] and NACCHO (unpublished data, April 1998).

Injury control programs grew from 40% in 1992-1993[10] to 49% in 1997 (NACCHO, unpublished data, April 1998). School-based clinics changed from 25% to 33% of all local health departments, and school health programs from 60% to 65%[10] (also NACCHO, unpublished data, April 1998). Given the tenacity of the substance abuse issue, the increase in substance abuse programs from 21% to 26%[10] (also NACCHO, unpublished data, April 1998) appears modest, although other providers in the communities could have increased their activity in this area.

The percentage of health departments providing many services has remained relatively constant. These services include other adult immunizations (influenza and tetanus), 92% and 87% in 1997; dental services at 44%; and HIV testing and counseling at 70%. Obstetrical services are provided or contracted for by 31%; sexually transmitted disease testing and counseling by 70%; sexually transmitted disease treatment at 64%; and laboratory services at 60% (NACCHO, unpublished data, April 1998).

Community outreach and education, recognized as essential services, have remained relatively constant, and in 1997, 88% of responding local health departments reported activity in this area. Health education/risk reduction is now provided by or contracted for by 87% of the health departments (NACCHO, unpublished data, April 1998).

Community Assessment

Community assessment, i.e. identifying the health problems and assets of a community, is one of the 10 essential elements. Many local health officials have been involved in facilitating community assessment and planning initiatives for many years. In the 1997 NACCHO study, 76% of local health departments responded that they directly provided, contributed resources to, or contracted for services related to community assessment. Although further study is needed to assess the depth of the involvement, community assessment typically is intended to be a public and inclusive endeavor, involving key members of a community as well as department staff. Their collaborative work includes prioritizing issues and developing a plan to meet the community needs. Several tools have been developed to assist local health departments and communities in carrying out these projects, including the Assessment Protocol for Excellence in Public Health (APEXPH), Planned Approach to Community Health (PATCH), Healthy Cities, Healthy Communities 2000, and Healthy People 2000. In addition, many states have developed state-specific tools, such as the Illinois I-PLAN. We can anticipate community assessment initiatives will continue to grow in the future, and they will broaden to include a wider range of community health-related factors.

Epidemiology and surveillance contribute to an understanding of a community's disease patterns and health needs. Eighty-three percent of local health departments reported that they directly provided, contributed resources to, or contracted out their epidemiology and surveillance services in 1997 (NACCHO, unpublished data, April 1998). Converting data into information is a core function of epidemiology, and local health departments have been increasingly challenged to develop information systems that not only perform surveillance functions but also assist in creating efficient health systems. The move toward integrated health information systems has developed as one way to meet the need for surveillance data at the local, state, and federal levels. Linkages between public and private data collection systems would allow for increased data sharing and improved reporting in the future. Data and information are cornerstones of epidemiology, and thus a challenge at the local level is to develop an information system that can be used for a variety of purposes, including surveillance. An integrated public and private system would meet several needs and is dependent on the willingness of providers of health care within an area to share health data.

Partnership Development and Collaboration

The importance of partnerships for the delivery of public health services and development of healthy communities has been widely promoted during the past 5 years. Thus, as part of the 1997 Profile, local health departments were asked if they have a specific partnership, or were currently considering the development of one, with numerous partners.

The greatest number of partnerships exists, or is being considered, with other government entities. Leading these are state health departments at 83%, followed by other local health departments at 72%, other state agencies at 68%, and other units of governments not at the state level at 62% (NACCHO, unpublished data, April 1998).

The next group most frequently cited as partners was other health providers. Hospitals were most often specified as partners or potential partners (67%); other providers such as private physicians were noted by 59% of responders, and community health centers/migrant health centers by 39%. Health insurance companies are engaged in partnerships or under consideration by 19% (NACCHO, unpublished data, April 1998).

The degree to which partnerships have been developed with community organizations is not reported as frequently. More than half (58%) did cite community and civic groups, such as the Chamber of Commerce, 44% noted businesses, and 37% the faith community (NACCHO, unpublished data, April 1998).

Universities and academic centers were noted by 52% of the responders, nonprofit and voluntary organizations by 64%, and professional associations by 53% (NACCHO, unpublished data, April 1998).

Several initiatives are encouraging the development of partnerships. For example, the Turning Point Project seeks to stimulate greater partnerships between the state and local health departments and the public and private sectors. As a result of this effort and others, changes in the types and number of partnerships among the sectors may be significant over the next 5-10 years; it will be important to observe the trends and their impact.

Use of Information Technology

The appropriate and effective use of information technology is critically important for local health departments. Access to accurate, comprehensive and up-to-date information is needed in order to operate effective surveillance and community assessment systems. However, anecdotal information has indicated that many local health departments have been operating without benefit of this technology. In order to assess the degree to which communication and information technology has been incorporated by local health departments, NACCHO conducted a random sample study in 1996. The results indicated that although electronic communications have taken on important roles in many local health departments, they have yet to be fully used in this group.

Almost all health departments appear to have access to a fax machine (96%), although the machine is not always located within the health department. Further, even though this technology has been widely available for over 10 years, it appears that more than 100 health departments still do not have routine or systematic access to this type of equipment.[12]

Eighty percent of responding health officials reported that they, as top agency executives, had their own work-related computer. About 50% of LHDs reported having dedicated support personnel to address hardware and software issues.[12]

Forty-seven percent of top agency executives use on-line services at work, although more than half of these rated their expertise using on-line services as little or none. Sixty-two percent of respondents indicated that at least one computer in the department had access to the Internet; conversely, almost 40% did not have any access. Given the wealth and speed of information available through the Internet, access by all health departments is necessary in order to assure the best safeguards to the public's health.[12]

Larger health departments usually had fewer computers per employee than did smaller health departments. This ranged from 1.75 employee per computer in health departments with five or less staff to 3.41 employees per computer for health departments with 700 or more employees.[12]

Challenges for Local Health Departments

This time of unprecedented change for the health and public health sectors involves questions of identity, credibility, need for recognition, and preparation for increasingly complex challenges with potentially greater consequences for very large percentages of the population. The mobile lifestyle of the world's population, great concentrations of populations, and the presence of very virile pathogens with no known cures characterize the public health challenges of the late 20th century.[13] Given this, as well as the changes in public health and health care delivery systems already discussed, the following issues are foremost on the agenda for local health department development.

Maintaining Professional Skills and Techniques

In order for local health staff to keep pace with the many demands and challenges, training is needed in management, programmatic and technical areas, and in the use of information technology. In 1996, 83% of responding local health departments reported a need to enhance their professional training and development in relation to electronic communications.[12]

In 1998, the US Senate recently asked for a report from the Centers for Disease Control and Prevention (CDC) concerning the training and technology needs of LHDs. Federal agencies and major health foundations also are taking these needs very seriously, which creates a sense of optimism that training needs of local health staff will be addressed in a systematic fashion.

Creating a Visible and Accountable Local Public Health System

While the concepts of measuring local public health performance and professional accreditation are not new, there is increased interest in establishing a comprehensive and systematic evaluation of performance and possibly a national system of voluntary accreditation for public health agencies. National performance measures would provide comparative data to be used in quality improvement, increasing accountability for dollars invested, and a greater level of credibility. The CDC, in conjunction with national and state-based public health organizations, is currently developing performance indicators and a national system for performance evaluation. Furthermore, drafts for a new chapter on public health infrastructure within the new Healthy People 2010: Objectives for a Healthy Nation include an objective concerning performance measures. Developments such as these over the next 5 years are likely to have a significant impact on health departments nationwide.

Developing Public Health Leaders

Demands for public health professional development have grown owing to the increased involvement of the private sector, the changing role of the public health sector, and the formidable challenge of retraining the public health work force. Federal, state, and local governments have been well aware of these needs and have created a number of programs to assist health officials in developing the visioning and strategic planning skills required to transform an industry / service.

CDC sponsors programs such as the Public Health Leadership Institute and the National Public Health Leadership Development Network, with the goal of making leadership development opportunities available to health professionals in every state. Several models are under development. Nine state and regional institutes are in full operation, and several others are under consideration. The Ohio Department of Health, for example, sponsors a year-long institute that includes public health professionals, as well as community teams of public health and key community leaders. New Jersey, Delaware, New York, Rhode Island, Vermont, New Hampshire, and Maine have established the Northeast Regional Public Health Leadership Institute. Other regional networks are now in operation. In 1998, it is estimated that 400 people will participate in the state and regional institutes now in operation. This is a significant increase from 25 participants in such programs in 1991.

Creating Healthy Communities in a More Challenging Environment

Problems threatening the health of the community continue to mount, yet resources to address these demands have not increased substantially, and in some areas, have decreased. Given this set of circumstances, health officials and others are taking a greater interest in using a systems approach to creating healthy communities. This brings a shift from focusing solely on the capacity of the public health agency itself, to a focus on the resources of the community as a whole, and to collaboration with other community agencies and providers at the local level. The establishment and popularity of organizations such as the Coalition for Healthy Cities and Communities demonstrate this growing interest. The Coalition includes a wide range of members and promotes the implementation of creative and collaborative approaches to achieving healthy communities.

In addition, new tools to obtain a community-wide perspective and partnerships are being developed. For example, NACCHO, in cooperation with the CDC, are developing a new tool, Assessment and Planning Excellence for Community Partners for Health (APEXCPH), to assist local health departments and communities to work together in several ways. These include creating a common vision, mobilizing the community, identifying community assets and needs, decision making about roles, securing needed resources, and managing the process of change. This document will also lay the groundwork for the development of public health performance measures.

A third effort and expression of this changing focus can be seen in the Turning Point Project which is currently sponsoring collaborative public health initiatives in a number of states and localities. Owing to the wealth of like-minded activity, it is reasonable to anticipate significant progress and success in improving public health practice through community-wide efforts.

Strategic Planning for Communities and Local Health Departments in Transition

The roles and responsibilities of local health departments are undergoing review by those internal and external to the organization. Health officials struggle with providing more essential services, though funding streams have not yet developed to support such activities. In many jurisdictions, the role of health departments in providing direct personal care is being debated. Some believe that the significant increase in managed care creates an opportunity for the health department to ease out of direct personal care, whereas, in other communities, this possibility has not arisen. In other jurisdictions, the health department has increased its provision of personal health services, as managed care plans end their involvement with Medicaid populations and no arrangements have been created to serve the medically indigent.

In our ever-changing environment, the breadth of responsibility of some local health departments has expanded, other departments have merged with other entities, and others have closed for lack of funding. These types of changes are likely to continue to occur. As issues are debated in various jurisdictions, it is critical that a systematic and strategic analysis be developed and implemented. This would include an assessment of a variety of options, critical analyses of their impact on the community's health, and planning for rational methods for implementation.

Conclusion

Local health departments contribute substantially to promoting the health of the public and achieving healthy communities. Nationwide, they provide a range of services responsive to the core functions and representative of the essential public health services. To meet the various challenges to improving the public's health, we have discussed several efforts underway to strengthen the local public health system. These include programs to develop performance indicators, leadership institutes, training and retraining opportunities, planning and assessment tools, and linkages between the local public health and medical sectors. By continuing to work together to strengthen partnerships and collaborations, the health of the public should be better served as we enter the new millennium.

References

1. Hanlon J. Is there a future for local health departments. *Public Health Rep.* 1973;88:898-901.
2. American Public Health Association. *The Model Standards for Community Preventive Health.* Washington, DC: American Public Health Association; 1979.
3. Institute of Medicine. *The Future of Public Health.* Washington, DC: National Academy Press; 1988.
4. US Department of Health and Human Services. *Public Health in America.* Washington, DC: US Dept of Health and Human Services; 1994.
5. Altman DE, Morgan DH. The role of state and local government in health. *Health Aff (Millwood).* 1983 Winter;2(4):7-31.
6. Mountin J, Flook E. *Guide to Health Organizations in the United States.* Washington, DC: US Public Health Service; 1953.
7. Miller CA, Brooks E, DeFriese G, Gilbert B, Jain S, Kavaler F. A survey of local public health departments and their directors. *Am J Public Health.* 1977:67(10);931-939.
8. National Association of Local Boards of Health. *National Profile of Local Boards of Health.* Atlanta, Ga: Centers for Disease Control and Prevention; September 1997.
9. National Association of County Health Departments. 1990. *National Profile of Local Health Departments.* Washington, DC: National Association of County Health Departments; 1990;20.
10. National Association of County Health Departments. *1992-1993 National Profile of Local Health Departments.* Washington, DC: National Association of County Health Departments; 1995;27.
11. Barry MA, Centra L, Pratt E Jr, Brown CK, Giordano L. *Where Do the Dollars Go? Measuring Local Public Health Expenditures.* Washington, DC: National Association of County and City Health Officials, National Association of Local Boards of Health, Public Health Foundation; March 1998.
12. National Association of County and City Health Officials. *Study of Electronic Communication Capacity of Local Health Departments.* Washington, DC: National Association of County and City Health Officials; 1996.
13. Woodall J. Stalking the next epidemic: ProMED tracks emerging diseases. *Public Health Rep.* 1997; 112(1):78-82.

Chapter 3

Contributions to Public Health by Organizations Other Than the Local Health Department

Local governmental health departments serve as the primary organizing and mobilizing forces for public health practice in most communities. These departments do not, however, act in isolation in performing core public health functions within the community. A broad range of other organizations and individuals contribute to public health activities in most communities, either independently or in collaboration with the local health department. These organizations include governmental agencies, private organizations, and an array of informal community associations and neighborhood groups.

This chapter reviews the major types of organizations that contribute to local public health practice and examines the extent and nature of their contributions. Observations are based on a study of local public health performance conducted with a nationally selected group of 63 public health jurisdictions during 1992-1993, together with detailed case studies conducted in a subset of these jurisdictions during 1994-1995.[1] This chapter begins by describing the types of organizations that contribute to public health and their motivations for doing so. Next, this chapter characterizes the extent and nature of these contributions using findings from a survey of public health performance in the 63 public health jurisdictions. Finally, the chapter examines some of the key policy and management issues that emerge from the contributions made to public health by various community organizations.

Organizations Contributing to Public Health

State Agencies

Beyond the official local health department, an array of other governmental agencies perform essential public health functions at the community level. State health agencies are clearly among the most important governmental contributors to public health. These agencies vary widely in their structure and authority, but they generally maintain responsibility for implementing public health policies and programs at the state level, largely through their relationships with local health departments. Consequently, state health agencies serve as important sources of funding and technical assistance for local health departments. In some states, state health agencies maintain direct administrative authority over the operations of local health departments, while in other states, the relationship between state and local health agencies is less centralized. Under these less centralized arrangements, state health agencies may assume direct responsibility for performing certain public health activities at the community level, while local health departments maintain this responsibility for other activities. Clearly, state health agency contributions to local public health practice vary widely across states and even within some states.

To further complicate matters, state governments may organize health and human service responsibilities in ways that divide public health authority into multiple state agencies. For example, a separate state agency for environmental quality may maintain responsibilities in monitoring and enforcing environmental safety issues. Similarly, a separate state Medicaid office (often located within human services departments (may administer responsibilities in assuring health care accessibility and quality for low-income and underserved population groups. State insurance departments are often given the lead authority for assuring consumer protection in managed care plans and other health insurance products, while state labor departments may carry out responsibilities in assuring occupational safety and health. Consequently, numerous state agencies may contribute to local public health practice. These contributions may include indirect activities such as funding and technical assistance as well as direct activities such as the performance of public health services in local communities.

Local Governmental Agencies

Other local governmental agencies beyond the health department make important contributions to public health practice. Local social services agencies administer important social support programs that often complement the efforts of health department services. These include programs that assure vulnerable and underserved populations with access to adequate food, housing, clothing, and medical products and devises. These agencies often provide services that are required by vulnerable populations in order to access needed public health and personal health care services, such as transportation, language translation, temporary child care, case management, and information and referral. Moreover, many communities are served by separate governmental agencies that administer programs for mental health and substance abuse. These programs often include components for prevention and health promotion that clearly fall within the domain of public health. Similarly, local governments may maintain separate agencies for carrying out environmental health functions such as assuring the safety and quality of water, air, soil, and food products. Governmental agencies also exist for serving the complex social and health needs of special populations such as children and the aged. Finally, local governments may operate special executive offices dedicated to specific health policy issues, such as a mayor's office on violence prevention or a county commission on child health. These types of government agencies often serve as important complements to the work of local health departments.

Local governmental agencies contribute to public health practice in a number of ways. First, they may assure access to needed health services by directly providing health-related services to community residents, either independently or in collaboration with the local health department. Second, they may contribute to the policy development process in public health by engaging in local health planning, priority-setting, and policymaking activities. Finally, these agencies may contribute to public health practice through efforts to assess health needs and investigate health threats among the individuals and communities that they serve.

Federal Agencies

Federal health agencies contribute to local public health practice primarily through the provision of funding, policy guidance, and technical assistance to the community organizations that are directly involved in implementing public health activities. In some cases, federal agencies may also engage in directly performing public health activities at the community level. Direct federal involvement in local public health practice typically occurs only for specific public health issues such as major health threats or for research and demonstration purposes.

Many of the federal agencies that contribute to local public health practice are organized within the US Department of Health and Human Services. Some of the most frequent contributors to local public health practice include the following:

- the Centers for Disease Control and Prevention (CDC), which operates 11 centers, institutes, and offices devoted to preventing and controlling specific disease risks and public health problems. One of these offices, the Public Health Practice Program Office, gives priority to assisting in the organization and operation of state and local public health agencies.
- the Health Resources and Services Administration, which administers federal programs for expanding public access to health care professionals and facilities, particularly in underserved areas. The Bureau of Primary Health Care within this organization provides funding and technical assistance to agencies that provide primary care services in medically underserved areas, including some local health departments. The Maternal and Child Health Bureau administers services and programs under the federal Maternal and Child Health Block Grant.
- the nation's two leading agencies for funding and administering health care research and demonstration initiatives: the National Institutes of Health and the Agency for Health Care Policy and Research. Both agencies conduct intramural as well as extramural research activities in areas of public health importance. These agencies may contribute to local public health practice by leading investigations of public health threats, conducting demonstrations of public health interventions, or supporting the public health research interests of local health departments and other community organizations.
- the Health Care Financing Administration, which administers the federal Medicare program and the joint federal-state Medicaid program for financing medical care services, as well as the newly developed Child Health Insurance Program (CHIP) for covering low-income uninsured children.

- the Indian Health Service, which administers programs that provide health services to federally-recognized American Indian and Alaska Native tribes.
- the Agency for Toxic Substances and Disease Registry, which operates programs to prevent and control exposure to hazardous wastes.
- the Substance Abuse and Mental Health Services Administration, which administers programs for the prevention, treatment, and control of mental illness and substance abuse.
- the Administration on Aging, which administers social and health services programs for older Americans.
- the Administration for Children and Families, which operates programs for the social and economic support of children and families.

A number of other federal agencies that are not included within the Department of Health and Human Services also contribute to local public health practice in some communities. These agencies include the following:

- the Department of Agriculture, which sponsors an array of health-related programs involving nutritional support, migrant health, food safety, and occupational exposure to pesticides;
- the Environmental Protection Agency, which supports and enforces an array of environmental health and safety policies and programs;
- the Department of Housing and Urban Development, which administers programs to address the health and social problems of populations residing in public housing facilities and in economically disadvantaged communities;
- the Department of Education, which supports programs in addressing the health education and health services needs of students;
- the Department of Labor, which administers programs to promote health and safety in the workplace.

These agencies make important contributions to local public health practice through direct community interventions and indirect contributions of funding and technical assistance.

Hospitals

Community hospitals have long been important contributors to local public health activities. The federal Hill-Burton program, which financed many hospital construction and capital improvement projects over the past half-century, required hospitals that used this funding to provide charitable services. Begun in the mid-1940s, this program established a strong tradition of charity care among community hospitals. As providers of uncompensated acute care services, hospitals continue to play invaluable roles in assuring access to health care for vulnerable and underserved populations. The charitable missions of many public and nonprofit hospitals motivate these organizations to engage in community health activities that extend beyond the realm of acute care. More recently, hospitals face pressures from policymakers and regulators to demonstrate the production of community benefits in order to retain their tax exempt status and their accreditation status. Additionally, the growth of managed care and capitated financing arrangements in many communities create financial incentives for hospitals to engage in public health activities as strategies for reducing costs and encouraging greater efficiency in hospital utilization. Similarly, hospitals are expanding their involvement in health promotion and disease prevention initiatives in order to attract the growing numbers of health care consumers and purchasers who value these activities.

Hospitals contribute to local public health activities in a variety of ways. In some communities, hospitals participate in directly providing community health services through efforts such as operating primary care clinics for underserved populations, sponsoring community health education programs; and conducting health screening fairs. Hospitals are also major contributors to community health assessment efforts. These contributions appear to be motivated in part by the Joint Commission on Accreditation of Health Care Organizations' recent decision to require its accredited hospitals to engage in community health assessment. Hospitals are important contributors to these efforts because of their unique positions within communities to observe disease effects and identify intervention areas. Finally, hospitals make important contributions to local efforts in public health planning and policy development. In many communities, hospitals wield significant political power through the substantial human and capital resources that they control. Consequently, hospitals can be powerful agents for mobilizing communities around public health issues and for organizing collaborative efforts to address these issues. Hospitals also maintain large administrative data systems that can offer remarkable insight into community health problems, through information such as age- and diagnosis-specific admissions and emergency room visits.

Ambulatory Care Providers

Ambulatory care providers also make important contributions to public health in many communities.

These providers include private physician practices as well as nonprofit health centers supported by federal, state, and local government subsidies. Private physicians often engage in public health activities through local and state medical societies. Medical societies vary widely in the extent of their involvement in public health activities. Some societies maintain only minimal involvement through participation in community health planning and policy development activities. Other medical societies are actively involved in designing and operating community health interventions such as free medical clinics, health fairs, and community health assessments. Private physicians may also contribute to public health activities independently, through such diverse efforts as volunteering in community health clinics, serving on local boards of health, or developing service agreements with local health departments for providing reduced-fee care to the uninsured.

Nonprofit health centers also play important roles in public health practice in the communities in which they operate. These centers include those that receive grants through one of the five federal health center programs (community health centers, migrant health centers, homeless health centers, public housing health centers, and school-based health centers), as well as those that are supported through state, local, or private funding. Some of these clinics offer comprehensive primary care services, while others specialize in areas such as family planning (i.e. Planned Parenthood clinics), pediatrics, or sexually transmitted disease services. In addition to assuring access to primary care services for vulnerable and underserved populations, these health centers serve as important sources for health education, counseling, and social support services. Often, health centers and local health departments develop reciprocal referral agreements and other collaborative arrangements for targeting health services to vulnerable populations. In some cases, health centers are directly operated by local health departments.

Managed Care Plans

Managed care plans are achieving a growing presence in many local communities. Some of these plans are making important contributions to local public health practice in the communities in which they operate. For some plans, these contributions are motivated by altruistic missions of community service, while other plans seek to achieve financial gains through these contributions by lowering overall medical care use and increasing market share. Many plans maintain the capacity for reaching large numbers of community residents and health care providers through their networks of enrollees and affiliated providers. Some plans use this capacity to encourage health promotion and disease prevention practices among their enrollees and to create incentives for affiliated providers to deliver appropriate clinical preventive services to their patients. Plans may also contribute to community health initiatives that target broad segments of the community population, as strategies for improving general population health and for promoting awareness of their organization among consumers, providers, and purchasers. For example, programs that distribute bicycle helmets to children or child safety seats to new parents have become popular strategies for managed care plans to achieve these objectives.

Managed care plans also participate in public health activities as strategies for obtaining information about community health risks and disease patterns. Plans use these types of information to anticipate health risks among their current and potential enrollees. In order to obtain this information, some managed care plans participate with other community organizations in community health assessment and surveillance efforts. Other plans conduct surveillance activities within their own enrollee populations and contribute this information to public health assessment efforts maintained by other community organizations.

Nonprofit Community Agencies

A range of other nonprofit community organizations engages in public health activities at the local level. Prime among these agencies are local chapters of national voluntary health associations such as the American Heart Association, the American Cancer Society, the American Diabetes Association, and the American Lung Association. These organizations implement public awareness campaigns and health education initiatives about disease risks and advocate for the public and private support of prevention, treatment, and control interventions. Similarly, local chapters of social service organizations such as the United Way, the Urban League, and Rotary International are often active in sustaining community-level efforts to identify health risks and to implement community health interventions. Through their active fund-raising efforts, these organizations often serve as important sources of local, nongovernmental revenues to support community-level interventions.

In addition to these national affiliates, many communities are served by locally developed organizations that have formed around community-specific needs and resources. These organizations include neighborhood associations, parent-teacher associations, church groups, and local environmental coalitions. These groups often participate in policy development activities such as community health planning activities and political lobbying efforts. In many communities, these groups also play important roles in implementing community health interventions, such as church- and school-based health education programs, and local environmental restoration projects.

Another type of community agency that has seen marked growth over the last decade is the community foundation. Acquisitions, mergers, and ownership conversions among local hospitals and health plans are generating substantial revenues that are being used to launch numerous new local health foundations.[2] In some communities, these foundations play important roles in developing and financing community health interventions. For example, some foundations sponsor extensive community health assessment activities designed to identify health risks and gaps in the health service delivery systems. Other foundations support the delivery of uncompensated health care to uninsured and underinsured community residents.

Universities

Universities and other institutions of higher education also make important contributions to local public health practice in many communities. Health profession schools such as schools of public health, medicine, and nursing are perhaps the most common contributors. Faculty from schools of public health often provide technical assistance to local health departments and other community organizations for activities such as conducting disease investigations, community health assessments, and community health planning activities. Additionally, health profession schools often collaborate with community health agencies in developing sites for internships and residencies for health profession students. These types of arrangements provide communities with additional clinical and administrative manpower that can be used to implement new community health interventions. Finally, universities may contribute to local public health practice by developing specialized training and continuing education opportunities for local health professionals. Recent advances in information and communication technology are facilitating the development of these opportunities through distance learning modalities.

It is important to note that health profession schools are not the only institutions of higher education that contribute to local public health practice. Other types of institutions (including liberal arts colleges, community colleges, and technical schools) also play important roles in contributing technical assistance, training, and educational expertise to community health interventions.

Other Organizations

A range of other organizations may contribute to public health activities in local communities. In some localities, employers are becoming active in promoting health within their workforces. Employer activities include efforts to reduce work-site health risks, promote healthy lifestyles and behaviors among employees and their families, and assist in the early identification and treatment of diseases. For example, employers may contribute to community health education campaigns in areas such as smoking cessation, physical activity, and nutrition. Similarly, employers may sponsor community health fairs and other initiatives designed to identify and address health risks within the community. Employers may undertake these activities independently or through associations such as business coalitions, local chambers of commerce, and economic development councils. Employers face compelling incentives for engaging in these types of activities, given their potential effects on employee productivity and costs incurred for health insurance and worker's compensation benefits.

Other organizations contributing to local public health practice include elementary and secondary schools, religious organizations, professional associations, and labor unions. These organizations vary widely in their involvement in public health issues and in their motivations for doing so. Nonetheless, their potential for making meaningful contributions should not be overlooked within individual communities.

The Extent and Nature of Public Health Contributions

To examine in greater detail the extent and nature of public health contributions by various community organizations, a study was conducted with a selection of 63 local public health jurisdictions during 1992 and 1993. This study used the Local Public Health Assessment Survey (described in Chapter 1) to produce measures of the proportion of total public health effort within a jurisdiction that is contributed by the official local health department and by other community organizations. This study also used the survey to pro-

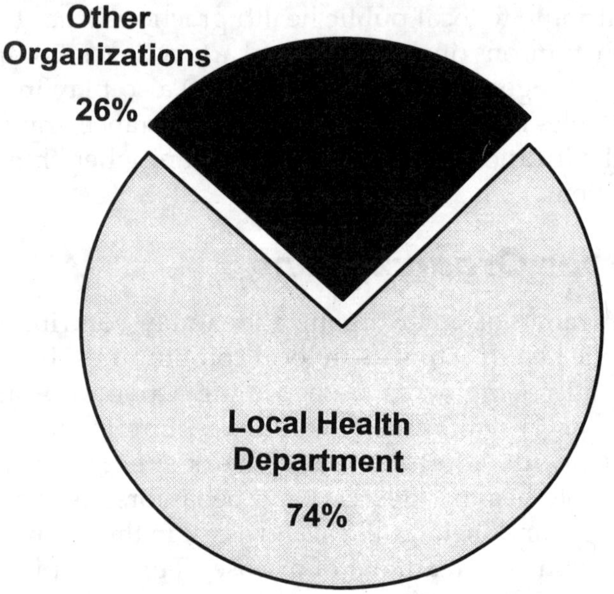

(Source: Data from Reference 1.)

Figure 1. Proportion of local public health activities contributed by the local health department and other organizations, 1992–93 (as reported by the local health official).

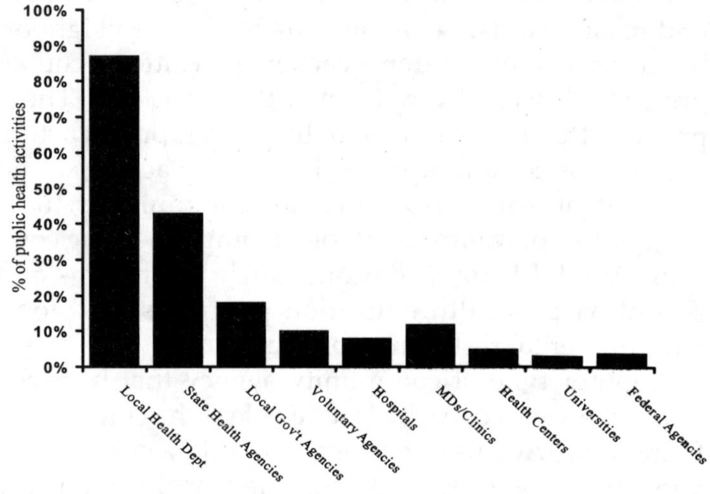

(Source: Data from Reference 1.)

Figure 2. Proportion of local public health activities in which selected organizations participate, 1992–93 (as reported by the local health official).

duce "participation rates" for each type of community organization, defined as the proportion of public health activities in which each type of organization participates. Both types of measures relied on the perceptions of the local health department director in each jurisdiction, who served as the key informant survey respondent. The 63 study jurisdictions represented a nonrandom selection of jurisdictions in 15 states that had participated in earlier studies of public health performance and included jurisdictions in Alabama (6), Arizona (2) California (2), Colorado (5), Maryland (6), Mississippi (6), North Carolina (5), New Jersey (7), New York (1), Ohio (2), Oregon (4), South Carolina (6), Tennessee (2), Washington (2), and Wisconsin (7). Results are therefore not generalizable to the full population of US local health jurisdictions, but they nonetheless provide useful insight into the roles played by community organizations in local public health practice.

Survey results indicate that on average, organizations other than the local health department contributed ~26% of the total community effort in public health within the study jurisdictions (**Figure 1**). The remaining 74% of effort was contributed by the local health department. Outside organizations contributed the largest share of effort to the core function of policy development (31%) and the smallest share of effort to the function of assessment (24%).

State agencies appeared to be the most frequent participants in public health activities, participating in an average of 43% of the 84 public health activities included in the survey (**Figure 2**). The average public health participation rate for local government agencies stood at 18%, compared with 12% for private physicians, 10% for community agencies, 8% for hospitals, and 5% for health centers. Universities were reported to participate in ~3% of public health activities, whereas 4% of activities were reported to involve federal agency participation. Only 2% of the activities were reported to involve participation from other types of organization not mentioned previously, such as managed care organizations, churches, and elementary and secondary schools. (The survey did not include specific categories for participation by these types of organizations, but rather it captured their participation through an open-ended "other" category. This may have resulted in significant underreporting of participation for these organization types, because respondents were not explicitly prompted for these organization types.)

When participation rates were separately computed for each of the three core public health functions, several interesting patterns emerged. State agencies were reported to participate in assessment activities more frequently than in policy development or assurance activities, as were federal agencies. In contrast, participation was reported to be highest for assurance activities among local government agencies, community agencies, private physicians, health centers, and universities. Only hospitals were reported to participate in policy development activities more frequently than in other types of activities.

Several interesting associations were observed between characteristics of local public health jurisdictions and contributions to public health by outside organizations. First, a strong positive association was identified between the overall level of public health performance in a jurisdiction and the proportion of effort contributed by outside organizations. This association appeared strongest for the public health functions of policy development and assessment. These results provide support for the view that contributions to public health by outside organizations can enhance local public health performance.

A strong relationship was also observed between state-local administrative structures and outside agency contributions. Outside agency contributions were significantly higher in jurisdictions where the local health department operated as a centralized administrative unit of the state health agency compared with jurisdictions having decentralized local health departments. Enhanced state agency involvement explains part but not all of the higher contributions observed in centralized health department jurisdictions. Another explanation for this trend may be that centralized departments benefit from higher levels of state funding and technical assistance, which they are then able to apply in developing stronger relationships with other community organizations. Centralized agencies may also be less susceptible to the local political issues and turf battles that challenge decentralized health departments.

Implications for Policy and Practice

This study documents the important public health contributions made by organizations other than the local health department. A broad array of organizations contribute to public health in most of the jurisdictions examined. State and local government agencies are responsible for the greatest volume of public health activities contributed by organizations other than the local health department. Most jurisdictions experience relatively limited contributions from private providers such as hospitals, physicians, and clinics.

Outside organizations appear to contribute less to assurance activities than to policy development and assessment activities. This trend appears somewhat inconsistent with the efforts underway in many communities to transfer responsibilities in personal health service delivery from public health agencies to other community providers. Clearly, outside organizations can play important roles in performing local public health activities. Nevertheless, public health managers and policymakers should consider the types of roles that these organizations are willing and able to take on before reallocating responsibilities in local public health practice. This study suggests that there may be important differences in public health contributions across different types of organizations and jurisdictions.

References

1. Halverson PK, Miller CA, Kaluzny AD, Fried BJ, Richards TB, Schenck SE. Performing public health functions: the perceived contributions of public health and other community organizations. *J Health Human Serv Admin*. 1996;6:288-303.
2. Lewin T, Gottlieb M. In hospital sales, an overlooked side effect. *New York Times*. April 27, 1997:1.

Chapter 4

Interactions Between Local Public Health Agencies and Other Health Organizations

Local public health practice is not the exclusive domain of a single type of organization or profession. As described in Chapter 3, a broad range of organizations contributes to local public health activities. These organizations complement the work performed by local health departments in promoting and protecting the health of communities. Contributions to public health may be carried out through a variety of mechanisms (both independent of and in collaboration with local health departments). This chapter examines the ways in which local health departments interact with other community organizations in carrying out core public health functions.

Background

Recent trends in health care delivery and financing in the United States suggest that improving the health of the public in the current environment requires strong linkages between public health and personal health care delivery systems. While the idea and the practice of collaboration in public health is not new, a number of recent developments provide new motivations for establishing such linkages. With the rapid growth of managed care plans and capitated financing arrangements, health care providers face compelling incentives for emphasizing traditional public health approaches in health promotion and disease prevention in order to reduce the need for more costly health services in their patient populations.[1,2] At the same time, public sector initiatives to contain health care costs create imperatives for public health agencies to work cooperatively with other community-based health providers to assure that health needs in the population are addressed in an era of restricted public funding.[3,4] Given these circumstances, collaboration between public health agencies and private health care providers should facilitate local public health practice as well as enhance personal health care delivery within managed care systems.

A recent study of local public health jurisdictions confirms that organizations other than the local health department contribute significantly to the public health activities performed in local communities.[5] This analysis does not, however, reveal whether or how public health agencies interact with these other organizations in performing public health activities. Evidence from the human services sector suggests that structural and functional characteristics of interorganizational relationships may have important effects on the performance of community-based service delivery systems.[6] In light of these earlier findings, we conducted a descriptive study to assess the extent to which local public health agencies currently interact with other organized health care providers and to examine the structural and functional characteristics of these interactions for a clearer understanding of their effects on local public health practice. This chapter presents findings from this study and identifies implications for local health departments, medical care providers, and public health policymakers. As such, this chapter offers a detailed examination of collaborative activities that, as Chapter 2 indicates, are occurring nationally among local health departments and other organizations.

Methods

The local public health jurisdictions examined in this analysis are part of a larger study of local health department structure and performance begun in 1979. Fourteen of the jurisdictions were selected for the original study because they were served by exemplary health departments, as determined by experts in the field.[7] Thirteen additional jurisdictions served by less developed health departments were matched by state to the 14 exemplary departments, using the recommendations of state health officials.[8-10] Finally, a survey of public health practices in all of the local health jurisdictions in six states was used to select the three highest and three lowest performing jurisdictions in each state, for a total of 36 additional jurisdictions.[11] While the cohort of 63 jurisdictions selected for the study is not a statistically random sample, it nonetheless includes substantial diversity with respect to population size, geographic region, degree of urbanization, managed care penetration, and performance of core public health practices.

Telephone Survey

A telephone survey of health department directors in each of the 63 local jurisdictions collected data on interactions between local public health departments and other health care organizations. Specifically, this survey focused on health department interactions with hospitals, managed care plans, and comprehensive primary health care centers. The survey inquired about contractual relationships as well as working relationships such as informal agreements and planning groups. We used data from a 1993 assessment of communitywide public health performance in the 63 jurisdictions to classify jurisdictions as low performing (below the median score) and high performing (at or above the median).[12] Each jurisdiction's assessment was based on the performance of core public health practices as identified by the Institute of Medicine,[3] including contributions made by the local health department and by any other organizations operating in the community. Fisher's Exact tests were used to test for differences in organizational interaction according to population size, geographic region, and public health performance level. To adjust for the effects of jurisdictional differences in the availability and accessibility of health care organizations, Fisher's Exact tests were computed separately on a subset of public health jurisdictions that were included only if managed care plans, hospitals, and health centers were physically located within the jurisdiction.

Case Studies

From the survey of all 63 jurisdictions, we selected a subset of 12 jurisdictions located in 11 states for in-depth case study analysis. These jurisdictions were chosen to achieve diversity with respect to the extent and type of interaction with other organizations, while also retaining diversity in jurisdiction size and geographic region. We conducted structured telephone interviews with the health department directors in each jurisdiction to probe for specific characteristics of health department interactions with other organizations. Interview responses were supplemented by review of health department documents including annual reports, mission statements, and strategic plans. As further validation of data collected from local health department directors, we conducted on-site interviews with the administrators of local hospitals and managed care plans in six of the case study jurisdictions. Interviews probed about the nature of interaction with local health departments and with other health care providers in the community. Content analysis was performed on transcribed interviews to validate survey results and to examine the structural and functional characteristics of interorganizational relationships.

Results

Survey Results

A total of 59 local health directors in 15 states participated in the survey (a response rate of 94%), reflecting substantial diversity in the types of jurisdictions served by local health departments (**Table 1**). Results confirm that the local health departments examined in this study are actively engaged in interactions with other types of health care organizations. The extent and nature of this interaction varies by type of organization. More health departments appear to maintain some form of interaction with hospitals (92%) than with community health centers (48%) or managed care plans (39%). This trend persists even when adjusting for the availability of organizations in the jurisdictions, because 95% of jurisdictions containing hospitals have health department/hospital relationships, 88% of jurisdictions containing health centers have health department/health center relationships, and 62% of jurisdictions containing managed care plans have health department/managed care relationships (**Table 2**).

The structure of health department interorganizational relationships varies by type of organization as well. Almost 83% of health department relationships with managed care organizations are formalized by contract compared with 56% of relationships with hospitals and 57% of relationships with health centers.

Table 1
Characteristics of Surveyed Local Health Department Jurisdictions

Characteristic	Percent (N=59)
Population Size[a]	
Under 25,000	13.6%
25,000-49,999	20.3%
50,000-99,999	13.6%
100,000-249,999	22.0%
250,000-499,999	15.3%
500,000 or more	15.3%
Jurisdiction Type	
City / town	13.6%
County or joint city / county	76.3%
Multicounty	10.2%
Availability of Health Organizations	
Jurisdictions served by hospitals	98.3%
Jurisdictions served by Federally Qualified Health Centers[b]	59.3%
Jurisdictions served by HMOs	64.4%
Jurisdictions served by Medicaid HMOs[c]	40.7%
Region[d]	
Western jurisdictions	23.7%
Midwestern jurisdictions	11.9%
Northeastern jurisdictions	13.6%
Southern jurisdictions	50.8%

[a]*Based on 1992 population estimates from the US Bureau of the Census.*[13]
[b]*Federally designated community or migrant health centers (Section 329 and Section 330 agencies).*
[c]*HMOs that are certified to enroll Medicaid beneficiaries that reside within the jurisdiction.*
[d]*The classification system used by the US Bureau of the Census is used to group jurisdictions by region.*[13]

Interorganizational relationships between local health departments and managed care plans appear more likely in jurisdictions with at least 100,000 residents than in smaller jurisdictions ($p = 0.003$). Much of this difference may be explained by the greater availability of health care organizations in more populous jurisdictions. Population-based differences in interorganizational relationships are much less pronounced when controlling for the availability of health care organizations (Table 2).

The prevalence of interorganizational relationships appears to vary by geographic region as well. When local jurisdictions in 15 states are grouped into four regional areas defined by the US Bureau of the Census,[13] interaction with managed care plans appears more common in western and midwestern jurisdictions, compared with southern and northeastern jurisdictions (Table 2). Some of this regional variation may again result from regional differences in the availability of health care organizations. Overall, regional differences in interorganizational relationships are less significant when controlling for this availability; however, regional differences in relationships with managed care plans remain significant ($p = 0.008$) (Table 2). Other organizational and community characteristics within local health jurisdictions may account for the remaining regional differences in interorganizational relationships, including such characteristics as local managed care market penetration and historical trends in the organization and financing of state and local health agencies.

The presence of organizational interaction in the surveyed jurisdictions varies somewhat with the level of performance in core public health functions and practices in the jurisdictions. Using data from a 1993 survey that scored each local jurisdiction on the proportion of core public health functions and practices adequately performed in the community,[12] jurisdictions are divided into low-performing jurisdictions (below the median performance score) and high-performing

Table 2
Local Health Department Interaction with Other Types of Organizations

Type of Interaction	Percent of Health Departments Having Interaction With:					
	Hospitals		Health Centers[a]		Managed Care Plans	
	In All Jurisdictions (N=59)	In Jurisdictions with Hospitals (N=57)	In All Jurisdictions (N=59)	In Jurisdictions with Health Centers (N=32)	In All Jurisdictions (N=59)	In Jurisdictions with MC Plans (N=37)
Any form of Interaction[b]	91.5%	94.7%	47.5%	87.5%	39.0%	62.2%
Contractual agreements only	50.8%	52.6%	27.1%	50.0%	32.2%	51.4%
In jurisdictions >100,000 population	93.5%	93.6%	52.8%	89.5%	58.1% ***	69.2%
In jurisdictions <100,000 population	89.3%	96.2%	39.3%	84.6%	17.9%	45.5%
In Western jurisdictions	92.8%	92.8%	57.1%	88.9%	85.7%	92.3%
In Mid-Western jurisdictions	10.0%	100.0%	14.3%	50.0%	42.9%	75.0%
In Northeastern jurisdictions	87.5%	100.0%	50.0%	100.0%	12.5% ***	33.3% ***
In Southern jurisdictions	90.0%	93.1%	50.0%	88.2%	23.3%	30.4%
In high-performing jurisdictions[c]	96.8%	96.8%	48.4%	100.0% *	29.0%	47.7% *
In low-performing jurisdictions[c]	85.7%	92.3%	46.4%	76.5%	50.0%	77.8%

[a]*Federally qualified community or migrant health centers (329 and 330 agencies).*

[b]*Any type of contractual or working relationship between organizations.*

[c]*Using data from a 1993 assessment of the performance of core public health functions and practices in the jurisdictions, we classify jurisdictions as high performing (at or above median score) or low performing (below median score).*

**significantly different at $p<0.10$ level.*

***significantly different at $p<0.05$ level.*

****significantly different at $p<0.01$ level.*

jurisdictions (at or above the median). The health departments in high-performing jurisdictions appear somewhat more likely to interact with health centers ($p = 0.10$) but somewhat less likely to interact with managed care plans ($p = 0.09$) (Table 2). Both of these associations approach statistical significance only when we control for the availability of organizations in the jurisdictions. In contrast, high- and low-performing jurisdictions interact with hospitals in similar proportions. These findings leave unexplored the possibility of performance-based differences in the structure and function of organizational interaction, which are examined further through case study analysis.

Case Study Results

Detailed interviews with the local health department directors in 12 jurisdictions help to explain the apparent lack of association between organizational interaction and public health performance by offering greater insight into the structural and functional characteristics of these interorganizational relationships. These interviews confirm that interaction occurs in variety of structural forms and for a diversity of functional purposes, all of which may modify the effects of interorganizational relationships on local public health practice. The sites selected for case study analysis include one jurisdiction in each of the states of Alabama, Arizona, California, Colorado, Maryland, North Carolina, Oregon, South Carolina, Tennessee, and Washington, and two jurisdictions in Wisconsin. Two of the jurisdictions are predominantly rural, eight jurisdictions are predominantly urban, and two jurisdictions contain both rural and urban areas. With respect to population size, three of the jurisdictions contain populations of less than 100,000 individuals, while nine jurisdictions contain populations of greater than 100,000. Medicaid managed care programs operate in eight of the jurisdictions.

Interviews with local health directors reveal substantial diversity in the mechanisms through which health departments interact with other organizations. Health department interaction with managed care plans and private physicians is most often structured around formal service contracts and agreements, a finding supported in the survey of all 59 jurisdictions. Joint ventures, defined as programs or services jointly administered by two or more organizations and requiring shared authority and control, are most commonly established with hospitals, health centers, and voluntary/nonprofit agencies. Interaction occurs through less formalized mechanisms in only a few jurisdictions.

Health department interactions with other organizations show diversity not only in their structure but also in their function. Interaction is observed in four primary functional areas: planning, program administration, service delivery, and community assessment. Voluntary/nonprofit agencies and hospitals are the most common collaborators with health departments for the purposes of joint planning. Managed care plan involvement in joint planning efforts occurs in fewer of the case study jurisdictions than does hospital and nonprofit involvement but in substantially more jurisdictions than does private physician and health center involvement. In many jurisdictions, organizations other than the local health department (particularly hospitals) take responsibility for initiating planning efforts.

Hospitals, health centers, and nonprofit agencies are also the most common collaborators with local health departments for program administration activities. These activities involve the sharing of program resources (most commonly staff) among organizations that maintain separately administered programs. Managed care organizations and private physicians participate in these types of relationships in only a few jurisdictions.

For service delivery activities, local health department interaction with managed care plans occurs in nearly as many jurisdictions as does interaction with other types of health care providers. Service delivery interaction with managed care plans is most often limited to client referral arrangements. By comparison, service delivery interaction with other types of health care providers commonly involves collaborative arrangements to produce services jointly (as in jointly operated programs or facilities) or to deliver services jointly (as in colocated services and coordinated delivery schedules).

Hospitals and nonprofit agencies are the principal organizations that interact with local health departments for community health assessment activities. Although all of the local health departments in the 12 study jurisdictions report involvement in some type of assessment effort, most of these departments do not interact with managed care plans, health centers, or private physicians in carrying out these efforts.

In all four functional areas, most health department relationships with managed care plans focus specifically on the Medicaid and medically indigent populations enrolled in these plans. Specifically, most of the managed care interactions encountered in this analysis occur for service delivery purposes and entail local health departments providing clinical health services to Medicaid enrollees in exchange for reimbursement from the health plans. Notable exceptions to Medicaid interactions exist, however. In three of the case study jurisdictions, the health departments and managed care plans engage in communitywide planning efforts that do not expressly focus on Medicaid beneficiaries. Health plans in four of these jurisdictions contribute staff and resources to communitywide health department programs that do not exclusively serve their own Medicaid enrollees. Finally, a health department in one jurisdiction maintains a contract to provide public health services to a health plan's commercial enrollees as well as its Medicaid enrollees. Interactions between health departments and managed care plans that do not focus exclusively on Medicaid enrollees appear to involve planning and program administration functions rather than service delivery functions. Most of these interactions do not involve reimbursements or exchanges of funds in contrast to the service delivery interactions for Medicaid enrollees.

Interviews with administrators of the major managed care plans and hospitals in local jurisdictions largely substantiate the information reported by health department directors on the extent and nature of health department interaction with their organizations. Interviews are conducted with 37 managed care plans and 32 hospitals in six jurisdictions, including one jurisdiction each in Colorado, Oregon, Tennessee, and Washington, and two jurisdictions in Wisconsin. Discrepancies between health director responses and managed care/hospital administrator responses are evident in only one instance, which most likely resulted from differential awareness about interactions occurring at operational (rather than managerial) levels of the organizations. These results suggest that health department directors provide valid information regarding their relationships with other organizations.

Implications for Policy and Practice

A survey of a nationally selected group of local public health jurisdictions reveals that interaction between local health departments and other key health care providers occurs in a substantial proportion of these jurisdictions and that the extent of this interaction varies widely. More than one third of the health departments surveyed maintain relationships with managed care plans, suggesting that these agencies are indeed responding to a changing health care environment that is increasingly reliant upon managed health care delivery. This finding, together with the finding that most existing relationships with managed care plans are formalized by contract, suggests a need among local health departments for model contracts and other forms of assistance in developing formal relationships with managed care plans. The need for such assistance is likely to be especially great in jurisdictions where managed care plans have only recently begun operation.

Case study analysis of interorganizational relationships in 12 local public health jurisdictions reveals important structural attributes that appear to vary by organization type. Highly collaborative forms of interaction involving shared authority and control (such as joint initiatives and jointly produced and delivered services) are not as common in health department relationships with managed care plans as they are in health department relationships with organizations having a more clearly defined community service mission such as nonprofit agencies, hospitals, and health centers. This trend is consistent with studies of organizational behavior that suggest that differences in organizational mission and culture may inhibit the development of interorganizational relationships.[14-17] Furthermore, this finding suggests a need for strategies to identify and emphasize the shared objectives of public and private health care organizations in local communities.[18]

The case study analysis also reveals important functional differences in interorganizational relationships that may affect the extent to which local communities are served by core public health functions. Interaction among all organization types appears relatively high for service delivery and program administration purposes. Both of these activities are essential components of the public health function of assuring that needed health services are available and accessible within the community, one of three core public health functions identified by the Institute of Medicine.[3] Interaction for the purposes of planning, a key component of the policy development function in public health, appears relatively low for some organization types, especially health centers and physicians. Similarly, interaction that focuses on assessment of health risks in the community, the Institute of Medicine's third core function, appears exceptionally low for physicians and managed care plans. Health departments may appear highly collaborative with respect to the overall level of interaction with other organizations, but the functional characteristics of interaction may be such that one or more core public health functions are not adequately addressed by these efforts. These findings suggest that communities could benefit from policies that support and encourage greater levels of interorganizational collaboration in the areas of communitywide planning and assessment.

In several states operating Medicaid managed care programs, policies are in place or under consideration that encourage the development of formal contracts and agreements between managed care plans and local public health agencies for the purpose of delineating service delivery roles and responsibilities.[14,19] Findings from this analysis support the need for these policies but suggest that such policies might be strengthened if they were to offer stronger guidance and incentives for developing coordinated efforts in public health practice. Interorganizational collaboration for delivering services to Medicaid populations appears strong and growing; policy action should now be aimed at supporting collaboration for population-based services that often lack stable funding sources in the public sector (particularly assessment and policy development activities).

The finding that hospitals and other organizations outside the formal public health system often initiate collaborative efforts may suggest a need for training and support in community leadership and coalition-building among local public health practitioners. In many jurisdictions, the leaders of private health care organizations may have more experience than their public health counterparts in forging multi-institutional partnerships. Programs that provide public health practitioners with education, training and support regarding interorganizational relationships may prove effective in encouraging not only a greater level of interaction in local communities but also a trend toward more communitywide, population-based efforts.[20]

This descriptive analysis of health department interactions confirms that interorganizational linkages in public health are occurring in an environment shaped by the forces of managed care and cost containment. Results indicate that the structure and function of these linkages vary greatly across organizations and may mediate the potential these interactions hold for improving local public health practice. Health departments and policymakers at federal, state, and local levels need to encourage and support linkages that effectively respond to core public health functions, especially those functions that may not be adequately addressed by existing health department programs and services. Though explored to some extent in this research, the types of linkages that are needed and the extent to which these linkages are feasible are not fully known and need to be further investigated from the perspectives of public health as well as other health care organizations.

References

1. Baker EL, Melton RJ, Stange PV, et al. Health reform and the health of the public. *JAMA*. 1994; 272:1276-1282.
2. Fielding J, Halfon N. Where is the health in health system reform? *JAMA*. 1994;272:1292-1296.
3. Institute of Medicine. *The Future of Public Health*. Washington, DC: National Academy Press; 1988.
4. Hatcher MT, Halverson PK, Kaluzny AD. Managed care and Medicaid: lessons and strategies for public health. *Health Care Manage Rev*. 1995; 2:1-10.
5. Halverson PK, Miller CA, Kaluzny AD, Fried BJ, Richards TB, Schenck SE. Performing public health functions: the perceived contribution of public health and other community agencies. *J Health Human Serv*. In press.
6. Bolland JM, Wilson JV. Three faces of integrative coordination: a model of interorganizational relations in community-based health and human services. *Health Serv Res*. 1994;29:341-366.
7. Miller CA, Moos M-K. *Local Health Departments: Fifteen Case Studies*. Chapel Hill, NC: American Public Health Association; 1981.
8. Miller CA, Moore KS, Richards TB, Kotelchuck M, Margolis L, Kaluzny AD. Longitudinal observations on a selected group of local health departments—a preliminary report. *J Public Health Policy*. 1993;14:134-150.
9. Miller CA, Moore KS, Richards TB. The impact of critical events of the 1980s on core functions for a selected group of local health departments. *Public Health Rep*. 1993;108:695-700.
10. Brooks EF, Miller CA. Recent changes in selected local health departments: implications for their capacity to guarantee basic medical services. *Am J Prev Med*. 1993;3:134- 141.
11. Richards TB, Rogers JJ, Christenson GM, Miller CA, Taylor MS. Public health core functions—Alabama, Maryland, Mississippi, New Jersey, South Carolina, and Wisconsin, 1993. *MMWR Morb Mortal Wkly Rep*. 1994;43:13-15.
12. Miller CA, Moore KS, Richards TB, Monk JD. A proposed method for assessing local public health performance. *Am J Public Health*. 1994;84:277-403.
13. US Department of Commerce, Bureau of the Census. *Statistical Abstract of the United States*. Washington, DC: US Dept of Commerce; 1994.
14. Halverson PK, Mays GP, Kaluzny AD, Richards, TB. Not-so-strange bedfellows: models of interaction between managed care plans and public health agencies. *Milbank Q*. 1997;75:1-26.
15. Fiol CM. A semiotic analysis of corporate language: organizational boundaries and joint venturing. *Admin Sci Q*. 1989;34:277-304.
16. Gulati R, Khanna T, Nohria N. Unilateral commitments and the importance of process in alliances. *Sloan Manag Rev*. 1994;35:91-70

17. Zuckerman HS, Kaluzny AD, Ricketts TC 3rd. Strategic alliances: a worldwide phenomenon comes to health care. In: Kaluzny AD, Zuckerman HS, Ricketts TC 3rd. *Partners for the Dance: Forming Strategic Alliances in Health Care.* Ann Arbor, Mich: Health Administration Press; 1995:1-18.
18. Mays GP, Halverson PK, Kaluzny AD, Norton E. Alliances between managed care plans and public health agencies: the effects of organizational, community, and market characteristics. Association for Health Services Research 18th Annual Meeting Abstracts. Washington, DC: AHSR; 1997.
19. Halverson PK, Mays GP, Miller CA, Kaluzny AD, Richards TB. Managed care and the public health challenge of TB. *Public Health Rep.* 1997;112:22-28.
20. Halverson PK, Mays GP, Kaluzny AD, House R. Developing leaders in public health: the role of executive training programs. *J Health Admin Educ.* 1997;15(2):87-100.

Chapter 5

The W. K. Kellogg Foundation Community-Based Public Health Initiative: *Observations and Experiences*

Contributed by Thomas A. Bruce and Steven Uranga McKane

An established and accepted tenet of public health is that the profession has ultimate responsibility for assuring the conditions by which people can be healthy.[1] However valid this may be conceptually, and however desirable it might be from a functional perspective, the capacity of those who practice public health often falls short of that vision. The system for addressing health and human service needs of people within the United States simply does not work well for all too many families and communities, and the public health profession does not have the proper resources, personnel, or clout to fulfill its responsibilities to make that system more appropriate.

In January 1991, the Kellogg Foundation announced a new initiative, called Community-Based Public Health (CBPH), designed to strengthen the practice and teaching of public health by creating formal partnerships with people in communities.[2] The vision was that of a discipline that achieves its goals of improved health and well-being through collaboration and coalition-building approaches rather than through simple formulae for additional services or more protocols of professional disease control. An underlying goal was to explore whether the addition of informed and engaged community partners might assist in addressing some of the limitations of the profession in carrying out some of its public mandates.

Fifteen consortia were selected from 108 applicants to participate in a year-long leadership and model development exercise. From this group, seven state consortia were selected in a competitive process to (1) reorient public health programs and services toward community needs and concerns and (2) allow community-based organizations to help shape a new local health services system, one in which the community partners would work in collaboration with health professionals to improve community health. The seven state consortia that developed these models (California, Georgia, Maryland, Massachusetts, Michigan, North Carolina, and Washington) were funded in September 1992, with individual awards between $1.4 and $2.25 million over 4 years. Individual project evaluations were supplemented with a major cluster evaluation carried out by staff from the Center for Urban and Regional Affairs at the University of Minnesota. The initial consortium awards were periodically supplemented to carry out special projects that grew out of the community health planning and development process.

Although each individual consortium had some unique goals and objectives, there was a common philosophic basis for them all. For the public health agency partners, the challenge was to become mission-driven, to improve outcomes by sharing responsibility with both the community and academic partners. The initiative was more ambitious than simply generating additional community services, however valuable that might be. It was also more than the simple promotion of public health practice or of implementing the Faculty/Agency Forum recommendations.[3] The CBPH initiative actually was about building the capacity of public health agencies to work in collaboration with academic partners and with the community, broadly defined, to carry out the core public health functions of assessment, policy development, and assurance. The

Table 1
Community-based Public Health Consortia

State	Public Health Agency	Public Health School	Other Health Schools	Community-Based Organizations
California	Alameda County Health Care Services Agency	UC Berkeley Sch. of Public Health	UC San Francisco Sch. of Medicine	21 neighborhood groups; 7 youth groups; 16 cbo's in East 14th Crossroads area of City of Oakland
Georgia	Fulton Co. Hlth. Dept.; Cobb Co. Bd. Health	Emory Univ. Rollins School of Public Health	Morehouse School of Medicine	Rose Garden Hills; Kennesaw Village; Fort Hill; and Roosevelt Circle – all in Marietta GA; initially two public housing units in Atlanta
Maryland	Baltimore City Health Department	School of Hygiene & Public Health, Johns Hopkins U.	Johns Hopkins Univ. Schools of Nursing and Medicine	Clergy United for Renewal of East Baltimore (CURE); Heart, Body & Soul, Health Care for the Homeless; Baltimore City Pubic Schools; The Family Place; The Julie Center
Massachusetts	Mass. Assoc. of Boards of Health; Mass. Dept. of Public Health	UMass School of Public Health & Health Sciences	UMass Medical Sch. Dept. of Family Medicine	Holyoke Latino Community Coalition; Northern Berkshire Community Coalition; Worcester Latino Coalition; North Quabbin Community Coalition
Michigan	Detroit Health Dept.; Genesee Co. Health Department	Univ. of Michigan Sch. of Public Health	Univ. of Michigan Sch. of Soc. Work; Wayne State Univ. Sch. of Soc. Work; Univ. Detroit-Mercy Sch. Health Sciences; Univ. of Mich-Flint	Agape House of Hartford Memorial Baptist Church; Barton McFarlane Neighborhood Assoc.; National Ctr. for Advancement of Blacks in the Health Professions; Flint Odyssey House; Genesee Area Skill Center; Genesee County CAA; Flint Area Cmty. Econ. Dvpt.; Flint Neighbor-hood Coalition
North Carolina	Chatham Co. Hlth. Dpt.; Orange Co. Hlth. Dpt.; Wake Co. Health Dept.; Lee Co. Health Dept.	Univ. of N.C. at Chapel Hill School of Public Health	UNC at Chapel Hill Area Health Educat. Centers	Joint Orange-Chatham Community Action; Orange-Chatham Comp-rehensive Health Services; Wake Health Services; Strengthening the Black Family, Inc.
Washington	Seattle-King County Health Dept.; Whatcom Co. Health Dept.	Univ. of Wash. Sch. of Public Health & Cmty. Medicine	Univ. of Wash. School of Nursing	Seattle Urban Health Alliance; Lummi Cedar Project; Group Hlth. Cooperative of Puget Sound

initiative required an extraordinary understanding of the community that is the substrate for health and wellness, as well as its spawning grounds for risky behavior and illness.

The Individual Consortia

California: Consortium members can be seen in **Table 1**. Activities of the California consortium have centered around a newly created "Community Health Academy," which is committed to the education and training of health professionals about community organization and development, as well as about cross-cultural competencies in realizing improved health outcomes. The Alameda County Health Care Services Agency has provided strong leadership for its partners by demonstrating those values in its own programming. The agency, moreover, has gone through a restructuring process to move away from a purely "services" approach. The new emphasis focuses on setting an agenda with coalition partners to achieve agreed-on objectives.

Georgia: Much of the activity of the Georgia consortium has centered on after school tutorial programs that include health education by peers and by public health graduate students; street outreach programs have been initiated to prevent violence and substance abuse. Community people have prepared themselves for political advocacy, and new leadership skills have been developed by community members to facilitate change and spawn local improvements. The Cobb County Board of Health has been exemplary in creating new neighborhood health centers to respond to community needs. The Fulton County Health Department has focused its efforts on some of the Atlanta public housing units, providing access to new preventive services and creating a new Male Responsibility Clinic.

Maryland: Most of the activities of this consortium have been centered in the East Baltimore neighborhood that surrounds the Johns Hopkins University Medical Center. Clergy members have taken leadership roles in building local social service networks through their churches, including health care services. Ministers preach health promotion and disease prevention from the pulpit, and congregations are involved in a broad array of community development activities. The Baltimore City Health Department has trained community people as lay health workers to carry out preventive services (e.g. diabetes and tuberculosis control, visual screening), and the Johns Hopkins health schools (public health, nursing, and medicine), in an effort to collaborate with the Health Department and church groups, have agreed to employ these individuals to carry out door-to-door research in the East Baltimore neighborhood.

Massachusetts: Activities have differed in four community sites in the western part of the state and include such things as Latino coalitions on community AIDS prevention in Holyoke; making use of the radio and print media for Latino health promotion in Worcester, training community people as health interpreters, and creating a national model for the role of community organizations in not-for-profit hospital conversions; and various women's and children's health projects in the two Berkshire sites. The only local health agencies for many small towns in the state are volunteer health boards, and the Massachusetts Association for Boards of Health has gone through a substantial training and development program in order to be a legitimate partner in the CBPH initiative. Its local units now link much more effectively with staff from the state health agency in carrying out community liaison programs in environmental and population-based health services.

Michigan: Activities are centered in three teams: in northwest Detroit a church-based health promotion program has served as the centerpiece, with an active school-based health careers club. Activities in Flint, where many retired auto union workers live, have focused on an array of local neighborhood health improvements (see profile of the Genesee County Health Department in the Section III case studies). In Ann Arbor, the faculty and students from the University of Michigan have committed themselves to modeling community-based approaches to teaching, research, and community service. The Detroit Health Department, in the midst of reinventing itself, has trained community health workers who become lay volunteers in rebuilding their neighborhood. The Genesee County Health Department has become a national model for community engagement and innovative approaches to reawakening pride in a city that has become a synonym for decay. The health department defines its role as much broader than simple health advocacy—it speaks out strongly for reasserting citizen ownership and responsibility for improving the quality of life and health for all who live within the city of Flint.

North Carolina: The targeted area includes one urban site (Wake County, home to Raleigh, the state capitol) and three rural counties. Activities include a water and sanitation project for a rural settlement, diabetes monitoring and weight management projects, economic development, and creation of a Neighborhood Computer Access Center, community drug patrols, and a variety of youth and recreational programs. All of these local health agencies (Wake County Health Department, Orange County Health Department, Chatham County Health Department, and Lee County Health Department) have served as models for linking local citizen groups with educational services, health services information, and community development expertise. More than just bridging to such programs, the local agencies have recruited and upgraded their own staff to model the approaches they are teaching to community residents.

Washington: Activities include programs on the Lummi Tribal reservation near the Canadian border and projects within the inner city of Seattle. The Lummi "Red Cedar" project has become nationally famous for its approaches to pulling their youth out of high-risk behaviors and immersing them in traditional tribal competitions in canoeing. In Seattle, inner city youth scholarships and community development minigrants have been used to expand opportunities for the education and training of community residents, with particular attention to youth. The Whatcom County Health Department has worked as a sister agency with the Tribal Health Authority in the Lummi Nation to address a spectrum of health care and public health issues. The Seattle-King County Health Department has strengthened its mastery of multicultural health approaches in response to the many immigrants who live in the inner city, and it has developed special collegial relationships and assistance programs for groups who want to build healthier neighborhoods.

Lessons Learned in the Initiative

Several of the lessons learned were quite general, reflecting the use of partnerships and coalitions to address health issues. The most important of these was that the community is at the heart of public health and that the protection and improvement of the community's health is best achieved by full participation of the community in the selection, design, and implementation of programs and services that traditionally have been launched by public health professionals.[4] There is, moreover, a specific body of knowledge for community-based approaches to public health practice, and core competencies can be identified.[5]

The W. K. Kellogg Foundation Community-Based Public Health Initiative showed that taking a community-based approach was not only possible but also that it advanced the goals of public health practice and education.[6-9] In those institutions that had had previous experiences in community health development, it was apparent that there were earlier evidences of community health improvement, and there was an accelerated rate of organizational change, i.e. new approaches to the way that the agency carried out its business. The people who worked in these collaboratives seemed to be motivated by both personal and professional reasons.

For the practice agencies, there was a shift from a services mindset[10] to a capacity-building and assets-based perspective.[11] Both the community members and the academic representatives became meaningfully involved in agency decision making, and structural reorganization of the department was quite common.

Defining the Community

It was impossible at the beginning of the initiative for the Kellogg Foundation to identify individual communities across the nation from its own knowledge, so it elected to work with the community groups that the local public health agency or the university recommended as being suitable or viable. Of the 18 participating CBPH communities, only one was built around a single existing community-based organization, Strengthening the Black Family, Inc. in Raleigh, NC. In another, about a dozen established community organizations formed the nidus in a multiethnic crossroads neighborhood (Oakland, Calif). There was a church-based community (Detroit, Mich) and a ministerial group (Baltimore, Md), a native tribe (Lummi), and a public housing association (Atlanta, Ga). In Worcester and Holyoke, Mass, the Latino coalitions took primary responsibility for defining the community. In three rural counties in North Carolina, it was small isolated neighborhoods or public housing units that had been active participants with a community action agency; in the Northern Berkshires and North Adams, Mass, it was a loose confederation of agencies and groups that had been identified by the state Area Health Education Centers system. In Cobb County, Ga, it was an isolated pocket of poor homes (Rose Garden Hills) and a private low-income housing complex (Kennesaw Village). In Seattle, Wash, it was two complex urban neighborhoods—one with many immigrant groups and the other a school district with low-income African-American families—both of these later merged to become "one" community (the Seattle Urban Health Alliance). Finally, in Flint, Mich, it was the area around a neighborhood public health facility that initially formed the community.

In those instances in which there had been no previous pattern of community cohesion or action, it was necessary to spend additional start-up time in building the community understanding of public health issues and of developing new ways that these groups could connect to existing health bureaucracies. We learned that the existing community-based organizations often did not speak for their broader communities, because they were service organizations rather than representative organizations (L. Brown, personal communication, 1994). Sometimes they were as derelict as some people in the agencies and universities in understanding the potential of vulnerable people to define and solve their own problems. We learned that it was a new discovery for most CBPH partners that community people bring strong assets to any collaborative endeavor, including a relevant history, knowledge, and the ability to relate positively with policymakers. We learned of an unexpected downside: that some of the community-based organizations that move most readily to partner with institutions run the risk of losing the identity of their own communities (M. B. Tuggle II, personal communication, 1995).

Every consortium developed some kind of community health worker as a part of its efforts[12] —recruiting, training, and employing people from the targeted communities to work in the health field either as advocates, technical assistants, or paraprofessionals in increasing access to health services, or, in East Baltimore, carrying out community research studies. Although the approach varied in each consortium, the collective judgment was that this is an important way to connect community people with complex health institutions. Moreover, the potential gains in community understanding about health issues and their buy-in to the health and prevention agenda argue strongly for continuing such an approach, even if job creation is not a major achievement (and in this time of welfare reform it often is!).

Local Public Health Agencies

In an apparent dichotomy, the local agencies started out in most of the consortia as silent partners,[13] seemingly distracted by other commitments and the usual array of day-to-day exigencies. Many were faced with serious external challenges: intensely political arenas, drastic reductions in budget, labor union challenges to changes that were needed, deeply divided governing boards, antigovernment public sentiment, personnel retirements and other changes in senior positions, and unprecedented changes in the health care environment, with removal of large blocks of Medicaid clients into managed care organizations.

Within a couple of years into the project, however, these seemingly troubled agencies had commonly become the centerpiece of many of the CBPH activities. The agencies contributed a considerable amount to the success of the project in nearly every site. They accepted and trained students, worked with community leaders on an ongoing basis, trained community people for various health roles, increased access to health services for the targeted neighborhoods, served as facilitators for community input and decision making, and worked behind the scene to empower others.[14] In one instance, the agency served as the fiscal and coordinating manager for the entire project (Cobb County Board of Health).

A lesson learned was that it was difficult to get all the agency personnel, even in the most involved and committed departments, informed and skilled in community-based work—in other words, the diffusion of the CBPH philosophy and know-how was not necessarily universal even in places where top leadership was supportive. In addition, it was a consensus that the boards of health needed to become more engaged in CBPH concepts.

Academic Partners

We were fortunate in bringing into the initiative some of the strongest and most respected schools of public health in the nation. One of the schools was quite new (Emory) and one was nontraditional in its educational programs (Massachusetts). All the schools had faculty and staff involved in the initiative in varying degrees, usually at about the 10% level. Faculties were drawn from all departments of the schools; however, the most common place was from the public health practice unit. Although some notable successes were seen in contact of faculty members with practitioners in the local agencies (see example in Section III case studies for the Genesee County Health Department), this was not as frequent as had been expected. It was a common observation that a dearth of faculty leaders was available who were acknowledged scholars in the field of community health.

Nearly every student in the graduate public health programs had some amount of contact with the CBPH project; in some instances, it was only through an introductory course, but for many students, it was an in-depth assignment to a local health agency or to a community learning experience. Many of these students became highly respected by their agency or community preceptors, and they helped plan and lead important new projects wherever they were assigned. For many agency personnel who were uncomfortable with the extent of new community involvement, the flow of bright and eager public health students into the work of the local health departments was the bright spot of the CBPH initiative.

Governance Structures That Linked the Partnerships

It seemed not to make a great deal of difference what kind of structure was created, so long as it was perceived to be fair and accountable. The most elegant and carefully designed governance structure demanded a great deal of time from the members but seemed to work well. The least structured consortium had no governing board and no by-laws, but it served nicely because of a series of overlapping teams that had compatible and constructive leaders. Two of the consortia went through traumatic changes in their governing structures after the partnerships disintegrated over resource and power issues, but these were reorganized after a period of delay and became quite functional. California had an advanced conceptual plan that vested all its resources in a new Community Health Academy, only to find that none of the key partners was fully supportive when the plan was put to the test. It was considered excessively competitive with their own organizations. In the end, the role of the academy was modified to complement the efforts of the partners, and its work of teaching community values and multicultural competency was able to proceed.

What is remarkable is that in spite of some structural defects and the lack of experience of many of the participants in collaboration, so much was achieved. Stories abound of how each of the partners was humbled by the experience, how each one had to learn to listen to the others, how each one was strengthened and empowered by the new insights that grew out of adversity and unexpected success. Not only were entire communities transformed during the course of the initiative (one thinks immediately of Rose Garden Hills and Kennesaw Village Ga), but in some instances, entire service and academic programs were restructured and organizational/institutional missions were changed to reflect the lessons that had been learned through shared leadership and community-driven health development.

Leadership

Leadership has been seen at every level of the initiative and in every consortium.[15] The senior cadre of leaders for the overall initiative was identified and trained during the initial Model and Leadership Development year, and it was a mistake not to have continued this period of training at each of the sites thereafter because of the continual entry of new, uninitiated people into the project. New leaders in place have emerged over time in each of the consortia, although in different contexts. In one of the projects in which the governance structure collapsed, it was new leadership in the local health agency, the university, and the community that pulled the project out of the doldrums. In California when the Community Health Academy was experiencing its rejection by the senior partners, it was new leadership that gave the project a fresh direction. In Georgia, it was the emergence of energetic neighborhood leaders that transformed the two communities.

One might have assumed that it would be professional leadership, particularly from the universities, that would have been the mainstay of the initiative. In some instances, that was so, and some of the public health agency representatives were clearly in the same category, but in the end, it was the community leadership that stood out as truly exemplary. Many of these community leaders emerged from obscurity, blossoming during the period of community building to become consortium leaders for the entire CBPH initiative.

Learning to Access Capital

Skill building, resourcefulness, entrepreneurial growth, and business expertise have exponentially increased throughout the project, more in some places than in others. All projects are approaching sustainability in one way or another. Some (the most primitive) are turning to other philanthropic support. Others are institutionalizing their projects within the bureaucracy of the health departments or the universities. One community is turning to corporate partners, another to the Empowerment Zone alliance. Still another is capitalizing on the new skills that have been learned about community/organizational teamwork in applying for neighborhood development funds.

Learning Citizenship and Civic Action

Evidence of the growing comfort across the groups with a common commitment to social change is accumulating. Broad community development in the sense of citizen engagement, civic responsibility, and local action is being seen regularly across the initiative. It is possible that the spin-off into other neighborhood projects, business enhancement, area beautification, voter registration campaigns, youth recreation, and the like will be one of the true measures of the CBPH achievements.

Health Outcome Improvements

These were not measured in a controlled fashion because that was not the intent of the initiative nor was it possible to determine such outcomes with the varied number of projects and the short time period of the efforts. Nonetheless, it is hoped that measurable health improvements will result. Examples of areas that may prove fruitful in the future are (1) rate of HIV seropositivity in Holyoke, Mass, where CEPA, the Latino coalition, is actively counseling community members about risk; (2) effectiveness of tuberculosis control, diabetes control, maternity outcomes, and entry into drug treatment programs in East Baltimore; (3) reduction in enteric infections in those North Carolina counties where access to clean water and sewage conduits have been achieved; (4) youth fitness indices in Raleigh neighborhoods; (5) elementary and middle school academic achievements for youth in Georgia where health and education have been linked in community efforts (it is notable that already there have been more honor students in the past two years than in the memory of the residents); (6) figures on violence and safety improvements in Detroit, metropolitan Atlanta, and Seattle neighborhoods; (7) lower incidence in drug-related crimes in East Baltimore and North Carolina; (8) evidence of improved access to health care in Worcester, Mass, where community interpreters have been active; also in the immigrant communities of

Oakland and Seattle where multiculturalism has been taught and practiced; and (9) evidences of healthier youth in the Lummi tribe and in most of the communities across the nation that focused their efforts on a healthier future for their young people.

Health Policy Formulation

In the beginning years of the initiative, it was very threatening to the community partners to think that they should begin to familiarize themselves with health policy issues. They simply were too deeply engaged in local activities and in trying to gain new skills in collaborative endeavors to think seriously about distant and unknown decision makers. As the initiative matured, however, there was increasing thought given to the system changes that would be needed to sustain the local efforts and to make corrections in the things that seemed at fault when plans did not work out well. At the outset, it became clearer that policy did not necessarily mean that national changes were needed in the way that things worked. Quite commonly, there was a growing realization that if the churches could institutionalize their new approaches to community development (Baltimore and Detroit), or if the public schools could adopt more of the trial programs (Atlanta, Baltimore, Detroit, and Seattle), or if the city governments could assist more with some of the neighborhood recreational or environmental programs (Detroit and Seattle), considerable headway could be made for the betterment of the people involved.

Led by some of the more visionary academic and health agency partners, it soon became clear, moreover, that health policy was more than local issues alone. As a result, a CBPH Policy Task Force was appointed that had community, agency, and academic representatives from each of the seven consortia. That Task Force deliberated often and hard over the course of a year. As a result of its efforts, a new national organization has been formed, called the Center for the Advancement of Community-Based Public Health. Its mission statement is as follows:

> (The Center) is committed to the advancement of community-based public health - the protection and improvement of community health through the full participation of the community. (It) seeks to improve the public's health by (1) building and maintaining local partnerships which include community-based organizations, universities, and public health agencies at the local level, and (2) influencing policy at all levels to promote community-based public health and the partnerships which carry it out (Center for the Advancement of Community-Based Public Health, unpublished information, 1998).

A parallel effort of the Kellogg Foundation that has strong policy significance is its initiative in Turning Point: Collaborating for a New Century in Public Health.[16] This new national initiative is being carried out in conjunction with the Robert Wood Johnson Foundation and is intended to create three types of new integrated partnerships: state health agency with local health departments, state coalitions of partners to advance the public's health, and broad local coalitions to do likewise. Public health stakeholders such as business and corporate groups; faith organizations; government agencies other than health; labor groups; schools; hospitals; medical, nursing, and dental practitioners; managed care organizations; insurers; and community-based organizations are to set up models in conjunction with the public health agencies that reflect a fundamental rethinking of the way that public health action can be best achieved. The project will begin with strategic planning efforts in selected states/communities that have been successful in a competitive selection process, and the activities were scheduled to begin in January 1998.

Summary

Since 1991, consortia have been formed in seven states of local public health agencies, communities, and academic public health and other health schools. The purpose has been to test the hypothesis that taking a community-based approach works better than standard professional approaches in improving the health of people in underserved and marginalized communities. It has been an explicit understanding, and one that has proven to be true, that participation in the Community-Based Public Health initiative significantly aids the public health agencies in gaining competency, visibility, relevance, and national stature during a period of unprecedented health system change. This initiative suggests that changes in the way that local health agencies perform their work in partnership with other professionals and with those individuals who are most at risk can be a valuable way of addressing contemporary health challenges.

References

1. Institute of Medicine. *The Future of Public Health.* Washington, DC: National Academy Press; 1988.

2. W. K. Kellogg Foundation. *Community-based Public Health Initiative, An Overview*. Battle Creek, Mich: W. K. Kellogg Foundation; 1992.
3. Sorensen AA, Bialek RG. *The Public Health Faculty/Agency Forum: Linking Graduate Education and Practice*. Gainesville: University Press of Florida; 1991.
4. Policy Task Force Report. *Community-Based Public Health Initiative*. Battle Creek, Mich: W. K. Kellogg Foundation; May 1996..
5. Bone LR, Competencies Task Force. Final report to the W. K. Kellogg Foundation of the Maryland CBPH Consortium. Battle Creek, Mich: W. K. Kellogg Foundation; March 1997.
6. Bruce TA, McKane SU, Grace HK. Community-based public health. In: *Proceedings of the Sun Valley Forum on National Health*. Chicago, Ill: The University in the Urban Community, Association of Academic Health Centers; 1995.
7. Bruce TA. Lessons learned: community-based public health initiative, In: *The 1996 Fred T. Foard Memorial Lecture*. Chapel Hill: School of Public Health, University of North Carolina; 1996.
8. Brownson RC, Riley P, Bruce TA. Demonstration projects in community-based prevention. *J. Public Health Manage Pract*. 1998:4(2);66-77.
9. Schmitz CC, Johnson CM, Himmelman AT, Wunderlich M. *Executive Summary: Cluster Evaluation of the Community-Based Public Health Initiative, 1996 Annual Report and Final Summary*. Battle Creek, Mich: W. K. Kellogg Foundation; October 1996.
10. Kears D. Comprehensive restructuring of the health and health care system in Alameda County, California, to incorporate CBPH principles and practice [transcript]. Battle Creek, Mich: W. K. Kellogg Foundation; August 1995.
11. Pestronk RM. Community-based practice, In: *Community-Based Public Health*. Bruce TA, McKane SU, eds. Washington, DC: American Public Health Association. In press.
12. Goetz C. *Indigenous Health Worker Models in Community-Based Public Health Consortia*. Cluster Evaluation Team Battle Creek, Mich: W. K. Kellogg Foundation; September 1995.
13. W. K. Kellogg Foundation. *Cluster Evaluation of the Community-Based Public Health Initiative: 1995 Annual Report*. Battle Creek, Mich: W. K. Kellogg Foundation; 1995.
14. Minutes, meeting of the CBPH practice directors. Raleigh, NC; June 1995.
15. Johnson CM. *Reflections on Leadership in Community-Based Public Health Consortia*. Battle Creek, Mich: Cluster Evaluation Team, W. K. Kellogg Foundation; September 1995.
16. W. K. Kellogg Foundation. *Turning Point: Collaborating for a New Century in Public Health, An initiative of the W. K. Kellogg and Robert Wood Johnson Foundations*. Battle Creek, Mich: W. K. Kellogg Foundation; 1997.

Chapter 6

Assessing the Performance of Local Public Health Systems: *Trends in the 50 States*

Efforts to define and evaluate public health services have substantially grown over the past decade. These efforts have emerged as public health practitioners face growing pressures to improve their systems for assuring community health and to demonstrate the value of these systems to policymakers, payers, providers, and the public at large. The Institute of Medicine's 1988 report on public health, which delineated three core functions for public health organizations, provided a rationale and a framework for many of these efforts.[1] In 1990, the US Department of Health and Human Services formalized the need for public health evaluative efforts in its Year 2000 objectives for the nation, challenging agencies to "increase to at least 90 percent the proportion of people who are served by a local health department that is effectively carrying out the core functions of public health."[2] To monitor progress toward this objective, public health agencies have begun to implement approaches for measuring local public health performance. In this paper, we examine the approaches adopted by state health agencies for measuring performance within local public health systems—defined broadly as the collection of public and private organizations contributing to public health at the local level. We present findings from a survey of state health agencies, a review of state performance assessment protocols, and a study of three illustrative cases.

Background

The Policy Context

Recent shifts in health policy lend urgency to efforts for assessing the performance of core public health functions. Federal, state, and local initiatives to privatize certain components of health services delivery are enabling private organizations to share responsibilities in providing many public health services with the public agencies that have traditionally provided these services. These initiatives (including Medicaid managed care programs, public-private partnerships, and public agency closures and ownership conversions) may have substantial effects on local public health delivery systems.[3] As a result, public health policymakers and practitioners require effective processes for monitoring local public health performance in the wake of these changes.

State health agencies assume a broad set of responsibilities for assuring health within their jurisdictions and therefore are uniquely situated to develop and maintain performance assessment processes for local public health systems. State health agencies vary widely in the statutorily defined administrative authority they maintain over local public health agencies.[4] Nonetheless, their responsibilities in providing funding, technical assistance, and advocacy for local public health organizations create unique opportunities to engage in performance assessment activities.

State health agencies face strong political and policy-related motivations to engage in public health performance assessment activities. Increasingly, state legislatures are demanding greater accountability for funds spent on public health and other publicly funded services. State health agencies are developing performance assessment approaches to meet these legislative mandates.[5,6] At the federal level, the US Department of Health and Human Services (DHHS) is rapidly moving toward implementation of "performance partnerships" grants with state health agencies, an outgrowth of the 1993 Government Performance and Results Act (GPRA).[7] This initiative, which is already underway in some states, allows state health agencies to establish action plans and performance objectives as part of their contracts with DHHS for federal public health funding. As part of this initiative, a special panel commissioned by DHHS recently identified performance measures that are appropriate for key public health, mental health, and substance abuse services.[8] This initiative places additional emphasis on the ability of state health agencies to measure public health performance at state and local levels and demonstrate accountability for federal funds. Finally, public health officials at all levels of government continue to explore the potential for developing national performance standards and accreditation programs for local public health agencies.[9] As these policy discussions progress, state health agencies face the additional incentive of developing performance measurement systems in anticipation of new policy initiatives.

Major Assessment Tools

In response to these incentives, a number of methods have been developed to assess the performance of public health systems. These methods range from self-assessment and planning tools to validated survey instruments designed to collect comparative data on performance across jurisdictions and over time. Two of the most popular self-assessment tools are the Assessment Protocol for Excellence in Public Health (APEX), developed by the National Association for County and City Health Officials and others;[10] and the Planned Approach to Community Health (PATCH), developed by the US Centers for Disease Control and Prevention.[11] Performance assessment survey instruments include those developed by researchers at the University of North Carolina at Chapel Hill[12] and by researchers at the University of Illinois[13] (both of which are based on the Institute of Medicine's three core public health functions, and on an associated list of 10 public health practices that were identified by a work group convened by the US Centers for Disease Control and Prevention.[14] Other performance assessment approaches have developed around a set of 10 essential public health services identified by the US Department of Health and Human Services and the Essential Public Health Services Work Group.[15-18] Additionally, many public health organizations have developed their own approaches for monitoring performance.

Survey Methodology

To examine the progress of state health agencies in developing and using local public health performance assessment methods, we conducted a survey of state health administrators. During March through June of 1997, investigators contacted representatives in each of the 50 state health agencies and the District of Columbia health department regarding participation in a survey of local public health performance assessment activities. Letters were sent to each agency's health director or state-local health liaison (where they existed), asking these officials to identify an administrator who could provide information on the agency's experience with and approaches to performance assessment for local public health systems. Structured telephone interviews were then conducted with the individuals identified through this process. Administrators were asked about the existence of initiatives within their state to assess the performance of local health departments and other organizations contributing to public health activities at the local level. Those agencies that reported such initiatives as "existing" or "under development" were queried about specific attributes of these initiatives. These agencies were also asked to submit copies of any written documentation regarding their assessment initiatives, such as assessment protocols, manuals, and reports. All respondents were asked to indicate their perceptions about potential barriers to state performance assessment activities.

We received a total of 50 responses and one refusal, yielding a 98% response rate. Twelve percent of respondents were state health directors, and 34% served as their agency's designated state-local health liaison. The remaining 54% of respondents served in a variety of senior administrative positions, including directors of quality assurance, planning, evaluation, and management.

We summarize the survey responses across all agencies, and across subgroups of agencies based on the type of administrative relationship that exists between state and local health agencies in each state. This subgroup analysis examines the extent to which state-local administrative relationships influence the design and implementation of local public health performance assessment efforts. Subgroups are based upon a typology developed in an earlier study of local health departments,[4] and include centralized administrative structures, in which local health units function directly under the state health agency's authority (SC, Fla, La, Miss, Ark, Vt, Va, Del, NM, Hawaii, RI, DC); decentralized structures, in which local health units operate solely under the authority of the local government and/or local board of health (NJ, Conn, Ind, Wis, Iowa, Mo, Neb, ND, Mont, Colo, Utah, Ariz, Idaho, Wash, Ore); shared structures, in which the state agency maintains authority for some functions performed by local health units, while other functions remain under local control (Minn, Ohio, Ky, WV, Md, NC, Ga); and mixed centralized and decentralized structures, in which some local health units operate as centralized agencies, while other units within the same state operate as decentralized agencies (Calif, Nev, Wyo, SD,

Table 1
Percent of State Health Agencies Involved in Performance Assessment Activities

Type of Involvement	All	Type of Agency: Centralized	Decentralized	Shared	Mixed
I. All Agencies	**(N=50)**	**(N=12)**	**(N=14)**	**(N=7)**	**(N=17)**
Any type of involvement in performance assessment (past, current, or planned)	88%	100%	93%	86%	76%
No involvement and no perceived need for involvement	8	0	7	0	6
No involvement but perceived need for involvement	4	0	0	14	12
II. Agencies Reporting Some Involvement	**(N=44)**	**(N=12)**	**(N=13)**	**(N=6)**	**(N=13)**
Stage of Implementation					
Past activity which is no longer active	20	8	15	17	38
Current activity which is active and ongoing	50	67	46	33	46
Planned activity which is currently under development	30	25	38	50	15
Scale of Implementation					
Implemented statewide	73	83	62	83	69
Implemented for geopolitical subdivision	27	17	38	17	31
Initiating Agency					
Process initiated by the state health agency	70	83	54	83	69
Process initiated by local health agencies	27	8	46	17	31
Process initiated by other organizations	3	8	0	0	0

Okla, Kan, Tex, Ill, Tenn, Ala, NY, Pa, NH, Mass, Mich, Me, Alaska). State agencies were classified into one of these four subgroups based upon information from the Center for Disease Control and Prevention's Profile of State and Territorial Public Health Systems.[19]

We also conducted a qualitative assessment of performance assessment activities based on a review of documents submitted by state health agencies. Documents were submitted by 18 agencies, representing approximately half (51%) of the agencies that reported an existing or planned assessment activity. Document reviews examined the types of measures used within state performance assessment activities, as well as the types of organizations targeted by these activities.

Results

Performance Assessment Involvement

Survey results suggest that state health agencies are heavily engaged in efforts to assess the performance of local public health organizations. Eighty-eight percent of respondents report that their department has some level of involvement in local public health performance assessment (**Table 1**). Of these departments, 50% maintain an ongoing performance assessment process that is currently active, 30% are engaged in developing a new or revised performance assessment process that is not yet active, and 20% report past involvement in a performance assessment process that is no longer active. Respondents from only four departments (8%) indicate that their department does not currently face a substantial need to assess the performance of local public health systems. Agencies with mixed state-local administrative relationships appear less likely than other types of agencies to report current or planned involvement in performance assessment activities.

Almost three quarters of the departments that report involvement in local public health performance assessment indicate that these activities are conducted on a statewide basis. The remaining 27% of these departments report that assessments are conducted only for specific geopolitical subdivisions within the state (most commonly the largest counties, cities, or districts).

Reasons for lacking statewide coverage in assessment activities include state agency requirements for pilot testing assessment activities before decisions are made on statewide implementation, state agency requirements for securing the participation and / or approval of local health agencies, and state agency reliance on local health agencies for initiation and / or implementation of performance assessment activities. Agencies reporting only past involvement in assessment activities appear much less likely to have used a statewide process, compared with agencies reporting current or planned activities (22% versus 86%).

Approximately 71% of the departments reporting involvement in assessment processes indicate that these activities are initiated by the state health agency. By comparison, 27% of these departments report that local public health agencies initiate these activities, and 2% indicate that other community organizations are responsible for initiation. State agencies that maintain decentralized administrative relationships with local public health agencies appear more likely to report that local agencies initiate performance assessment activities, compared to agencies with other types of administrative relationships. Moreover, agencies reporting current or planned involvement in assessment activities appear substantially more likely to have initiated the activities, compared to agencies reporting only past involvement (80% versus 33%).

We find only modest differences in operational characteristics between agencies that report existing or planned performance assessment processes (assessment agencies) and those that do not (nonassessment agencies) (**Table 2**). Assessment agencies appear to have somewhat smaller per capita staffing levels and per capita expenditures than nonassessment agencies. Assessment agencies also oversee somewhat larger numbers of local public health agencies compared to nonassessment agencies. With regard to administrative relationships between state and local health agencies, both centralized and decentralized relationships appear more common among assessment agencies. Nonassessment agencies appear more likely to maintain mixed relationships which are centralized for some local public health agencies decentralized for other local agencies. Assessment agencies serve states with somewhat larger populations and somewhat poorer socioeconomic and health status indicators, compared with nonassessment agencies. Poverty, infant mortality, low birthweight births, and teen births all appear somewhat more common within states served by assessment agencies.

Performance Assessment Development

Of the 44 departments reporting involvement in performance assessment activities, 36% indicate that these activities were exclusively developed from internally established performance measures, policies, and guidelines (**Table 3**). Another 45% of these departments indicate that their performance assessment processes were derived purely from externally developed tools and protocols. The remaining 18% of departments report that their assessment processes were developed by combining externally developed tools with internally developed methods. Among those agencies reporting only past involvement in performance assessment activities, externally developed tools appear more commonly used than internally developed tools or combined methods (89% compared with 0% and 11%). In contrast, agencies with current or planned involvement in assessment activities report the use of internally developed methods (46%) more commonly than externally developed tools (34%) or combined methods (20%). The most commonly used external assessment tools include APEX (41%), PATCH (14%), and survey instruments developed by universities (14%). Several states also report using the assessment processes developed by other state health departments such as those in Washington, Missouri, Minnesota, and West Virginia.

Half of the agencies reporting involvement in performance assessment activities indicate that these activities were developed to reflect performance levels for the Institute of Medicine's three core public health functions (assessment, policy development, and assurance). These agencies report that the core function concepts were useful for such activities as selecting appropriate performance measures, delineating domains of performance, and evaluating the findings of performance assessment efforts. One quarter of the agencies with performance assessment processes indicate that these processes were designed to measure performance for the 10 essential public health services identified by the US Department of Health and Human Services. Several of these agencies report that their performance assessment processes were carried out in conjunction with a larger, multistate study of public health expenditures for the 10 essential public health services, conducted by the US Public Health Service and the Public Health Foundation during 1996. Almost half of the agencies with performance assessment processes report that they used neither the Institute of Medicine's core function concepts nor the DHHS's essential public health services framework in establishing these processes.

Table 2
Selected Characteristics of States with and without Performance Assessment Activities

Characteristic	Current or Planned Assessment Activity? No (N=15) Mean	No (N=15) St. Dev.	Yes (N=35) Mean	Yes (N=35) St. Dev.	Signif.[a]
Average number of state FTE employees in health (1000s, FY 1993)[b]	12.2	14.1	13.8	13.4	
Average population per state health employee[b]	425	210	437	250	
Average state health expenditures ($ Millions, FY 1994)[b]	422	414	691	1,051	
Average state health expenditures per capita ($)[b]	121	71	106	42	
Average number of local public health agencies (1990)[c]	49.1	56.0	60.4	39.1	
% of states with centralized state-local administrative relationships (1990)[c]	6.7	25.8	31.4	47.1	*
% of states with decentralized state-local administrative relationships (1990)[c]	13.3	35.2	31.4	47.1	
% of states with shared state-local administrative relationships (1990)[c]	13.3	35.2	14.3	35.5	
% of states with mixed state-local administrative relationships (1990)[c]	66.7	48.8	22.9	42.6	**
Average resident population (1000s, 1995)[b]	4,310	5,140	5,570	6,080	
Average % of population below federal poverty level (1995)[b]	11.9	3.3	13.9	4.3	*
Average % of population lacking health insurance coverage (1994)[b]	14.3	4.1	13.6	3.6	
Average number of Medicaid beneficiaries (1000s, 1994)[b]	512	673	745	941	
Average % of population receiving Medicaid (1994)[b]	10.9	2.5	13.1	3.6	**
Average infant mortality rate, per 1000 live births (1995)[b]	7.1	1.4	8.0	2.0	*
Average % of births low birthweight (1995)[b]	6.7	1.3	7.3	1.8	
Average % of births to teens (1995)[b]	12.2	3.4	13.3	3.4	
% of states in West census region[d]	33.3	48.8	22.9	42.6	
% of states in Midwest census region[d]	6.7	25.8	31.4	47.1	*
% of states in Northeast census region[d]	26.7	45.8	14.3	35.5	
% of states in South census region[d]	33.3	48.8	31.4	47.1	

[a]*Differences are assessed using Cochran-Cox t-tests for continuous variables and Fisher's Exact tests for dichotomous variables: **p<0.05 *p<0.10.*

[b]*Source: US Bureau of the Census. Statistical Abstract of the United States, 1997.*

[c]*Source: US Centers for Disease Control and Prevention. Profile of State and Territorial Public Health Systems: 1990, 1991.*

[d]*Regions are as defined by the US Bureau of the Census.*

These agencies base their assessment processes on statutorily defined public health activities or internally developed concepts of public health practice. Agencies reporting only past involvement in performance assessment activities appear somewhat less likely to use one or more of these established frameworks, compared with agencies reporting current or planned assessment activities (44% compared with 51%).

Overall, 68% of the agencies reporting involvement in performance assessment activities indicate having significant unmet needs regarding these activities (Table 2). Unmet needs are reported by half of the agencies with no involvement in performance assessment activities, by 56% of the agencies with past involvement only, and by 71% of the departments with current or planned involvement. Frequently mentioned unmet needs include the identification and measurement of valid outcome indicators for public health services (seven agencies), the ability to assess the public health activities performed by nongovern-

Table 3
Selected Trends in Performance Assessment System Development Among State Agencies with Involvement in Local Public Health Performance Assessment

Trend	All (N=44)	Centralized (N=12)	Decentralized (N=13)	Shared (N=6)	Mixed (N=13)
		Type of Agency			
I. Performance Assessment Methods					
Used only internally developed methods	36%	42%	31%	50%	31%
Used only externally developed methods	45	33	54	33	54
Used both internally developed and externally developed methods	18	25	15	17	15
II. Performance Assessment Frameworks					
Used IOM core function framework only	25	33	31	17	15
Used DHHS essential services framework only	2	0	8	0	0
Used both IOM and DHHS frameworks	23	17	23	17	31
Used neither IOM nor DHHS framework	50	50	38	67	54
III. Unmet Needs in Performance Assessment					
Experienced unmet needs in assessment	68	58	69	83	69

Table 4
Selected Trends in the Use of Performance Assessment Results Among State Agencies with Involvement in Local Public Health Performance Assessment

Trend	All (N=44)	Centralized (N=12)	Decentralized (N=13)	Shared (N=6)	Mixed (N=13)
		Type of Agency			
Used for state-level planning and policy development	39%	50%	31%	50%	31%
Provided to local public health agencies for use in local planning and policy development activities	20	17	31	17	15
Used to allocate state health agency funds across programmatic areas and local jurisdictions	16	25	8	0	23
Used to inform budget appropriation decisions made by state legislature	7	17	8	0	0
Used for evaluation of public health programs	5	8	0	17	0

mental organizations (five agencies), the identification and measurement of efficiency indicators for public health services (four agencies), the ability to make valid comparisons across local public health jurisdictions (four agencies), the ability to assess levels of community involvement in public health activities (three agencies), and the ability to assess the competence and training needs of local public health staff (three agencies).

Use of Performance Assessment Results

When queried about how performance assessment results are used by state agencies, 39% of the agencies having involvement in assessment processes report that their results are used for state-level planning and policy development activities (**Table 4**). These activities include developing new training and technical

Table 5
Percent of State Health Agency Representatives Reporting Selected Issues as Barriers to Local Public Health Performance Assessment Activities

Issue	All	Type of Agency			
		Centralized	Decentralized	Shared	Mixed
	(N=50)	(N=12)	(N=14)	(N=7)	(N=17)
Cost of conducting assessment activities	68%	67%	69%	43%	80%
Securing qualified staff for conducting assessment activities	60	58	77	57	50
Obtaining appropriate methods for assessing performance	58	58	46	57	69
Securing the participation of local public health agencies in assessment activities	27	20	23	14	40
Lack of perceived need for performance assessment activities within organization	9	0	8	14	13

Each number represents the proportion of respondents who reported that they "agree somewhat" or "strongly agree" that the issue is a substantial barrier to their organization's performance assessment efforts.

assistance projects for local health departments, modifying state contract requirements and programmatic objectives to respond to areas of low performance, and developing new state-sponsored public health programs and policies in areas of low performance. Agencies that maintain centralized and shared administrative relationships with local health departments appear more likely to use assessment results for these purposes. Twenty percent of agencies with performance assessment processes report that results are fed back to the local public health agencies to assist them with local planning and policy development activities. Agencies with decentralized administrative structures appear somewhat more likely than other types of agencies to use results for this purpose. Agencies in seven states, or 16% of the states with performance assessment processes, indicate that results are used to allocate state agency funds among programmatic areas and among local public health jurisdictions. Three other state agencies (7%) report that performance results are used to inform the budgetary decisions made by their state legislatures. Finally, two agencies (5%) indicate that performance results are used to evaluate the effects of public health programs, policies, and services on community health.

Agencies reporting only past involvement in performance assessment activities appear less likely to have used the results for state-level planning and budgeting purposes, compared with agencies reporting current or planned involvement. Among agencies with current or planned performance assessment activities, 49% report that the results are (or will be) used for state agency planning, and 20% report that the results are used to allocate funding across program areas and local jurisdictions. Among agencies reporting only past involvement in assessment activities, none indicate that the results were used for state agency planning or funding decisions.

Perceived Barriers to Performance Assessment

Among a list of potential barriers, financial, staffing, and methodological issues are most frequently perceived to present challenges for state health departments in conducting local public health performance assessment activities (**Table 5**). More than two thirds of respondents agree that the cost of conducting performance assessment activities is a major challenge for their organization. By comparison, ~60% of respondents agree that securing qualified staff to conduct performance assessment activities is a major challenge for their organization. Fifty-eight percent of respondents report the lack of appropriate methods for assessing the performance of local public health systems as a major challenge. Somewhat surprisingly, only a minority of respondents (27%) indicate that securing the participation of local health agencies is a major challenge to their department's performance assessment activities. Agencies with decentralized administrative structures appear no more likely to report this barrier than other types of agencies.

Agencies reporting current or planned involvement in performance assessment appear somewhat less likely to indicate cost and local participation as barriers, compared with agencies reporting no involvement or past involvement only. Cost is reported as a barrier by 65% of the agencies with current or planned involvement, compared with 77% of the agencies without this involvement. Local participation is reported as a barrier by 25% of the agencies with current or planned involvement, compared with 31% of those without this involvement. Conversely, agencies with current or planned assessment involvement appear somewhat more likely to report securing qualified staff as a barrier, compared with agencies having past or no involvement (68% compared with 43%).

Performance Assessment Designs

A review of written protocols from 18 (51%) of the agencies reporting existing or planned performance assessment systems reveals several important design characteristics that may warrant further attention as these systems are refined and expanded over time. First, relatively few of the systems reviewed here include measures of health outcomes (especially those which are likely to be sensitive to local public health interventions). Most of these activities are constructed around indicators of public health structure and process, such as measures of service availability, capacity, and accessibility. For example, a structural measure used by one agency indicates whether or not the local health department has a publicly available policy agenda and strategic plan. Several other agencies use a process measure to indicate whether or not a community health needs assessment has been conducted by the local health department. By contrast, outcome measures indicate the extent to which public health interventions are having a desired impact on health. Only three of the assessment systems reviewed here incorporate these types of measures. All three systems use community-level measures of health status, such as the prevalence of behavioral risk factors or the incidence of vaccine-preventable diseases within the community. One of the assessment systems also uses outcome measures that are targeted at specific public health services, such as the proportion of family planning clinic clients who become pregnant. Whether communitywide or service-specific, outcome measures enable performance assessment systems to inform resource allocation decisions at both state and local levels on the basis of the effectiveness of alternative public health interventions.

Another prevalent design characteristic of state assessment systems is a focus on local health department activities and performance. Recent studies have documented the substantial public health contributions made by organizations other than the local health department.[21] Nonetheless, few of the assessment systems examined in this study include public health performance measures for other organizations, such as hospitals, community health centers, private physician practices, and managed care plans. Public health performance assessment systems should strive to measure the contributions made by these other organizations, especially in light of the growing responsibilities being transferred to them through contracts, managed care programs, and other privatization initiatives.

A final and related design characteristic of performance assessment systems involves the ability to evaluate the roles played by public health agencies in monitoring and enforcing public health responsibilities carried out by other organizations in the community. In many communities, public health agencies are reducing their involvement in direct service provision and acquiring expanded responsibilities in monitoring and evaluating the services provided by other organizations. Despite these trends, most of the performance assessment systems examined in this study include only cursory measures of activity in monitoring, evaluation, and oversight. Performance assessment systems need to place added emphasis on these roles, which are becoming critical responsibilities of public health agencies in the current health care environment.

Illustrative State Assessment Practices

The diversity of performance assessment practices underway within state health agencies can be illustrated through the experiences of three individual states. The states chosen as illustrative cases follow one of three basic strategies for developing performance assessment systems: (1) assessment processes that rely primarily on externally developed methods; (2) assessment processes that rely primarily on internally developed methods; and (3) and assessment processes that integrate externally developed and internally developed methods. As the cases illustrate, these three development strategies are not completely pure in practice. Internally developed approaches are unlikely to be developed without any knowledge of externally developed methods; likewise, assessment approaches using external methods are unlikely to be implemented without some degree of customization and adjustment. Nonetheless, the three development strategies provide a useful framework for comparing alternative state experiences in developing and implementing performance assessment systems. The cases selected for illustration here show differences not only in the development strategy used but also in the types of measures and assessment methods used. We derive examples of each approach from documents supplied by the state health agencies in Wisconsin, Washington, and Florida.

An Assessment Process Using Externally Developed Methods

The local public health performance assessment process underway in Wisconsin illustrates an approach for using externally developed assessment methods to construct an effective process for monitoring local public health practice and encouraging improvement within a decentralized state-local administrative structure. State public health legislation passed in 1993 requires all local health departments within the state to implement a performance assessment process in 3-year cycles in order to remain eligible for state public health funding. Pursuant to this legislation, the state Bureau of Public Health has implemented a policy requiring local health departments to use an externally developed assessment tool, APEX, every 3 years. The APEX process includes an internal performance assessment that enables agencies to evaluate their own capacities and service levels, and an external assessment that enables these agencies to evaluate the contributions made to public health by other community organizations. Local health departments report the results of their assessments to the state Bureau of Public Health, which then uses these findings for state-level planning and programming. To facilitate this process, the state Bureau of Public Health provides each local agency with annual reports of health status and health risks for the population residing within its jurisdiction. This agency also provides annual training sessions and ongoing technical assistance to local health departments regarding the correct methods for implementing APEX.

Interestingly, during early 1994 Wisconsin's state hospital association developed a community health assessment process designed for hospital use that draws heavily upon the APEX process. As a parallel effort to the Bureau of Public Health's activities, the Wisconsin Hospital Association provides training sessions and technical assistance to its member hospitals regarding implementation of their assessment process. Hospitals are encouraged to work collaboratively with local health departments in conducting their assessments. Likewise, the state bureau encourages local health departments to conduct the external assessment component of their APEX processes in collaboration with local hospitals. To facilitate collaboration at the local level, the state bureau and the state hospital association coordinate both the content and the timing of their regional training schedules. This strategy insures that local health departments and hospitals in the same region receive training in similar performance assessment techniques at about the same time. This strategy encourages collaboration not only between health departments and hospitals but also between neighboring health departments.

Wisconsin's state health agency makes use of a well-established, externally developed assessment tool that has already been used by one third of the nation's local health departments. Nevertheless, the agency administers an innovative process through which the assessment tool is used by local agencies. By encouraging collaboration among local health departments and hospitals, the state health agency hopes to insure improved compliance with the statewide assessment mandate and to encourage comprehensive, carefully executed assessment processes. The coordinated training and technical assistance efforts provided by the state health agency and state hospital association offer additional ways of insuring the quality of local assessment processes.

An Assessment Process Using Internally Developed Methods

Washington state's local public health performance assessment process developed from a larger state initiative begun in 1993 to improve the public health services delivered through Washington's state health agency and its decentralized collection of local health departments. State legislation passed in that year required the state health agency to prepare a comprehensive public health improvement plan to be updated every 3 years. As part of this process, the state health agency was charged with identifying the core public health functions that local public health agencies should perform, and developing systems for measuring this performance. The agency began this task by reviewing existing approaches to conceptualizing and measuring public health activities, but was unable to find an externally developed framework that adequately captured the extent and nature of public health activities in Washington. Through a collaborative process that included participation from health care organizations at all levels of government and the private sector, the state health agency derived its own unique set of 88 core public health activities that public health organizations in Washington should perform.

These activities were organized under five broad public health functions: assessment, policy development, administration, prevention, and access and quality. The agency also identified four public health capacity elements that were presumed to be necessary for adequately performing core public health functions: (1) the presence of supportive organizational structures and policies; (2) a skilled public health workforce; (3) a effective public health information and communication system; and (4) active involvement with the public, community providers, and elected officials.

During 1995, the state health agency developed a measurement tool to assess local public health performance in the core function and capacity areas that were previously identified. The tool was designed to assess performance in each of the five core function areas and in each of the four capacity areas. In June 1996, the agency sent this assessment tool to all 33 of the local health departments operating within the state. While strongly encouraging local health departments to complete the assessment tool, the state health agency allowed responses to be voluntary. In total, 85% of the local health departments returned their responses, allowing the state health department to obtain performance measures in the jurisdictions where 95% of the state's population reside. Responding departments confirmed that the assessment tool accurately captured their jurisdictions' capacities and performance levels. Results from the survey suggested that the core functions of prevention and administration were being performed at higher levels than the functions of assessment, policy development, and access and quality. Among the core public health capacities, structure and policies were found to be most fully developed in local jurisdictions, followed by skills and resources, community involvement, and information and communication. During midyear 1996, the state health department adapted the performance assessment tool for use with tribal communities and administered it to the state's 26 tribes. A 73% response rate was achieved for this survey. Performance results appeared remarkably similar to those of the local health department survey.

The state health department plans to use the results of its performance assessment in several important ways. First, feedback from local health departments suggest that the core function of access and quality should be divided into two separate dimensions for the purposes of performance measurement and improvement. Second, the state health department plans to use findings from the survey to inform its contracting activities with local health departments. Findings regarding public health capacity are expected to be particularly useful in determining the feasibility of specific state-supported programs and services in local jurisdictions. Ultimately, the department hopes to be able to use the performance assessment process as part of a performance-based contracting system that will allow the department to issue contracts and grants based on expected improvements in local public health core function performance and capacity. Finally, the state health department hopes to use findings from its assessment process to identify "best practices" in local public health activities and to develop guidelines for supporting these practices among local public health organizations. These guidelines would be designed to assist local organizations in linking public health practices to improved community health outcomes.

Washington's experience with local public health performance assessment illustrates the value to be gained from internally developing a measurement and reporting system that adequately captures unique characteristics and perspectives within the state. By developing its own assessment system through a collaborative interorganizational and intergovernmental process, the state agency secured critical support and buy-in for the system from a wide range of organizations (including those that eventually would be evaluated through the system). State administrators report that the benefits of their internally developed system largely outweigh the costs that were incurred through substantial development time and effort.

An Assessment Process Integrating External and Internal Methods

The performance assessment process maintained by Florida's state health agency operates as part of a larger initiative designed to enhance the effectiveness and efficiency of local public health services. In Florida, these services are delivered through a centralized network of county public health agencies that are organized and administered through regional districts. Florida's Statewide Public Health Quality Improvement System draws on the core concepts of continuous quality improvement (CQI) and total quality management (TQM) methods, which have gained popularity in industrial sectors and, more recently, the health care field. In operating a performance assessment process to support its quality improvement system, the state agency employs a wide range of indicators to track the performance of local public health jurisdictions over time and in comparison with each other. These indicators include a collection of health status measures that are used to monitor the health outcomes of local public health services. These health status measures were largely chosen from those included in the US Department of Health and Human Services' Healthy People 2000 objectives for the nation, and the American Public Health Association's Healthy Communities 2000 model standards. The state health agency also uses a group of indicators to measure local public health structures and processes, drawing mainly on the indicators used in the APEX and PATCH assessment tools. The agency combines indicators from these externally developed planning and assessment tools with additional measures that are sensitive to the specific attributes of local public health services in Florida. These additional measures include routinely collected programmatic data regarding local public health service delivery characteristics and utilization information, as well as data gleaned from chart audits, client satisfaction surveys, and employee satisfaction surveys that are conducted periodically in each local public health jurisdiction.

The state agency conducts a performance review process in partnership with each local health department using a 1-year cycle for large jurisdictions and a 2- to 5-year cycle for smaller jurisdictions. As part of this process, each local department establishes a goal for each performance indicator. The state health agency collects and analyzes the performance indicators for a given local jurisdiction and then conducts an on-site review with the local department. During this review, the state health agency and local health department evaluate the progress that has been made in meeting the goals established by the local department. Staff from the state and local agencies use the process specified in the APEX protocol to examine problem performance areas in detail and develop a plan for improvement. Each on-site review ends with a concluding workshop and a performance report issued by the state health agency.

Florida's public health assessment system has successfully operated since 1990, with frequent revisions and improvements made to the process along the way. The state health agency has made ample use of existing performance assessment methods in designing its process, but it has also found it necessary to add components that address unique characteristics and concerns of Florida's public health system (such as utilization and delivery measures for specific programs and services, and measures of client and employee satisfaction). State officials report that the costs of maintaining this process are substantial but worthwhile, given the improvements in public health effectiveness that are likely to be gained.

Summary And Discussion

Results reveal a diversity of initiatives underway at the state level for assessing the performance of local public health systems. That a substantial majority of state health departments report these initiatives as operational or under development is reassuring (suggesting high levels of state involvement in monitoring and improving local public health practice). These initiatives represent active, state-level efforts to address an important component of the US Department of Health and Human Service's Year 2000 objectives for the nation. Below we note several policy implications that stem from specific findings about performance assessment efforts.

Tailored Methods

Survey results suggest that, despite the existence of a growing number of public health performance assessment tools and protocols, only a minority of state health agencies adopt and implement these methods in unmodified form. Many states develop their own methods of assessing public health performance based on the unique capacities and priorities of state agencies and their constituents and on the local arrangements for public health delivery found within these states. Other agencies use externally developed assessment tools in combination with internally developed methods. Such a strategy allows agencies to make use of tested and validated assessment instruments while also insuring that their assessment process encompasses state-specific characteristics and concerns. Given clear variations in conceptualizing and practicing public health across states and localities, flexibility in measuring local public health performance appears to be a prudent approach.[26]

External approaches to defining core public health activities (such as the core public health functions identified by the Institute of Medicine or the essential public health services identified by the US Department of Health and Human Services) are used in some but not all of the state performance assessment activities identified in this survey. The general framework delineated by the Institute of Medicine is more widely used among state agencies than the more focused list of 10 essential services. No department indicates the use of either framework without substantial modification to capture the unique ways of defining and performing public health activities within its state.

State-Local Relationships

When performance assessment activities are examined according to the type of state-local administrative relationship, we find some variation in the extent of health agency involvement but little variation in the nature of the assessment activity. Agencies with centralized relationships appear somewhat more likely to have a current or planned activity underway and are somewhat more likely to have initiated this activity. Reasons for this difference in involvement are not immediately clear, because centralized agencies do not appear any less likely to face financial or procedural barriers to performance assessment in comparison to other types of agencies.

Health Resources and Needs

Performance assessment involvement does not vary in expected ways with general operational characteristics of state health agencies. Agencies with current or planned involvement in assessment activities do not appear to benefit from greater human and financial resources. However, agencies that report such involvement do appear to face greater socioeconomic and health status needs. This finding suggests that these agencies may face greater pressures for performance improvement from policymakers, providers, and the public at large. These agencies may also maintain an enhanced awareness of the need for performance improvement.

Sustainability

Several important differences emerge between agencies reporting past involvement in performance assessment and those reporting current or planned involvement. Agencies with only past involvement are more likely to report a limited scale of implementation and a reliance on externally developed methods. Moreover, these agencies are less likely to report using assessment results for state planning and budgeting purposes. These findings are consistent with several factors that have proven effective in enhancing the adoption of innovations within organizations: (1) broad and consistent implementation to enhance the potential for impact; (2) the participation of key organizational stakeholders in developing and implementing the innovation to insure sufficient buy-in; and (3) linking the innovation with core organizational processes in order to emphasize its utility and centrality.[25]

Design Features

Our review of performance assessment protocols reveals several important design features that merit further attention as states expand and improve on their assessment activities. One of these features, the lack of relevant outcome measures, may be addressed by incorporating routinely collected health status measures into the assessment metric. Several health agencies use this strategy, including one examined as an illustrative case (Florida). The use of such outcome measures, however, must be tempered with the understanding that straightforward causal relationships between local public health practices and community-level health status measures do not always exist. Innovative ways of analyzing and interpreting such outcome measures exist,[5,27] but public health agencies must be willing invest the time and resources in fully developing these methodologies.

Another common design limitation involves the lack of measures for public health contributions made by organizations other than the local health department. Several methodologies exist for constructing such measures;[21,28] however, our results indicate that they have not been widely adopted in practice. Another promising source for such measures appears to be the emerging information systems maintained by state health data organizations. A recent review of these systems reveals that they maintain an expanding array of information from public and private health organizations.[29] Many of these systems are designed to facilitate service delivery and coordination across multiple community providers. Despite the growing availability and accessibility of these systems within states, few are being linked to local public health performance assessment activities. Nonetheless, these systems exist as promising sources of information about public health activities performed by other community organizations.

A final design limitation stems from public health agencies' growing roles in monitoring and enforcing the public health responsibilities of other health organizations. The growing importance of these roles demands mechanisms for assessing the adequacy of their performance. Several state Medicaid agencies have developed mechanisms for reviewing the adequacy of service agreements established between local health departments and managed care plans. These same approaches may prove useful in assessing the comprehensiveness and enforceability of health department agreements with other organizations that assume responsibilities in performing specified public health functions, such as hospitals and physician clinics.

New Policy Initiatives

The current heterogeneity in state performance assessment systems poses some challenges for new public health policy initiatives such as federal performance-based contracting efforts and national programs for accreditation and performance standards. At least in the short run, these initiatives cannot depend upon the widespread availability of a uniform set of performance measures that can be used to characterize local public health practice across the nation. In pursuing these new initiatives, policymakers may need to accept approaches that preserve some degree of flexibility and variation in the measures and methods used to assess performance, much like the approaches currently taking shape in the heterogeneous managed care industry.[30,31] Over time, these approaches should yield the evidence needed to support more standardized methods for measuring public health performance.

On balance, we find the observed variation in local public health performance assessment methods to be healthy rather than problematic. The science of public health performance measurement is still young, and ideas about what constitutes effective public health practice remain fluid. Despite the uncertainties inherent in these assessment efforts, states are recognizing the urgent need to measure public health performance and are devising viable approaches to address this need. These approaches are all worthy of examination and encouragement as the field of public health attempts to converge on valid, reliable, and feasible measures of performance.

References

1. Institute of Medicine, Committee for the Study of the Future of Public Health. 1988. *The Future of Public Health*. Washington, DC: National Academy Press; 1988.
2. US Department of Health and Human Services. *Healthy People 2000: National Health Promotion and Disease Prevention Objectives*. Washington, DC: DHHS; 1990.
3. Halverson PK, Kaluzny AD, Mays GP, Richards TB. Privatizing health services: alternative models and emerging issues for public health and quality management. *Qual Manag Health Care*. 1997;5:1-18.
4. DeFriese GH, Hetherington JS, Brooks EF, et al. The program implications of administrative relationships between local health departments and state and local government. *Am J Public Health*. 1981;71(10):1109-1115.
5. Nelson DE, Fleming DW, Grant-Whorley J, Houchen T. Outcome-based management and public health—the Oregon Benchmarks experience. *J Public Health Manag Pract*. 1995;1(2):8-17.
6. Griffin SR, Welch P. Performance-based public health in Texas. *J Public Health Manag Pract*. 1995;1(3):44-49.
7. US General Accounting Office (GAO). *Performance Budgeting: Past Initiatives Offer Insights for GPRA*. Washington, DC: GAO; March 1997.
8. US Department of Health and Human Services, Panel on Performance Measures and Data for Public Health Performance Partnership Grants. *Assessment of Performance Measures for Public Health, Substance Abuse, and Mental Health*. Washington, DC: National Academy Press; 1997.
9. Turnock, BJ, Handler A. Is public health ready for reform? The case for accrediting local health departments. *J Public Health Manag Pract*. 1996; 2(3):41-45.
10. National Association of County and City Health Officials (NACCHO). *Assessment Protocol for Excellence in Public Health*. Washington, DC: NACCHO; 1991.
11. Greene LW. PATCH: CDC's Planned Approach to Community Health, an application of PRECEED and an inspiration for PROCEED. *J Health Educ*. 1992;23(3):140-147.
12. Miller CA, Moore KS, Richards TB, McKaig C. A screening survey to assess local public health performance. *Public Health Rep*. 1994;109:659-664.
13. Turnock BJ, Handler A, Hall W, Potsic S, Nalluri R, Vaughn EH. Local health department effectiveness in addressing the core functions of public health. *Public Health Rep*. 1994;109:653-658.
14. Dyall WW. Ten organizational practices of public health: a historical perspective. *Am J Prev Med*. 1995;11:6-8.
15. Baker EL, Melton RJ, Stange PV. Health reform and the health of the public: forging community health partnerships. *JAMA*. 1994;272:1276-1282.
16. Eilbert K, Barry M, Bialek R. *Measuring Expenditures for Core Public Health Functions*. Washington, DC: Public Health Foundation; 1996.
17. Eilbert KW, Barry M, Bialek R, et al. 1997. Public health expenditures: developing estimates for improved policy-making. *J Public Health Manag Pract*. 1997;3(3):1-9.
18. Grason HA, Guyer B. *Public MCH Program Functions: Essential Public Health Services to Promote Maternal and Child Health in America*. Baltimore, Md: The Johns Hopkins University School of Hygiene and Public Health; 1995.
19. US Centers for Disease Control and Prevention (CDC), Public Health Practice Program Office. *Profile of State and Territorial Public Health Systems: United States, 1990*. Atlanta, Ga: CDC; 1991.
20. US Centers for Disease Control and Prevention (CDC). Estimated expenditures for essential public health services—selected states, fiscal year 1995. *MMWR Morb Mortal Wkly Rep*. 1997;46(7): 150-152.
21. Halverson, PK, Miller CA, Kaluzny AD, Fried BJ, Richards TB, Schenck SE. Performing public

health functions: the perceived contribution of public health and other community agencies. *J Health Human Serv Admin*. 1996;18(3):288-303.

22. National Association of County and City Health Officials (NACCHO). *Special Report: Planning Activities of Local Health Departments*. Washington, DC: NACCHO.
23. Washington State Department of Health. *Public Health Improvement Plan: A Blueprint for Action*. Olympia: Washington State Department of Health; 1996.
24. Speake DL, Mason KP, Broadway TM, Sylvester M, Morrison SP. Integrating indicators into a public health quality improvement system. *Am J Public Health*. 1995;85(10):1448-1449.
25. McLaughlin CP, Kaluzny AD. *Continuous Quality Improvement in Health Care: Theory, Implementation, and Applications*. Gaithersburg, Md: Aspen Publishers; 1994.
26. Miller CA, Halverson PK, Mays GP. Flexibility in measurement of public health performance [editorial]. *J Public Health Manag Pract*. 1997;3(5):vii-viii.
27. Schenck SE, Miller CA, Richards TB. Public health performance related to selected health status and risk measures. *Am J Prev Med*. 1995;11(suppl 2):55-57.
28. Miller CA, Moore KS, Richards TB, Monk JD. A proposed method for assessing the performance of local public health functions and practices. *Am J Public Health*. 1994;84(11):1743-1749.
29. Mendelson DN, Salinsky EM. Health information systems and the role of state government. *Health Aff (Millwood)*. 1997;16(3):106-119.
30. Schroeder J, Lamb S. Data initiatives: HEDIS and the New England Business Coalition. *Am J Med Qual*. 1996;11(1):S58-S62.
31. Joint Commission on Accreditation of Healthcare Organizations (JCAHO). *Performance Measurement Systems: Evaluation and Selection for Project ORYX*. Chicago, Ill: JCAHO; 1997.

CHAPTER 6 APPENDIX:
Queries Used in the Telephone Survey of State Health Agencies

1.0 To your knowledge, has your organization been involved in any initiatives to assess the performance of local public health agencies or to assess the availability and/or adequacy of public health services delivered at the community level? (PROMPT: This includes planning for future implementation of such an initiative).

NOTE: If no, skip to question 2. If more than one initiative, repeat questions 1.1 through 1.10 for each initiative.

1.1 Is this initiative: currently active and ongoing; completed and currently inactive (date completed: ______); or planned for future implementation?

1.2 When did [will] this initiative begin?

1.3 Was [will] this initiative [be] developed internally by the organization[s] involved, or was [will] it based on established protocols for performance assessment?

1.3.1 What is the name of the protocol that was [will be] used?

1.3.2 Was [will] this protocol [be] implemented intact, or was [will] it [be] modified or changed in any substantial way? If modified, describe they ways in which it was [will be] modified.

1.4 Do you have any documentation on the protocol that you could send to us, such as the protocol itself and any manuals, reports, or papers describing the methodology and results?

1.5 Was [will] the protocol [be] implemented on a statewide basis (i.e. for all local public health jurisdictions), in an individual jurisdiction, or in some other geographic area?

1.6 Which organization was the primary initiating agency in implementing the performance assessment initiative: state health agency, local health agency, other organization (specify)?

1.7 Was this initiative based on the three core public health functions originally identified by the Institute of Medicine in its 1988 report (Assessment, Policy Development, and Assurance)? If so, how?

1.8 Was this initiative based on the ten essential public health services that have been identified by the US Department of Health and Human Services (Baker et al. 1994)? If so, how?

1.9 How were [will] the results of this initiative [be] used (mark all that apply):

_____used for state planning and policy development activities

_____ provided to local public health agencies for use in local planning and policy development activities

_____ used to allocate state funds across programmatic areas and/or local jurisdictions

_____ used to inform budget appropriation decisions in state legislature

_____ used for evaluation of public health programs and services

_____ other (specify).

1.10 Are there plans to conduct another performance assessment initiative in the future?

2.0 Do you have any performance assessment needs related to public health that are not addressed by existing tools and protocols? If so, describe.

3.0 Please rate the following set of statements in terms of your level of agreement with them, using the following scale: (1) strongly disagree, (2) disagree somewhat, (3) neither agree nor disagree, (4) agree somewhat, (5) strongly agree.

_____ a. My organization does not currently face a significant need to conduct an assessment of the performance of local public health organizations, programs, and structures.

CHAPTER 6 APPENDIX:
Queries Used in the Telephone Survey of State Health Agencies *(con't)*

_____ b. The cost of conducting a public health performance assessment initiative is a major challenge to my organization.

_____ c. The ability to secure the participation of local public health organizations in performance assessment activities is a major challenge for my organization.

_____ d. The lack of reliable and accurate performance assessment methods is a major challenge to my organization.

_____ e. The lack of qualified staff to conduct performance assessment activities is a major challenge to my organization.

4.0 What other barriers does your organization face in assessing local public health performance?

Chapter 7

Longitudinal Observations of Local Health Departments: *Structure, Function, and Interaction*

Background

Local health departments have weathered dramatic changes in their environments over the past two decades. Changes in health and social policy, newly emerging and resurgent health threats, demographic shifts, macroeconomic cycles, and marketplace trends in health care delivery are but a few of the forces that have shaped the demand for and provision of public health services during this period. Local health departments have proven remarkably adaptable and responsive to these forces.

By adapting to community-specific capacities and needs, local health departments have become as heterogeneous as the communities they serve. This variability in local public health practice might lead some observers to conclude that public health is in disarray.[1] However, a detailed examination of local trends has suggested that practice variation in public health often reflects the worthy efforts of health departments to assure community health in the context of public and private resources that vary widely across communities.[2,3] In this view, public health practice variation often stems not from gaps in effective local public health decision making but rather from the underlying variation in community health resources and needs.

This chapter examines how local health departments change over time in response to these resources and needs by using a series of longitudinal observations made on a group of 15 local health departments during the period from 1979 to 1997. The analysis presented here extends an earlier study of these same departments over the period from 1979 to 1992 by adding yet another period of observation.[2,3] The 15 health departments were originally selected for study in 1979 by an expert panel of public health officials. These organizations were selected as exemplary health departments, particularly with regard to the delivery of personal health services. The selected group included two departments each from Washington, California, and Oregon, and one department from each of the states of Arizona, Colorado, Michigan, New Jersey, New York, North Carolina, Ohio, South Carolina, and Tennessee. Five of the departments served jurisdictions with large rural populations, whereas the remaining 11 departments served predominantly urban and suburban jurisdictions. Three of the departments served jurisdictions with less than 100,000 residents, whereas 12 departments served larger jurisdictions.

Detailed case studies of these departments were conducted for each department during 1979, based on site visits and interviews with key departmental officials.[3] During 1991 and 1992, a follow-up study was conducted with these same departments. Structured telephone surveys were administered to each health department director, collecting information on health department organization, structure, and performance in core public health functions.[2,4] Five years later, during the spring and summer of 1997, semistructured telephone interviews were conducted with the directors of these same departments to assess changes in organizational structure and function.

Observations from the 1997 interviews are examined and compared with earlier observations to assess changes in local health department operations and to identify implications for local public health practice. This chapter begins with a review of the major demographic and health resources changes that have occurred within the jurisdictions served by the 15 departments, as well as a summary of health director perceptions regarding the most pressing public health issues faced by the departments. This chapter continues by examining longitudinal trends in health department organizational structure, financing, scope of services, and interorganizational relationships. We conclude by identifying a set of durable themes and policy implications that emerge from the longitudinal trends examined in this selection of local health departments.

Community Characteristics

The demographic characteristics of the communities served by the 15 health departments changed markedly during the period from 1979 to 1997. Most of the communities served by these jurisdictions increased substantially in population size. Three jurisdictions experienced net decreases in population during this period, and one other jurisdiction increased in size by less than 2%. The remaining communities experienced population growth of 5% or greater during this period, with five communities showing increases of more than 20%. Nine communities experienced growth in the proportion of nonwhite residents. Many communities also experienced marked growth in the number of non-English speaking residents, creating special challenges for assuring access to needed health services for these population groups.

Health resources changed substantially in many of these communities as well. Eight communities experienced net decreases in the number of hospitals operating within the jurisdiction, whereas four communities experienced increases in hospitals. Physicians increased in number within all of the communities, but population growth outpaced physician growth in four communities. Membership in health maintenance organizations increased dramatically in all but one community.

When queried about the most pressing public health issues facing their departments, a majority of the health directors mentioned illicit drug abuse and community violence as among the top issues in 1997. Tobacco use and access to primary care services were also commonly mentioned public health issues. When asked about the most dramatic changes in public health issues that had occurred within their jurisdictions over the past 15 years, health directors commonly cited decreases in infant mortality (three departments) and increases in community violence and substance abuse (four departments). Other changes that were mentioned included increases in childhood immunization rates, decreases in childhood infectious diseases, and increases in morbidity and mortality due to HIV / AIDS. Despite the occurrence of new and resurgent health threats over the past two decades, most health directors felt that overall health status within their jurisdictions had increased during this time period.

Organizational Structure and Administration

Nonmedical administrative leadership has become increasingly prevalent among the 15 health departments since 1979. Physicians served as the senior administrative official in only five departments in 1997, down from 12 departments in 1979. Of the 10 departments with nonphysician health directors in 1997, all are served by physician-trained medical officers who report to the director. The number of female health directors increased from two to six during the 18-year period. Turnover in health department senior leadership occurred in all but 2 of the 15 health departments during this period. Five health departments experienced turnover in leadership during the period from 1992 to 1997.

The number of health departments served by local boards of health has remained static over the past 5 years. Eight departments operated under separately appointed boards of health in 1997, and an additional four departments operated under city or county legislative commissions that were empowered to serve as the local board of health. Three departments reported no board of health.

Only one of the 15 local health departments under study has undergone major changes in jurisdictional boundaries. During the mid-1980s, Thurston County (Washington) discontinued its involvement in a jointly operated, two-county health district and developed its own single-county health department. This change was initiated to address difficulties in financing and decision-making within the former two-county intergovernmental structure.

Seven of the 15 local health departments have undergone major changes in organizational structure since 1979. These changes have assumed one of three forms: integration of new operational units, disaggregation or discontinuation of former operational units, and reorganization of existing operational units. Four of these departments have integrated new operational units into their organization either by creating new units or by merging with existing, formerly separate units. For example, during the early 1980s Contra Costa County (California) integrated its public health department, county hospital, and network of primary care clinics into a single department in an effort to enhance coordination in health services and realize operational efficiencies. Two other health departments developed managed care plans for serving Medicaid beneficiaries during the 1990s. A fourth department assumed operation of a federally funded homeless health center during the early 1990s after it encountered financial difficulties.

A second group of health departments has lost major organizational units over the past two decades through disaggregation or discontinuation. For example, in Maricopa County (Arizona), a network of primary care centers was separated from the local health department and integrated with the county hospital system. This reorganization occurred under Arizona's Medicaid managed care program begun in 1982 in an effort to facilitate coordination between ambulatory care and acute care services. A similar effort to disaggregate public health and primary care operational units occurred in Yolo County (California) during 1992. In this effort, a formerly consolidated department of health services was divided into four separate county departments for public health, primary care services, mental health services, and alcohol and drug services. This effort was undertaken primarily to reduce administrative complexity.

A third group of health departments has undergone efforts to reorganize or redistribute existing operational units in order to realize improvements in effectiveness and efficiency. In Newark (New Jersey), a separate division of environmental health was carved out of the larger health department during the 1980s. This action was taken to enhance the visibility of environmental health functions within the department and to improve management and accounting systems for this operational area. In Denver (Colorado), the integrated public health and hospitals agency was reorganized from a county government agency to a state-recognized independent health care authority in early 1997. This effort was undertaken to give the agency greater flexibility in operations such as contracting, financing, and personnel management.

The number of departments that are integrated with public hospitals has remained small among our selection of local health departments. One of the two departments that was organized in this manner in 1979 became independent of its hospital during the 1980s when the county hospital was sold to a state university. Another health department that remained independent of its county hospital in 1979 was later integrated with the institution during the 1980s in an effort to foster greater coordination and administrative efficiency. A third department has remained administratively consolidated with its county hospital since the early part of the 20th century.

Integrated health and human service agencies have also remained relatively rare among the selection of 15 local health departments. In 1979, four departments operated as consolidated health and human services agencies that provided both public health and social services to local residents. Three of these departments were later disaggregated through the creation of separate public health and human service agencies during the 1980s. During this same time period, one health department that had operated as a separate agency in 1979 was consolidated with its local social services agency.

Scope of Services

Personal Health Services

A majority of the 15 local health departments continue to offer a comprehensive array of primary care services in addition to population-based public health services. In six departments, a single operational unit provides both primary care services and population-based public health services. In two other departments, separate divisions for delivering primary care and public health services exist, but they are consolidated within a single department. In two cases, responsibilities for delivering primary care services have been transferred from the public health agency to a separate governmental department since 1979. The remaining five local health departments in this study have continued to operate in jurisdictions that are not served by comprehensive primary care programs maintained by local government agencies.

All 15 departments provide an array of categorical personal health services that includes immunizations, family planning, tuberculosis control services, and sexually transmitted disease services. Four departments, however, report declining involvement in personal health services delivery due to the growth of Medicaid managed care. One department has discontinued the delivery of well child services because all eligible children now receive services through a new managed care program for Medicaid beneficiaries and the medically indigent. Three other departments have reported decreasing utilization of family planning and sexually transmitted disease services in the wake of similar managed care programs. In contrast, two health departments have reported an increased involvement in providing personal health services over the past 5 years. Both departments attribute this increase to service agreements they have established with Medicaid managed care plans.

Six health departments provide school health services, although only two of these departments operate comprehensive school-based primary care clinics. Both of these comprehensive school health providers have expanded their numbers of clinic sites and staff over the past 5 years. Two departments operate home health agencies, both of which have experienced increases in utilization over the past 5 years. These increases are attributed primarily to the growth in home health use among Medicare beneficiaries. One department has added hospice services to its array of personal health services during the past 5 years in response to community demand. Four departments provide substance abuse services, most of which have undergone expansions in service delivery over the last 5 years.

Population-Based Services

All 15 departments report involvement in providing the population-based services of health education, health promotion, and epidemiological surveillance. Ten departments report involvement community health needs assessment activities, and three of these departments report increased emphasis on these activities over the past 5 years. All three departments attribute this emphasis to the involvement of other community organizations in the assessment process, including hospitals, voluntary agencies, and managed care plans. Two departments indicate increased involvement in providing case management, information, and referral services over the past 5 years. Both of these departments cite their service agreements with Medicaid managed care plans as the sources of this increased activity.

Responsibilities in environmental health services are maintained by all of the 15 local health departments. During the 1980s, one of these departments separated its public health and environmental health functions into two distinct administrative divisions within a larger department of health and human services. Nonetheless, environmental health services remain an integral part of the public health activities performed by the departments in this study.

Public Health Financing

Funding for local public health services has dramatically increased over the past two decades. An earlier study of these 15 local health departments finds that funding increased more than threefold between 1979 and 1992 (from $7.6 million to $24.4 million in nominal dollars) for the average department.[2] Data for fiscal year 1997 suggest that health department budgets have continued to increase during the 1990s to an average of $33.3 million in nominal dollars. Health director reports of financing trends suggest that public health funding continues to rise and that a diversity of factors is contributing to this growth.

Fee Revenue

Fee revenue has become a dominant source of funding for local health departments over the past two decades. In 1997, the average department received 38 percent of its revenue from fees compared with 29% in 1992 and 13% in 1979. Five departments reported growth in fee revenue over this 5-year period, with most of this revenue derived from the delivery of personal health services. Two of these departments reported that they now depend on fees for 50% or more of their total departmental revenue. One department attributed its fee growth primarily to the delivery of home health care and categorical personal health services. Three other departments reported significant growth in fee revenue owing to their contracts with Medicaid managed care plans. All three of these organizations provided comprehensive primary care services as well as case management services for Medicaid beneficiaries enrolled in managed care plans. Three other departments reported sizable losses in fee revenue as a result of Medicaid managed care plans. These departments did not secure contracts with managed care plans, and consequently they have sustained losses in the numbers of Medicaid clients they serve.

Local Governmental Funding

Local government contributions play diverse roles in financing local health department activities. In three of the departments examined in this study, local revenues comprise the primary source of funding. All of these departments are city government agencies. None of these departments report substantial changes in funding levels from local government sources over the last 5 years. In two other departments, local government revenues have declined over the last decade and currently comprise less than 5% of the total health department budget. For the majority of health departments in this analysis, local revenues exist as an important but not dominant source of funding, accounting for between 10 and 30% of the total health department budget. For these departments, local funding levels have remained relatively stable over the past 5 years.

State and Federal Funding

State government represents an important funding source for most of the health departments included in this study. Pure estimates of state support are difficult to obtain because health department staff often do not know when federal funds are passed through states to local agencies. When state funds and federal passthrough funds are considered together, the case study departments received an average of 22% of their funding from state sources in 1997, down from 30% in 1992 and 28% in 1979. This decline appears attributable to increases in fee revenue rather than to decreases in state awards. Three departments reported that state revenues have increased significantly over the last 5 years, while no department reported substantial decreases in state funding. State funding mechanisms included contracts, grants, and general revenue sharing agreements. The two departments reporting the highest shares of revenue from state sources (46 and 45%) received dedicated shares of state sales and motor vehicle tax receipts.

Federal funding sources are difficult to measure because federal passthrough funds are often indistinguishable from state funds. Nonetheless, five departments indicate receiving direct federal grants in support of public health services (down from eight departments in 1979 and six departments in 1992). The department most dependent on direct federal funds reports receiving 25% of health department revenue from federal grant sources. All of the departments receiving federal grants report that this funding has fluctuated over the past 5 years. Most indicate that these funds support short-term research and demonstration initiatives maintained by the health department rather than established, on-going public health programs.

Interorganizational Relationships

Hospitals

Local health department relationships with other organized health care providers appear to have grown over the past several decades. Only two departments report little or no collaborative activity with hospitals serving their jurisdictions. Planning and needs assessment activities appear to be the most common reasons for collaboration with hospitals. Thirteen departments indicate that they work collaboratively with at least one of the hospitals serving their jurisdiction for these purposes. Ten departments maintain service agreements, contracts, or joint programs with local hospitals for the purposes of providing health services to individuals and populations. More than half of these departments indicates that their collaborative relationships have developed only within the past 5 years. Health departments appear to interact more often with public hospitals than with private hospitals and with not-for-profit hospitals more often than with investor-owned hospitals.

Three health departments report that competitive pressures have deteriorated relationships with some of the hospitals in their jurisdictions. One of these departments competes with a hospital in providing home health care services. Two other departments indicate that the competitive pressures stem from their involvement as providers in competing managed care networks.

Private Physicians

Seven health departments report close working relationships with the private medical community (most frequently through the local medical society). These relationships primarily involve activities for community planning and needs assessment, provider education, and data sharing and surveillance reporting. Health officers in four departments actively participate in the local medical society. One health officer reports that the health department's participation in Medicaid managed care networks has strengthened its relationship with the local medical community because of the need to coordinate care with the private physicians that now serve managed care enrollees. Another health department reports that medical community relationships have been strained by the rapid acquisition of private physician practices by local hospitals. These acquisitions are perceived to have exacerbated physician competition and reduced communication and collaboration around communitywide health issues.

Community Health Centers

Health departments maintain strong and growing relationships with the community health centers that operate within their jurisdictions. Six of the health departments now operate health centers as a result of mergers and newly initiated clinics (up from two departments in 1979 and three departments in 1992). Seven other departments serve jurisdictions that contain health centers operated by nonprofit organizations or other agencies of local government. Most departments report interacting with health centers for the purposes of shared funding, joint community health planning, and patient referrals.

Medicaid managed care programs appear influential in the relationships between health departments and community health centers. Five departments indicate that their interaction with health centers has expanded as a result of the managed care programs implemented in their jurisdictions over the past 5 years.

Three departments developed formalized referral agreements and care coordination plans with health centers as part of their participation in managed care networks. Two other departments developed their own Medicaid managed care plans in collaboration with local community health centers. In contrast, one department reports that interaction with health centers has deteriorated with the growth in Medicaid managed care. In this jurisdiction, competition between health centers and the department for managed care contracts has caused earlier cooperative efforts to be dismantled.

Managed Care Plans

Health department relationships with managed care plans have rapidly grown during the last two decades. In 1979, only two of the health departments in this study maintained relationships with prepaid health care delivery systems. By 1997, 13 departments interact with managed care plans to some degree (12 of which maintain formal contracts with these plans for delivery of specified public health and personal health services). All of these service contracts are with managed care plans that serve Medicaid beneficiaries or state-designated medically indigent populations. Seven departments report interacting with managed care plans for the purposes of community health planning, and four departments indicate interaction for community health assessment. Two departments report interacting with the full population of managed care plans serving their jurisdiction, including those that serve only commercial and Medicare populations. Two departments that operate their own managed care plans indicate that competitive relationships with private plans limit the extent of interaction with these other plans. A third department that operates its own plan appears to maintain successfully collaborative relationships with other plans for the purposes of joint planning and community health assessment.

Other Organizations

Health departments interact with a broad range of other community organizations in carrying out public health functions. Four departments report that collaborations with nonprofit and voluntary organizations have intensified over the past 5 years, primarily for the purposes of community health assessment, planning, and community-level prevention. Organizations such as the United Way have initiated broad-based efforts in health and human services assessment in several jurisdictions. Local chapters of national organizations such as the American Heart Association and the American Cancer Society have become major sponsors of community-level education and health promotion efforts in local communities. Community-based associations and neighborhood groups have also become important contributors to public health interventions in areas such as violence prevention, environmental health, minority health, and adolescent pregnancy prevention. Several local health departments report that university relationships continue to be important to local public health activities. These relationships most commonly involve projects for technical assistance and health professions training sites rather than the arrangements for shared staff, facilities, and funding that proliferated in 1979.

Policy and Managerial Implications

The trends noted in these 15 case study departments cannot be reliably generalized to the full population of public health agencies, but they nonetheless offer insight regarding the evolving nature of local public health practice. Longitudinal observations reveal that virtually all of the departments included in this study have undergone substantial changes in structure and operation over the past two decades. Several implications for public health policy and management emerge from these observations.

First, the wide variation in health department organizational structures that existed in 1979 remains despite the fact that many organizations underwent substantial structural changes during the intervening years. Some departments moved to disaggregate personal and population-based health services, while others consolidated activities that were previously separate. These trends suggest that there continue to be little consensus regarding an "optimal" organizational structure for local health departments. Any arrangement entails advantages and disadvantages that must be evaluated in relation to local resources, political and market dynamics, and community health needs. The observations presented here demonstrate that local health department organizational structures can be fluid and responsive to changes in context and perspective.

Similarly, the local health departments included in this study are successfully operating under a variety of financing arrangements. Variation in funding sources and levels across departments appears to have grown markedly over the past two decades. A number of departments now rely heavily on fee income, which offers much more flexibility in how funds can be used than most governmental grant sources. Some of these departments even assume and manage financial risk under prepaid, or capitated, financing arrangements with managed care plans. Other departments continue to depend heavily on local and state government appropriations or on direct federal grants. Whatever the source, local health departments have secured substantial funding increases throughout the past two decades. The extent to which these increases can be maintained over time remains uncertain (especially given the uncertainties of the managed health care industry). What does appear clear is that, despite substantial changes in funding sources and mechanisms, successful health departments have aggressively pursued viable funding options to support and expand their essential public health activities. This almost entrepreneurial approach to public health funding may prove be an important public health strategy for weathering the changes yet to come in an increasingly market-driven health care system.

On the whole, the local health departments included in this study appear successful in adapting to the dramatic health policy and marketplace changes that have occurred at federal, state, and local levels. Managed care growth, Medicaid reform, hospital closures and mergers, and public health privatization initiatives are but a few of the challenges that these health departments have faced over the past two decades. In the wake of these changes, some health departments have maintained and even expanded the range of personal health services they provide. Other departments have successfully refocused their organizations around population-based activities and health services not sufficiently available from community providers. A key component of both strategies appears to be increased interaction with other community organizations. Many departments have used relationships with other organizations to expand their capacity for community health assessment and planning activities. Similarly, departments with continuing involvement in personal health services delivery have developed relationships with managed care plans in order to sustain these activities under new Medicaid programs. Some departments have even joined together with other community providers to form their own managed care plans. In a variety of ways, local health departments are using interorganizational relationships to address the challenges posed by policy and marketplace changes.

No single strategy or set of guidelines can be identified to assist local health departments in managing the challenges posed by shifts in health needs, resources, and priorities. Successful health departments appear able to monitor these local shifts and to mobilize the unique set of community institutions and resources to address them. Variation in local public health structure and practice should therefore be expected (both across health departments and over time). Such variation may indicate successful public health performance rather than disarray.

References

1. Institute of Medicine. *The Future of Public Health*. Washington, DC: National Academy Press; 1988.
2. Miller CA, Moore KS, Richards TB, Kotelchuck M, Kaluzny AD. Longitudinal observations on a selected group of local health departments: a preliminary report. *J Public Health Policy*. 1993; 14(1):34-50.
3. Miller CA, Moos M-K. *Local Health Departments: Fifteen Case Studies*. Chapel Hill, NC: American Public Health Association; 1981.
4. Miller CA, Moore KS, Richards TB, Monk JD. A proposed method for assessing the performance of local public health practices and functions. *Am J Public Health*. 1994;84(11):1743-1749.

Part II:

Case Studies in Local Public Health Practice

Chapter 8

Case Studies in Local Public Health Practice: *Selection, Methodology, and Organization*

Local public health practice in the United States has evolved into an intricate and varied collection of institutions, professionals, skills, and technologies. Local health departments, together with the many other organizations contributing to public health, use a variety of approaches for addressing their communities' unique health needs. To be sure, local variation in public health practice is not new. Differences in local resources, priorities, and health needs have given rise to important structural and functional differences in public health agencies throughout their history.

By examining the variation in local public health practice in detail, observers can gain valuable insight regarding the strengths, weaknesses, opportunities, and challenges facing public health organizations and the communities they serve. Case studies provide a powerful method of obtaining and analyzing these detailed observations both within and across communities. Case studies offer an in-depth view of the structures and processes used in, and the outcomes resulting from, local public health practice. As such, case studies can assist in examining key public health policy and managerial issues and in identifying promising new models of practice that may be suitable for implementation in other communities. Caution must be used in applying case study findings to other settings, because generalizability and representativeness of findings cannot be assured. Nevertheless, case studies offer a unique view of the dynamic and complex inner workings of local public health systems, providing valuable insight for public health managers, policymakers, researchers, and students.

This chapter provides an overview of the case studies in local public health practice that are included in this book. First, the criteria used for selecting the cases are described. Second, the methodology used in constructing the case studies is discussed. Finally, this chapter provides an overview of how the case studies are organized.

Case Selection

The chapters that follow present detailed case studies of eight local public health jurisdictions. In selecting these jurisdictions, our primary purpose was to identify communities that were exemplary both in the performance of core public health functions and in the extent of collaboration with other community organizations. This purpose reflects the increasingly apparent view that community health partnerships are essential to the continued success of the nation's public health system, given the policy and marketplace changes taking shape within the larger health system.[1,2] Cases were selected in part to help answer the following questions:

- What types of collaborative public health arrangements are achieving success?
- What are the organizational and environmental factors that appear to facilitate and inhibit the success of these arrangements?

Cases were selected from a larger collection of 63 local public health jurisdictions that have been the subject of ongoing study over the past two decades. Fourteen of the jurisdictions in this larger collection were identified by a national expert panel as having exemplary local health departments, particularly in the area of personal health care services.[3-6] Thirteen additional jurisdictions were included because they were located in the same states as the 14 exemplary departments but were served by less-developed health departments. Finally, a survey of public health practice in all of the local health jurisdictions in six states was used to select the three highest and three lowest performing jurisdictions in each state for a total of 36 additional jurisdictions.[7] While this larger cohort of 63 jurisdictions is not a statistically random sample, nonetheless, it includes substantial diversity with respect to population size, geographic region, degree of urbanization, managed care penetration, and performance of core public health practices.

Cases were selected from this larger cohort using the following criteria. First, we selected all jurisdictions that scored above the median score on a survey of local public health performance that was administered to the health directors in all 63 jurisdictions during 1992-1993.[8] We then used information from a 1994 survey of local health departments to select those jurisdictions served by health departments that maintained collaborative relationships with at least two of the following three types of organized health care providers: hospitals, community health centers, and managed care plans. With this subset of 15 local public health jurisdictions, we conducted telephone interviews with the local health department director in each jurisdiction to obtain further information about the nature of public health collaboration within the community. On the basis of this information, a subset of six public health jurisdictions were purposefully selected so as to include a wide array of collaborative public health arrangements and to preserve some diversity with respect to geographic location and population size.

Two additional cases were added to the collection of public health jurisdictions selected for study, based on the recommendations of public health experts. These two cases were not part of the original 63 jurisdictions that had been the subject of earlier investigations, but they were regarded as being sufficiently innovative and distinctive so as to merit inclusion in the current case study analysis. One jurisdiction was selected because of the unique approach being used to privatize certain local public health responsibilities. Another jurisdiction was selected because of an innovative public health collaboration that had developed with the support of the W. K. Kellogg Foundation.

Eight jurisdictions from six different states and four different US census regions were selected for detailed case analysis (**Table 1**). These jurisdictions are Denver, Colorado; Multnomah County, Oregon; Milwaukee, Wisconsin; Beloit, Wisconsin; Thurston County, Washington; Southwest Washington Health District, Washington; Genesee County, Michigan; and Memphis-Shelby County, Tennessee. Five of the jurisdictions are counties or joint city-county areas, two are cities, and one is a multicounty district. One jurisdiction contains less than 100,000 residents, while four jurisdictions contain between 100,000 and 500,000 residents. The remaining three jurisdictions contain more than 500,000 residents. Two jurisdictions encompass rural areas within their borders, while six jurisdictions serve primarily urban and suburban populations.

Case Study Methodology

The unit of analysis for these case studies is the local public health jurisdiction rather than the official local public health agency. We use public health jurisdictions as proxies for the true focus of public health practice (the community). This approach allows us to capture the array of efforts undertaken by both public and private entities that contribute to the health of a defined population. The public health jurisdiction provides a convenient way of defining a population and identifying the institutions, resources, and interventions that contribute to this population's health. Official local public health agencies figure prominently in the case studies because of their governmental charge to "assure the conditions in which people can by healthy" within these jurisdictions.[9] However, we also examine the public health contributions of other community organizations (both those made independently of and those made in collaboration with the local health department.

We used a multiphased process for collecting information about each public health jurisdiction selected for study. Some information about the jurisdictions had already been collected through earlier studies. During 1992 and 1993, health department directors in six of the jurisdictions had participated in a telephone survey regarding the performance of core public health functions in their jurisdictions. These same six departments participated in a 1994 telephone survey regarding the extent of health department collaboration with hospitals, community health centers, and managed care plans. These prior studies provided baseline measures of public health performance and interorganizational collaboration for most of the cases under study.

During the spring and summer of 1995, extensive site visits were conducted in seven of the local public health jurisdictions. The site visit for the eighth jurisdiction was completed during the spring of 1997. During these site visits, investigators conducted semi-structured interviews with the local health director and a collection of senior administrative officials at the local

Table 1
Characteristics of Selected Public Health Jurisdictions

Characteristic	Beloit, WI	Denver, CO	Genesee, MI	Memphis-Shelby, TN	Milwaukee, WI	Multnomah, OR	Southwest Washington, WA	Thurston, WA
Jurisdiction Type								
County			X			X		X
City	X				X			
Joint City-County		X		X				
District							X	
Population of Jurisdiction								
Less than 100,000	X							
100,000-499,999		X	X				X	X
500,000 or more				X	X	X		
Rural Component Within Jurisdiction							X	X
Separate Local Board of Health								
Policy/budgetary authority		X					X	
Advisory authority only	X		X					
Community representation on board			X					
Health Department Service Delivery								
Direct provision of comprehensive primary care services		X		X		X		
Direct provision of categorical/screening services only	X		X		X		X	X
Health Department Interaction with Managed Care Plans								
Operates a managed care plan		X				X		
Contracts with managed care plans for clinical services	X			X	X	X		
Works with managed care plans on community health issues		X	X	X	X	X	X	X
Health Department Interaction with Community Hospitals								
Integrated with a public hospital		X						
Contracts with community hospitals for clinical services	X		X	X	X	X	X	
Works with hospitals on community health issues	X	X	X	X	X	X	X	X
Health Department Interaction with Community Health Centers								
Operates a community/migrant health center	*	X				X	*	*
Contracts with health centers for clinical services	*	X	X		X	X	*	*
Works with health centers on community health issues	*	X	X	X	X	X	*	*

* No community health centers operate in these jurisdictions

health department serving each jurisdiction. Interviews collected information about the structural and operational characteristics of the health department, the contributions to public health made by other community organizations, and the nature of health department relationships with other community organizations. Each health director was also asked to complete a self-administered survey regarding public health performance within the jurisdiction (the same survey that most departments completed during 1992 and 1993).

In-person interviews were also conducted with the chief administrators and/or medical directors of the major hospitals and managed care plans that operated within each jurisdiction. These interviews collected information about involvement in public health activities and relationships with the local health department and other community health organizations. In most communities, interviews were also conducted with a range of other community organizations, such as community heath centers, voluntary health associations, and social service agencies. Interviews that could not be completed in person were conducted via telephone following the site visit.

Interviews of 1 to 2 hours in duration were conducted with between 12 and 25 organizations in each jurisdiction. In total, interviews were completed with 10 local health departments, 34 hospitals, 43 managed care plans, and 12 other community organizations. All interviews were audiotaped, transcribed, and analyzed for content using computerized text analysis software.

Key organizational documents were also requested from the local health departments and other community organizations serving each of the public health jurisdictions. These documents included annual reports, strategic plans, community health assessments, mission statements, community benefit reports, and contracts for public health services. These documents were reviewed for relevant content.

During the fall of 1997 and spring of 1998, telephone follow-up interviews were conducted with the health department directors in each of the eight public health jurisdictions. These interviews collected information on major changes that had taken place in the local public health system since the time of the original site visit.

Case Study Organization

A separate case study has been constructed for each public health jurisdiction. A standard format is used to present detailed information and analysis about public health practice in each jurisdiction. A description of each of the major headings included in the case studies is given below.

Community Characteristics

An array of demographic and health-related information is summarized for the population residing in each jurisdiction. Basic demographic and socioeconomic data are obtained from the US Department of Commerce, Bureau of the Census, and state and local economic development agencies. Community health status measures are obtained from local and state community health assessment reports, as well as federal surveillance systems such as the National Center for Health Statistics' vital statistics system. Measures include disease-specific death rates, birth outcome information, prenatal care information, and infectious disease rates (where available). Information on community health resources and manpower is obtained from a variety of sources. Physician availability is obtained from the American Medical Association; hospital statistics are obtained from the American Hospital Association; community health center information is obtained from the Bureau of Primary Health Care, US Health Resources and Services Administration; and managed care plan data are obtained from the American Association of Health Plans (formerly, Group Health Association of America). Other health resource information is directly obtained from community respondents.

The Local Health Department

Information regarding the organizational and operational characteristics of the official local health department is presented in this section. A description of the health officer and senior staff is provided, along with a discussion of major organizational units within the department. This section also examines the major types of services performed by the department, along with information on service volume and capacity (where available). A description of the health department's infrastructure and resources is provided, including an analysis of funding sources and levels.

Other Contributors to Local Public Health Activities

This section profiles the range of community organizations that contribute to local public health practice either independently or in collaboration with the local health department. Separate subsections are devoted to state agencies, hospitals, managed care plans, community health centers, and other community organizations. Information for this section derives from interviews with the various organizations and reviews of organizational documents.

Measures of Local Public Health Performance

This section presents results of the Local Public Health Performance Assessment Survey, a structured survey instrument designed for administration to local public health officials.[8] The survey instrument contains queries about the availability and perceived adequacy of 84 public health activities in the local jurisdiction. Each of these activities is linked to one of the three core

Table 2
Three Core Functions[a] and 10 Core Practices[b] of Public Health

Assessment

1. Assess the health needs of the community
2. Investigate the occurrence of health effects and health hazards in the community
3. Analyze the determinants of identified health needs

Policy Development

4. Advocate for public health, build constituencies and identify resources in the community
5. Set priorities among health needs
6. Develop plans and policies to address priority health needs

Assurance

7. Manage resources and develop organizational structure
8. Implement programs
9. Evaluate programs and provide quality assurance
10. Inform and educate the public

[a]*As defined by the Institute of Medicine.*

[b]*As identified by Centers for Disease Control and Prevention consensus conferences.*

public health functions identified by the Institute of Medicine in 1988,[9] and also to one of 10 public health practices identified by a Centers for Disease Control and Prevention work group in 1991 (**Table 2**). On the basis of responses to this survey, local public health performance summary scores are computed for all activities as well as for each of the three core functions and each of the 10 public health practices separately. Separate scores are also computed that reflect total performance in the jurisdiction, as well as the proportion of total performance that is contributed by the local health department. Finally, questions are included on the survey that allow measurement of the proportion of public health activities in which various types community organizations participate. These participation rates can be computed for state agencies, local government agencies, federal agencies, hospitals, private physicians, community health centers, other voluntary and nonprofit agencies, and other types of organizations.

For most jurisdictions, performance measures were obtained at two different time points (1992-1993 and 1995-1996), allowing an analysis of changes in performance over time. For two jurisdictions, measures were obtained at only one time point. Performance scores are displayed for the total jurisdiction (community performance) and for the local health department (health department performance) using figures specifically designed for this purpose (**Figures 1 and 2**). Figures 1 and 2 express each score as the proportion of the maximum possible score. For each year of observation, performance scores for each of the public health practices are separately plotted, and connected with a line. Separate figures display community performance scores and local health department scores. **Figure 3** displays participation rates for each of the major types of community organizations that contribute to public health. These rates are separately computed for each of the three public health functions.

Figure 1 indicates a general increase in community performance between 1993 and 1997 for most public health practices, with the exception of the practices *investigate* and *evaluate*. Figure 2 shows an increase in local health department performance, with the exception of the public health practice *evaluate*. Figures 1 and 2 show substantial variation in performance across the 10 public health practices and across the three public health functions. The numbers shown below Figure 2 express local health department performance as a percentage of total community performance (a measure of relative health department contributions). These numbers suggest that the largest increases in local health department contributions occur within the assessment function. Figure 3 indicates increases in public health participation by most types of community organizations. Figure 3 also indicates that most types of organizations participate more in policy development activities than in assessment or assurance activities.

Future Prospects and Projections

In this final section, case study findings are used to identify a set of policy and managerial implications for the local jurisdiction. Key opportunities and challenges for local

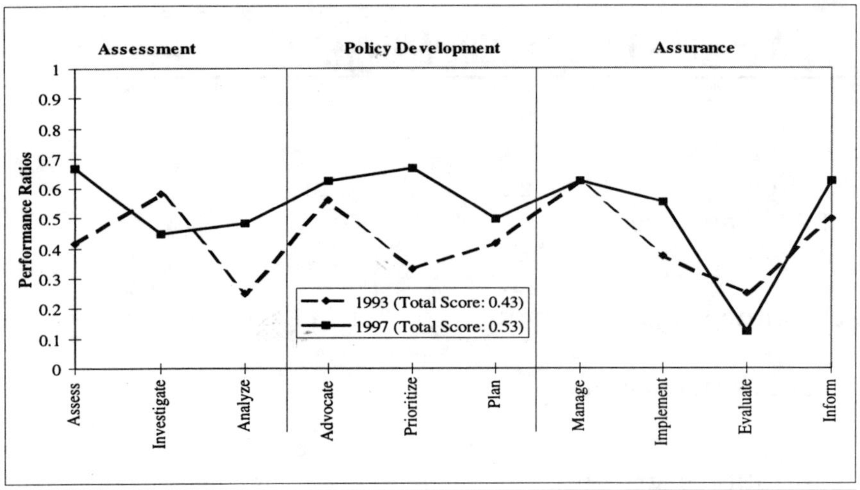

Figure 1. Example community public health performance scores.

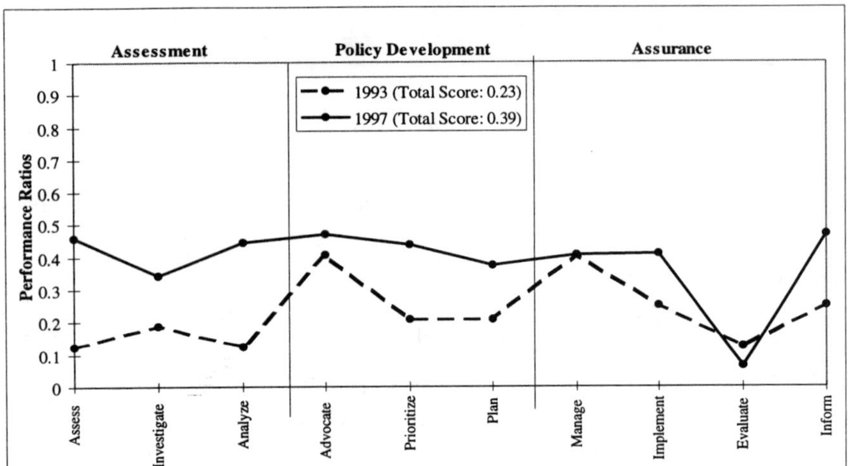

Health department performance score as a percentage of community score

	Assess	Investigate	Analyze	Advocate	Prioritize	Plan	Manage	Implement	Evaluate	Inform
1993:	30%	32%	50%	72%	62%	50%	65%	67%	50%	50%
1997:	69%	76%	92%	75%	66%	75%	65%	74%	50%	75%
Chg:	+129%	+138%	+83%	+04%	+05%	+50%	0%	+11%	0%	+50%

Figure 2. Example local health department performance scores.

public health practice are identified through comparisons of organizational capacities with political, economic, social, and health status trends. The prospects for public health improvement are assessed in light of these issues.

Overview of Part II

Case studies are presented in alphabetical order in the next eight chapters. Chapter 9 describes the public health system serving the small city of Beloit, Wisconsin, which has sustained an array of successful interventions through the joint efforts of the local health department, hospital, physician group, and other community organizations. Chapter 10 examines public health activities in the much larger jurisdiction of Denver, Colorado, which is served by a combined health and hospitals agency that now operates as an independent health care authority. Active groups of hospitals, managed care plans, and community health centers add richness and complexity to Denver's local public health activities. Chapter 11 provides an analysis of the Genesee County, Michigan, public health system, which has been shaped by community-based efforts assisted through a W.K. Kellogg Foundation initiative, and by interorganizational efforts led by the community's largest employer and union. Chapter 12 describes how the extensive primary care and public health system in Memphis and Shelby County, Tennessee, has adapted to recent changes created by Medicaid reform and managed care growth.

The Milwaukee, Wisconsin, local public health system, which is detailed in Chapter 13, illustrates how long-standing relationships among the local health department, hospitals, health centers, and managed care plans can successfully evolve with changes in market dynamics and community health needs. Chapter 14 describes how the public and private organizations serving Portland and Multnomah County, Oregon, balance competition and collaboration in performing public health activities within the community. A unique arrangement for privatizing the delivery of many public health services is examined in the study of the Southwest Washington Health District surrounding Vancouver, Washington, in Chapter 15. In the final case study, Chapter 16 presents an analysis of the Thurston County, Washington, local public health activities, which are sustained through unique collaborative activities among a local health department, hospital, and managed care plan. Chapter 17 identifies several overarching themes and implications from the case studies that offer insight for practice, management, and policy making in local public health.

References

1. Baker EL, Melton RJ, Stange PV, et al. Health reform and the health of the public. *JAMA*. 1994; 272:1276-1282.
2. Lasker RD, and the Committee on Medicine and Public Health. *Medicine and Public Health: The Powers of Collaboration*. New York: The New York Academy of Medicine; 1997.

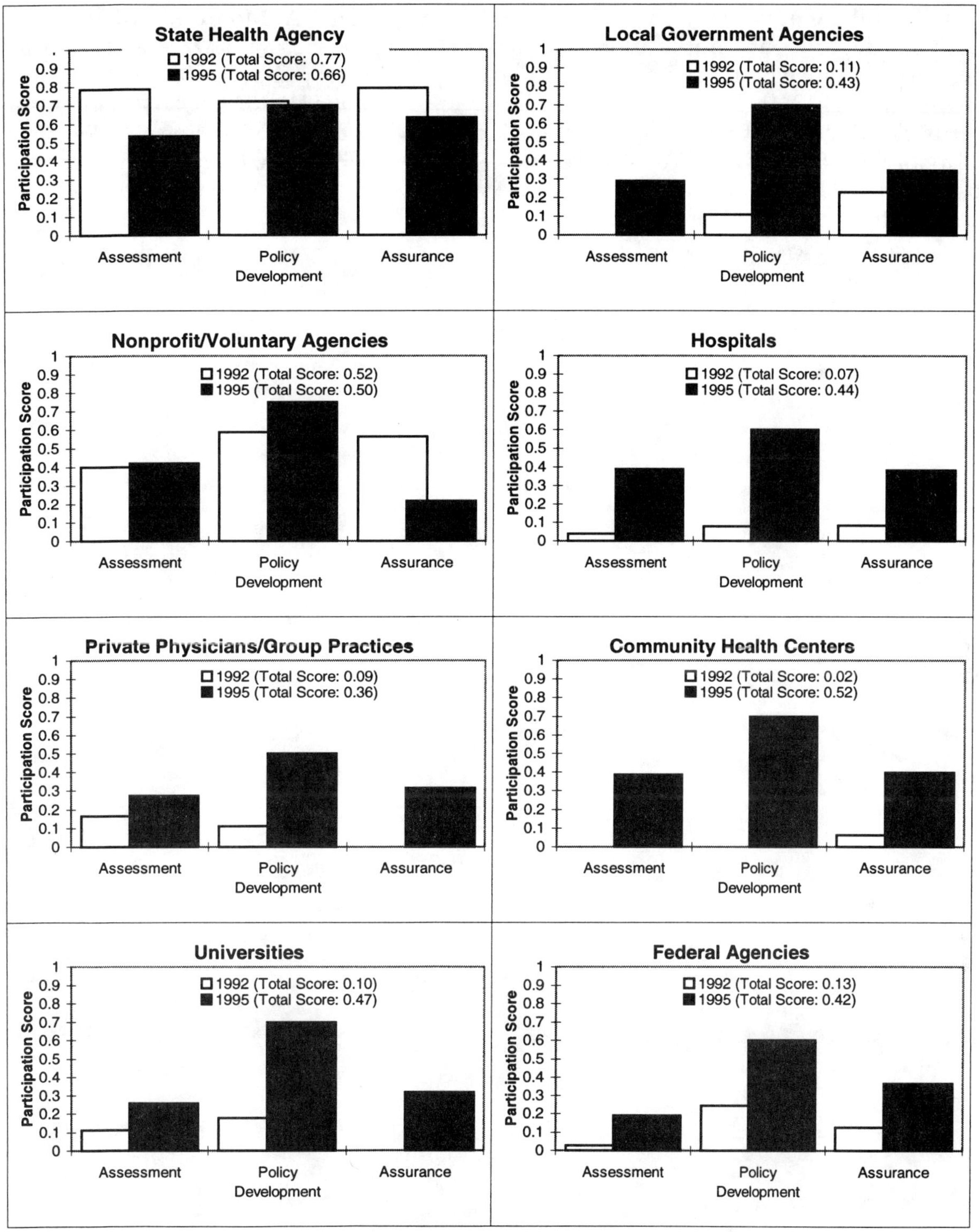

Figure 3. Example participation in public health activities by other organizations (as reported by the local health director).

3. Miller CA, Moos M-K. *Local Health Departments: Fifteen Case Studies*. Chapel Hill, NC: American Public Health Association; 1981.
4. Miller CA, Moore KS, Richards TB, Kotelchuck M, Margolis L, Kaluzny AD. Longitudinal observations on a selected group of local health departments—A preliminary report. *J Public Health Policy*. 1993;14:134-150.
5. Miller CA, Moore KS, Richards TB. The impact of critical events of the 1980s on core functions for a selected group of local health departments. *Public Health Rep*. 1993;108:695-700.

6. Brooks EF, Miller CA. Recent changes in selected local health departments: implications for their capacity to guarantee basic medical services. *Am J Prev Med*. 1987;3:134-141.
7. Richards TB, Rogers JJ, Christenson GM, Miller CA, Taylor MS. Public health core functions—Alabama, Maryland, Mississippi, New Jersey, South Carolina, and Wisconsin, 1993. *MMWR Morb Mortal Wkly Rep*. 1994;43:13-15.
8. Miller CA, Moore KS, Richards TB, Monk JD. A proposed method for assessing the performance of local public health functions and practices. *Am J Public Health*. 1994;84(11):1743-1749.
9. Institute of Medicine. *The Future of Public Health*. Washington, DC: National Academy Press; 1988.

Chapter 9

Case Study of Beloit, Wisconsin

Key Attributes

- Systems for integrated health and social services delivery
- Successful responses to diminishing grant funds
- Balance of collaborative and competitive relationships among community providers
- Limited managed care involvement

Community Characteristics

Demographic and Socioeconomic Characteristics

The city of Beloit is located in southeastern Wisconsin just north of the Illinois state line and ~50 miles from the state's capitol in Madison. Census data from 1992 indicate that the city contains ~36,000 residents, making it the second largest municipality within Rock County. Compared with state and national averages, a larger proportion of Beloit residents are under 25 years of age, and a smaller proportion are between 25 and 64 years of age. The city contains a more racially and ethnically diverse population than those of the surrounding county or state, with 80% of the population being White, 16% African American, 2% of Hispanic origin, and 1% Asian (**Table 1**). Approximately 5% of the population speak a language other than English at home. Educational attainment among Beloit residents lies below state and national levels, with 72% of the population having at least a high school degree, and 11% holding bachelor's degrees or higher educational levels. Income among Beloit residents also exists below state and federal levels, with 17.5% of the population estimated to live below the federal poverty level in 1990. Manufacturing companies employ the largest share of Beloit workers, followed by wholesale and retail trade industries, and health services industries. The unemployment rate stood at 7.8% in 1990, exceeding both the state and federal averages.

Community Health Status Indicators

Vital and health statistics for Rock County, which encompass the city of Beloit, suggest that community health status exceeds national norms in a number of important areas. Statistics for infant mortality, teenage births, low birth weight births, and births without timely prenatal care are all lower in Rock County than in the nation as a whole (**Table 2**). This county-level information, however, masks substantial health problems and risks that are specific to the population of Beloit. Vital and health statistics for the years 1991 through 1995 suggest that Beloit residents exceed state and national trends in the prevalence of many health status problems and risks. Infant mortality for the city stands at 8.9 deaths per 1000 live births during this 5-year period, exceeding the statewide rate of 7.8 and

Table 1
Demographic Characteristics: Beloit, Wisconsin

Population (1990)	35,573
Percent of metropolitan area population	
Median age in years	31.1
Percent 65 years and older (1990)	13.5
Percent non-White (1990)	18.2
Percent speaking a language other than English at home (1990)	4.5
Percent completing high school degree (1990)	72.4
Percent of individuals below federal poverty level (1989)	17.5
Median household income (1989)	$25,859
Average percent unemployed (1992)	9.7

Source: US Department of Commerce, Bureau of the Census.

Table 2
Health Status Indicators: Rock County, Wisconsin, 1996

	County	US
Infant mortality rate per 1000 live births	5.6	7.3
Percent of births to mothers age 10-17	4.5	5.1
Percent of infants with low birth weight	6.9	7.4
Percent of births with prenatal care later than first trimester	13.4	18.1
Deaths per 100,000 population, crude rates	864.2	876.0
Cancer, all types	197.4	203.4
Lung cancer	52.4	59.3
Female breast cancer	19.5	35.9
Heart disease	264.6	276.4
Cerebrovascular diseases	65.8	18.7
Chronic obstructive pulmonary diseases	48.3	11.9
Suicide	14.1	11.6
Pneumonia and influenza	44.3	31.6
HIV/AIDS	1.3	11.7
Diabetes mellitus	16.8	23.3
Homicide	3.4	7.9

Source: Wisconsin Department of Health and Family Services, 1997; National Center for Health Statistics, 1998.

national rate of 7.2. During this same period, 8.0% of all births to Beloit residents were low birth weight (less than 2500 g), compared with 6.1% statewide and 7.4% nationally. Similar to state and national trends, one fifth of all pregnant women in Beloit did not initiate prenatal care during the first trimester, while 5% of these women initiated care during the third trimester or not at all. Contributing to Beloit's problems with birth outcomes, almost 21% of births were to teenage women, compared with 10% statewide.

Age-adjusted mortality rates for the period from 1991 to 1995 suggest that Beloit exceeds the statewide average in deaths from lung cancer, other cancers, ischemic heart diseases, and chronic obstructive pulmonary diseases. Leading causes of death in Beloit include ischemic heart diseases (231 deaths per 100,000), other cancers (165 per 100,000), lung cancer (78 per 100,000), and cerebrovascular diseases (74 per 100,000). When deaths are examined as a function of years of potential life lost, premature births and suicide exceed all causes of death among Beloit residents except cancer.

Sexually transmitted diseases remain problem for many Beloit residents. During 1994, community providers detected and treated a total of 133 cases of gonorrhea, 266 cases of chlamydia, and 34 cases of herpes. When expressed as a proportion of Beloit's total population, these case rates exceed state and national averages. Nine individuals tested positive for the HIV antibody during this time period. Other communicable diseases appear less problematic in Beloit, with no reported cases of tuberculosis, measles, mumps, rubella, or pertussis during 1994. Nonetheless, substantial proportions of the community population remain at risk for childhood diseases. An estimated 55% of Beloit children aged 2 years and under were up-to-date on immunizations with the basic (4:3:1) series in 1994, compared with 76% statewide and 75% nationally.[1]

Local Health Resources and Manpower

Beloit Memorial Hospital, a 148-bed nonprofit community hospital, is centrally located within the city. During 1994, the hospital served ~5000 inpatients and more than 104,000 outpatient visits through its network of specialty clinics and ambulatory surgery center. The hospital also operates a growing preferred provider organization (PPO) that provides health care coverage for the employees of local businesses, in collaboration with a group of local physicians. Another major source of hospital services for Beloit residents is the Mercy Health System, located in the neighboring city of Janesville 10 miles north of Beloit. This nonprofit sys-

Table 3
Health Resources: Rock County, Wisconsin

Number of nonfederal physicians (Number per 100,000 population) 1992[a]	218 (153)
Family practice	19 (13)
General practice	7 (5)
Internal medicine	40 (28)
Obstetrics / gynecology	10 (7)
Pediatrics	15 (10)
Number of community hospital beds (FY1995)[b]	454
Beds per 100,000 population	318
Number of community hospitals (FY1995)	3
Number of HMOs (1994)	6
Number of federally qualified health centers (1994)[d]	0
Total number of clinic sites	0
Local public health expenditures for Beloit only (1997)	$2,062,180
Percent from direct federal sources	0%
Percent from state sources (including federal pass-throughs)	33%
Percent from local sources	25%
Percent from Medicaid	9%
Percent from Medicare	0%
Total federal funding for community health centers (1996)[e]	0
Total federal funding for migrant health centers (1996)[e]	0
Total federal block grant funds for preventive health services (1996)[e]	0
Total federal block grant funds for maternal and child health services (1996)[e]	0
Total federal block grant funds for substance abuse services (1996)[e]	$996,542
Total federal funding for homeless health services (1996)[e]	0
Total federal funding for National Health Service Corp (1996)[e]	0

[a]*American Medical Association Physician Masterfile, 1992.*
[b]*American Hospital Association, 1997.*
[c]*Group Health Association of America, 1995.*
[d]*US Bureau of Primary Health Care, 1994.*
[e]*US Department of Commerce, 1997.*

tem includes a 241-bed community hospital, several free-standing ambulatory care clinics providing both primary care and specialty services, and an HMO that serves both commercial groups and Medicaid beneficiaries. One of Mercy's clinics is located within the city of Beloit. In 1994, the system served ~9000 inpatient admissions and 317,000 outpatient visits. Tertiary care facilities are available at the University of Wisconsin Medical Center in Madison, which is ~50 miles from Beloit.

Approximately 218 nonfederal physicians practice in Rock County, which encompasses the city of Beloit (**Table 3**).[2] Fifty-six of these physicians practice within the city of Beloit, most of whom practice as part of a group practice organization known as the Beloit Clinic. These numbers produce population-to-physician ratios of 655:1 for Rock County and 635:1 for Beloit. Primary care physicians practicing within the city include 13 family / general practitioners, six pediatricians, 10 general internists, and five obstetricians / gynecologists. No federally qualified health centers operate within the city, although Rock County is designated as a federal health professions shortage area for primary care, mental health, and dental health care providers.

Primary care services delivered by private providers are supplemented by several community health programs that target vulnerable and underserved populations within the community. Several of these programs are operated by Beloit's local health department in partnership with other community organizations. The Merrill Center, a community health center jointly supported by the health department, Beloit Memorial Hospital, and the Beloit Clinic, provides childhood immunizations, medical screenings, and well child examinations under the federal Early and Periodic Screening, Diagnosis, and Treatment (EPSTD) program for Medicaid beneficiaries. The Fourth Street Clinic, operated by a nonprofit nutrition and health services corporation in partnership with the local health department, provides services including pregnancy testing, nutrition counseling and assistance under the federal Special Supplemental Food Program for Women, Infants, and Children (WIC), prenatal care case management, and eligibility screening for Medicaid and other publicly supported health programs. The local health department also operates a public health clinic that offers targeted services for health promotion, disease prevention, and communicable disease control. All of these community clinics are staffed by advance-practice nurses and supervised by local physicians. Additionally, local chapters of the Salvation Army and United Way operate a free health clinic in partnership with the Rock County health department and Mercy Medical Center. Although this clinic is located several miles outside the city limits of Beloit, substantial numbers of Beloit residents receive primary care services through this clinic. This clinic operates 2 to 3 days per week and is staffed by volunteer physicians from Mercy Medical Center and other private providers.

Managed care organizations are small but growing components of Beloit's local health care resources. Local health care administrators estimate that 15 to 20% of the residents in Rock County are enrolled in managed care plans. Both area hospitals operate PPOs, and one also operates a staff-model health maintenance organization (HMO). In addition to the hospital-based plans, at least four other HMOs report operating in Rock County, all of which are based in the surrounding metropolitan areas of Madison or Milwaukee. Medicaid managed care is expanding rapidly in Wisconsin, with mandatory HMO enrollment now in effect in the state's five urban counties for beneficiaries who receive assistance through the federal Temporary Assistance to Needy Families program (TANF, formerly Aid to Families with Dependent Children), and for low-income children and pregnant women. Less populated areas, including Beloit, operate under a system of voluntary HMO enrollment which is expected to grow as the state's 19 Medicaid-certified HMOs expand their operations into less populated areas of the state. Currently, only one of the HMOs operating in Rock County is certified to enroll Medicaid beneficiaries, but several others indicate that they plan to seek certification once mandatory enrollment is implemented within the county. Additionally, both Mercy Health System and Beloit Memorial Hospital hope to develop HMOs products for serving Medicaid beneficiaries once mandatory enrollment is implemented.

The Local Health Department

The Beloit Health Department maintains a long history of providing both personal and population-based health services to residents of the city. Local public health services in Wisconsin historically were organized around cities and towns, rather than counties. County health departments have emerged more recently in some areas, as a strategy to promote efficiency through consolidation and to secure a broader base of financial support. A full-service county health department developed in Rock County in 1980, but the city of Beloit chose to remain distinct from this organization and continue to operate its own health department. City administrators report that this decision was made largely to insure that the unique health risks and concerns of city residents—who are more culturally diverse and more socioeconomically challenged than the residents of many other areas within the county—receive adequate attention and resources. Rock County's health department therefore developed to cover areas of the county outside the city limits of Beloit.

Organizational Structure

The Beloit Health Department is one of seven municipal departments within the city's administrative structure. The department is headed by a full-time administrative director/health officer who reports to the city manager and an elected city council. The city manager is appointed by an elected city council, which makes budgetary decisions for the health department and establishes its broad operating policies. Until 1996, a separate local board of health did not exist in Beloit, as city legislation in 1955 had abolished this body and transferred its functions to the city council. An executive advisory board consisting of the city manager and the department heads of other city departments had provided the health department director with guidance and assistance in general managerial and governmental issues. In early 1996, the state health department adopted the requirement that all local health departments must maintain a board of health with community representation. Beloit complied by forming a seven-member advisory body, which comprises city officials and community members appointed by the Beloit city council.

Claudette Cummings maintains a 24-year history as the administrative leader of the department. Educated with a master's degree in community health, Ms. Cummings originally joined the city to help salvage a struggling visiting nurse association and merge the entity with the city's existing health department. Once this merger was complete, she worked in tandem with the department's part-time physician-trained health officer in overseeing the department's programs and services. In 1996, Ms. Cummings assumed the position of health officer in response to a state law requiring such positions to be filled by full-time administrators. As the health officer, Ms. Cummings maintains overall responsibility for enforcing health regulations, overseeing clinical staff and personal health services within the department, and maintaining professional relations with the private medical community. Dr. Donald Burant, MD, who served as Beloit's part-time health officer for more than 12 years, continues to assist in the clinical programs of the department. A board-certified pediatrician, Dr. Burant maintains a 33-year private practice as part of the Beloit Clinic, and serves on the faculty of the University of Wisconsin's medical school. Additionally, since 1995, Dr. Burant has served as vice president for medical affairs at Beloit Memorial Hospital. Through these diverse roles, Dr. Burant has maintained strong, collaborative relationships between the health department and the local medical community.

Health department activities are organized and performed through four administrative divisions. A division of public health nursing houses all of the department's clinical services programs, including those for sexually transmitted diseases, immunizations, lead screening, and prenatal care coordination. Four public health nurses staff this division, with oversight from the health officer. A community resources division houses the department's community outreach and support services, many of which are implemented in partnership with other community organizations. Services include a neighborhood drug and violence prevention project, and a range of health promotion, education, and prevention programs implemented through the city's two community health centers. An environmental health division maintains the department's programs for food safety inspections, housing code enforcement, vector control, and epidemiological investigation. Until 1996, the department also operated a home health nursing division that housed functions that the department assumed from the local visiting nurse association when it closed in 1973. These functions included in-home skilled nursing and rehabilitative care, personal (custodial) care services, and home companion services for elderly and disabled persons. This division was sold to Beloit Memorial Hospital in 1996.

Service Areas

Personal Health Services

Immunization services. A broad array of health promotion and disease prevention services are provided through the department's public health nursing division. An active childhood immunization program holds immunization clinics at the health department office and at three community locations. Over 4300 immunizations were delivered through this program during calendar year 1994. Using funds acquired through a grant from the state health agency, this program has subcontracted with a local nonprofit health and nutrition organization to support a community health nurse's activities in encouraging timely immunization delivery. These activities include providing reminder telephone calls and letters to the families of children believed to be at-risk for underimmunization; providing follow-up contact with families after initial reminders; conducting home visits with families who have chronic problems with underimmunized children; providing immunization referrals to underimmunized children who are treated at the hospital emergency department; and conducting educational sessions with local providers regarding strategies for monitoring immunization status and encouraging utilization.

The health department also operates an active senior influenza vaccination program that provides vaccinations during the fall of each year at several community locations. As a Medicare provider, the health department is able to directly bill Medicare for these vaccinations and therefore provide the services at no cost to Medicare beneficiaries. The department administered 2300 influenza vaccinations through this program in 1994.

Maternal and child health services. The department maintains several innovative maternal and child health programs that have become models for other jurisdictions within the state. Using a state grant from the federal Maternal and Child Health Block Grant, the health department operates a "one-stop shopping" maternal and child health center in collaboration with a local nonprofit organization, Nutrition and Health Associates. The Fourth Street Center, as this program is called, provides case management services to low-income pregnant women and their infants through a team of public health nurses. Case managers assure timely access to and utilization of prenatal care services, as well as access to other needed health and social services such as nutritional support, family planning services, clothing, housing, and substance abuse services. After birth, public health nurses visit the home at least once per month during the first 2 months postpartum, providing education and training to new parents and conducting infant health examinations. In-home well child examinations, funded through the federal Early and Periodic Screening, Diagnosis, and Treatment (EPSDT) program, are conducted by the nurses at 3 and 10 months postpartum. Begun in 1989 in Beloit, this program was implemented statewide in 1993 as a basic benefit for Medicaid beneficiaries. During calendar year 1994, 184 women received prenatal care coordination services through this program in Beloit, generating approximately $38,000 in reimbursement from the Wisconsin Division of Medical Assistance.

Another maternal and child health service operated by the health department provides outreach to low-income pregnant women who do not have access to other sources of health care coverage and are therefore eligible for a state program that provides this coverage. The health department's outreach initiative identifies potential beneficiaries of the state program through personal contacts made by public health nurses at health department clinics, community centers, health fairs, and other community presentations. Once eligibility determination is made, health department nurses provide referral and follow-up through the prenatal care coordination program insure that beneficiaries receive needed care.

Perhaps one of the department's most comprehensive and all-inclusive maternal and child health programs is a newborn visits program, which provides all Beloit residents with in-home newborn health checks as well as education and training for new parents. Public health nurses conduct these home visits within 24 hours after discharge from the hospital. Almost 300 newborn visits were conducted during 1994.

Women's health services. The department operates a monthly women's health clinic which provides free Pap smears and instructions on self-administered breast examinations. For low-income, underinsured women age 50 years of age and older, the department provides referral to local private physicians who have agreed to provide mammograms, clinical breast examinations, Pap smears, and pelvic examinations through a state program funded by the US Centers for Disease Control and Prevention.

Other personal health services. The department operates a clinic that provides sexually transmitted disease testing and treatment services, as well as family planning services, to area residents. Services are rendered using a sliding scale fee schedule, with free care provided to individuals without ability to pay. Anonymous HIV/AIDS education, testing, and counseling services are also offered through this clinic, which is staffed by health department nurses. During 1994, ~725 individuals were screened for sexually transmitted diseases, and 236 individuals were counseled and tested through the anonymous HIV/AIDS testing program. Tuberculosis (TB) testing services are also provided through the health department clinic using the Mantoux skin testing program. As part of the department's TB control program, identified cases are provided with medically indicated tuberculosis drugs and monitored monthly for side effects and compliance with treatment.

The department also collaborates in maintaining a health screening and assessment program for individuals who are eligible for medical care services under the state's general relief program for uninsured individuals. Through this program, a community health nurse is stationed in one of Beloit's community centers to screen uninsured individuals for identifiable health needs, provide basic diagnostic and preventive health services, and refer individuals to appropriate community providers. Eligible individuals are provided with a state-funded voucher to cover the cost of services provided by private practitioners. The health department collaborates with the Beloit Memorial Hospital and the Beloit Clinic in funding and managing this program. A 1994 evaluation of the program suggests that substantial cost savings are realized in the form of reduced emergency room utilization at Beloit Memorial Hospital.

The health department's home health nursing program provides services to residents in a three-county area surrounding Beloit. Departmental staff directly provide skilled nursing services, custodial care, and in-home companion services through this program. The department maintains a contract with Beloit Memorial Hospital for providing in-home ancillary services through the program, including the services of physical and occupational therapists, clinical social workers, enterostomal therapists, and nutritionists. A total of 16,609 patient visits were delivered during 1994, of which 86% were to Medicare beneficiaries, 7% to Medicaid beneficiaries, and 5% to commercially insured individuals. The remaining 2% of services were delivered to self-pay, veterans administration, and state general assistance clients.

Finally, the department operates a home companion registry that is designed to provide respite care, support, and assistance to community-dwelling elderly and disabled individuals to prevent the need for institutional care. Program staff maintains a registry of companions who have received training in basic home care techniques, many of whom are unemployed and/or low-income city residents. Through the program, clients contract directly with trained companions for a $6 per hour fee. Approximately 300 clients are annually served through this program.

Community Health Services

In addition to personal health services, the health department maintains a range of community health programs that are designed to address larger socioeconomic determinants of health among Beloit residents. Most of these services are provided in collaboration with other community organizations, through a network of three multiservice neighborhood centers that were originally established with funding from the Robert Wood Johnson Foundation. These centers offer a "one-stop shopping" source for health and human services in low-income and underserved neighborhoods of the city. Services provided through these centers include the following:

- the Safe Place program, an after-school drop-in center for elementary school children, led by a licensed elementary school teacher and aided by area college students who serve as youth mentors. This program provides age-appropriate social and health education services in areas such as violence prevention, school drop-out prevention, drug abuse prevention, injury prevention, and health and physical fitness promotion. Thirty to 45 students participate in these activities daily.
- the Family Self Sufficiency program, a case management service mandated by the US Department of Housing and Urban Development for beneficiaries of Section 8 housing assistance. The case manager provides referral and follow-up to ~21 families regarding employment counseling and other needed health and social services.
- the Nonviolent Conflict Resolution Program, which provides counseling and arbitration for both adolescent and adult community residents, and holds community workshops in nonviolent dispute resolution techniques.
- the Teen Self-Sufficiency Program, which works to facilitate school attendance among pregnant and parenting adolescents, and to encourage appropriate family planning techniques among these youth. Services provided through this program include transportation and child care assistance, homemaker assistance, parenting education and training sessions, and family planning counseling and follow-up.
- an adolescent pregnancy prevention program, which matches at-risk adolescent women with youth mentors for conducting activities that emphasize self-esteem and healthy decision-making in areas such as sexual activity, substance abuse, and school performance.
- the Parent Support Services program, which provides child abuse and neglect prevention services to at-risk families. Services include stress management training and education, parenting skills training, and case management and referral services for other health and human services needs. Services are provided through a parent aide who is matched with each at-risk family.
- the neighborhood drug use and crime prevention program, which supports part-time outreach workers in two of the community centers. These outreach workers provide counseling to community members regarding substance abuse awareness and crime prevention techniques, and implement community awareness projects within at-risk neighborhoods and local elementary and junior high schools.

Community Health Assessment

The health department is engaged in several efforts to assess health needs within the city and evaluate the health resources and capacities available within the community to address them. As part of a statewide initiative sponsored by the state health agency, the department is in the process of conducting a self-assessment of its organizational strengths and community needs and resources using the Assessment Protocol for Excellence in Public Health (APEX), developed by the National Association of County and City Health Officials and collaborating agencies. Departmental staff participated in APEX training sessions conducted by the state and are in the process of implementing the protocol.

The health department also collaborates with the county health department and several local chapters of the United Way in conducting a countywide human services needs assessment. This assessment was completed in June 1998 and identified five major health concerns for Beloit: access to health care, chronic diseases, maternal and child health, substance abuse, and adolescent suicide and pregnancy. The department is now forming task forces around each of these areas to implement plans and programs for community health improvement.

Environmental Health Services

Beloit's environmental health division conducts state-mandated routine health inspections in a variety of public institutions, including food service establishments, child care facilities, schools, hotels, and swimming pools. The department administers the Code

Enforcement Team, an program designed to respond rapidly to chronic housing problems by including representation from multiple municipal agencies, such as the police department, the local housing authority, and the department of public works. An active food-sampling program operates within the environmental health division, which routinely monitors retail food products for potential health risks. Samples from a local supermarket during 1994 resulted in an US Food and Drug Administration investigation and the statewide recall of a prepared food item. Other environmental health programs include a lead poisoning prevention and control program that evaluates the residences of children found to have elevated blood lead levels; an electromagnetic field testing program, a residential radon testing program, and a noise pollution complaint investigation program. The division contracts with the local chapter of the Humane Society for animal control activities.

Infrastructure and Resources

Health department programs and services are provided through a central office located in central Beloit, a satellite clinic located near the Illinois state line, and through the network of three community centers that are owned by area nonprofit organizations. The department employs a total of 83 full-time equivalent (FTE) staff positions for maintaining these programs. Staff include 17 FTE nurses (10 of whom are dedicated to the home health program), one health educator, one environmental health inspector, and numerous other administrative, outreach, and support staff.

Excluding the home nursing program, the department's calendar year 1994 expenditures totaled $1,216,087. A total of 43% of these funds were derived from city and county appropriations, representing a 3% increase over the previous year. Thirty-two percent of revenues were derived from federal and state government categorical grants-in-aid; 19% from private grants and donations; 3% were derived from personal health service fees; and three percent from environmental health fees and licenses. Approximately 2% of the total Beloit city tax levy ($476,292) was allocated to health department programs. Of this amount, ~21% is allocated for personal health services delivered through health department clinics and community centers; 47% supports public health nursing services delivered in the home and community, such as newborn home visits and maternal case management; 19% supports environmental health activities; and 13% supports the department's community support services, which are carried out through community centers in partnership with other local organizations.

Many of the department's community support services were initiated in 1991 with the support of Robert Wood Johnson Foundation demonstration grants for integrated health and human services delivery. These funds were gradually phased out over the three years that followed, but the department was successful in securing funds to continue and expand these programs through a variety of sources, including a local foundation, the local United Way chapter, the state health agency, and Beloit Memorial Hospital.

The department's home health program generated an additional $1,124,046 in revenue during 1994. Revenue increased 28% and service volume increased 24% from the previous year.

Other Contributors to Local Public Health Practice

State Health Agency

Local health departments in Wisconsin are decentralized units of local government, and their relationships with the state health agency primarily involve funding and technical assistance. Beloit's local health department maintains a close working relationship with Wisconsin's state health agency, which is housed within a larger health and human services agency known as the Department of Health and Family Services. This consolidated state department manages all state programs and services related to public health, medical care, long-term care, mental health, substance abuse, public assistance, and child protection. The state division of health is one of five divisions within this umbrella agency. The division of health is further divided into programs for medical assistance (Medicaid), disability services, health statistics, and public health. Within this division, the state's bureau of public health manages programs in six areas: maternal and child health, communicable disease, occupational health; environmental epidemiology, chronic disease prevention and health promotion, and emergency medical services.

Beloit health department's most frequent interaction occurs with the state bureau of public health. This state agency is an important funding source for many health department programs and services, such as the maternal and child health services delivered through the Fourth Street Center and the screening services delivered through the department's women's health clinic. As a medium-sized local health department that is representative of many other departments within the state, Beloit has served as a pilot for several state public health interventions initiated by the bureau of public health. Beloit's Fourth Street Center was initially funded as such a pilot project in 1989. During the center's initial years of operation, the state bureau of public health worked closely with the Beloit health department in conducting a rigorous evaluation of the program's "one-stop shopping" approach to delivering maternal and child health services. Results from this evaluation eventually led to the program being passed as a statewide Medicaid benefit in 1993.

Even for programs that do not receive state funding, the Beloit health department serves as a model for the state in implementing collaborative interventions in public health. Administrators within the state bureau of public health indicate that they continually monitor Beloit's experience with programs such as the integrated health and human service programs funded by the Robert Wood Johnson Foundation and the case management program for general medical assistance beneficiaries that is sustained through collaboration among the local health department, Beloit Memorial Hospital, and the Beloit Clinic. The state agency uses Beloit's experiences as examples to motivate and facilitate similar efforts in other local public health jurisdictions within the state. State administrators suggest that, because of the close working relationships maintained between Beloit's local health department and the private medical community, the locality serves as an incubator for collaborative public health interventions that potentially can be exported to other local jurisdictions.

Beloit also works closely with the state health agency for the purpose of local public health assessment. The bureau of public health maintains a policy of having each local public health jurisdiction implement the Assessment Protocol for Excellence in Public Health (APEX) in 3-year cycles. The bureau conducts regional training sessions with local health departments regarding appropriate strategies for implementing APEX and encourages local health departments to collaborate with neighboring departments as well as with other community organizations in conducting these assessments. As part of this process, the state bureau requires local health departments to report their jurisdiction's priority health issues as identified through the APEX process, along with a plan for achieving improvements in these issues. The state bureau offers local health departments ongoing technical assistance in implementing the APEX assessment process and in designing and implementing plans for improving on priority health issues. To facilitate the process of health assessment, the state bureau of health statistics provides each local public health agency with an annual report of health status and health risks within their populations. This agency also equips each agency with a computer that can be used to track and report vital and health statistics, as well as to analyze trends in health status and health risks within their jurisdiction.

County Health Department

As a provider of public health services to county residents outside the city of Beloit, the Rock County Health Department faces many of the same health needs and risks as the Beloit health department. As a result, interaction between the two public health agencies is growing. The county health department maintains a staff of ~27 full-time equivalent positions and a budget of approximately $1.4 million for serving the 107,000 Rock County residents who live outside the city limits of Beloit. Historically, Beloit's unwillingness to consolidate its city health department within the newly emerging county health department created some animosity between the two organizations. Competitive pressures have also fueled some conflict between the organizations. Both organizations operate home nursing programs in the area and have traditionally competed to provide newborn home visits to the patients of local hospitals. Intense competition between the two local hospitals has added additional strain to health department relationships. Beloit's health department maintains a long history of collaboration with Beloit Memorial Hospital, while Rock County's health department works closely with Mercy Medical Center. Additionally, the county and city health departments are often required to share state and county public health funds. The methods used to allocate funds among county and city public health programs occasionally create tension between the two health departments.

Despite these areas of potential conflict, the two health departments are experiencing success in forging partnerships that address public health issues of common concern. Both departments serve on countywide and multicounty task forces addressing such public health issues as communicable disease control and adolescent pregnancy prevention. The two departments are also collaborating in conducting a countywide community health assessment process in cooperation with local United Way chapters. Most of the interaction between the two departments involves planning and assessment activities; however, the organizations are also initiating efforts to collaborate for service delivery. The county health department is now supplementing the capacity of its own home nursing service by contracting with Beloit's program.

Hospitals

Beloit Memorial Hospital

Beloit Memorial Hospital maintains an active and growing involvement in community health issues. Much of this involvement derives from the hospital's longstanding mission as a nonprofit, community-based organization governed by its board of community representatives. The hospital serves as an important source of care for vulnerable populations, with more than 10% of its patients being Medicaid beneficiaries, and 5% receiving uncompensated care. As competition from nearby Mercy Medical Center has increased, Beloit Hospital administrators report that their involvement in community health issues has become a central component of their organization's strategy for growth and survival. To differentiate the organization from its competitor, administrators are attempting to move the hospital beyond the delivery of traditional medical services and to offer a more comprehensive range of programs and services to meet the health needs of Beloit residents. In carrying out this effort, the hospital relies heavily on its long-standing relationships with the other organized health care providers in the community, including Beloit's local health department.

Along with the local health department and the Beloit Clinic, the hospital is a primary sponsor of the community health nurse program that provides health screening, assessment, and referrals for low-income uninsured individuals who are eligible for the state's general relief program. A community health nurse employed by the hospital staffs the program and the hospital's division of nursing provides administrative support and oversight for the program. In addition to providing expanded access to health care for uninsured individuals, the program appears to reduce utilization of the hospital's emergency room, thereby freeing hospital resources for other activities.

Hospital and health department staff also collaborate in operating the health department's maternal and child health programs. As part of the department's prenatal care coordination program for at-risk mothers, health department nurses follow their clients during their delivery in the hospital and communicate with the hospital's medical and nursing staffs about postpartum health needs that should be monitored after discharge from the hospital. Similarly, as part of the health department's newborn home visitation program, the hospital's nursing staff assists health department staff in assessing education and training needs of new parents and in identifying maternal and child health issues that should be monitored after discharge.

Beloit Hospital also served as an important collaborator in the local health department's home health nursing program before it was sold to the hospital in 1996. Interestingly, this program had historically created some tension between the hospital and the health department, as a result of the hospital's desire to acquire a larger role in managing and operating the program. Hospital administrators indicated that the home health program offered the organization an effective avenue for becoming more involved in community-based service delivery. Nevertheless, administrators suggested that the health department's expertise in public health nursing is a critical component of the existing program, which could not be duplicated by the hospital if it were to initiate its own home health service. Initially, the hospital and the city of Beloit discussed the possibility of co-ownership for the growing home health program. Such an arrangement would have allowed the health department to retain its involvement in an important community service and revenue source, while also taking advantage of the hospital's substantial expertise and infrastructure in medical management. Ultimately, the city chose to sell the nursing program to the hospital in 1996. This decision allowed the health department to focus its resources more intensively on population-based services, while continuing to collaborate with the hospital on community health issues.

The hospital is currently exploring another possible avenue of engagement in community-based health services—the operation of a family practice residency program as part of a hospital-affiliated community health center. The proposed center would be designed to serve primarily Medicaid and uninsured individuals and staffed by residents from the University of Wisconsin's department of family medicine. Both the local health department and the local Beloit Clinic would play central roles in managing the health center. Historically, the Beloit Clinic has remained unconvinced of the need for additional primary care resources. However, some clinic administrators now acknowledge the potential benefits of an expanded supply of Medicaid primary care providers under the state's impending Medicaid managed care initiative. Dr. Donald Burandt, who serves as the hospital's vice president of medical affairs as well as the health department's health officer, has taken the lead role in developing this proposal in collaboration with the Beloit Clinic and the University of Wisconsin. In July 1998, Beloit was designated a federal primary care site and awarded a $1 million grant to establish a community health center.

In addition to its involvement in personal health services, the hospital serves on several community health planning and advisory bodies that have convened to address pressing health issues within the community. The hospital founded the countywide Maternal and Child Health Coalition, which brings together multiple health and human service organizations within the county on a regular basis to identify outstanding health issues and track available community resources. Hospital administrators report that this program has kept the participating organizations informed of potential referral sites and aware of possible health risks that should be investigated. Additionally, the hospital serves in an advisory capacity to several community health interventions, including programs for promoting effective parenting skills and for improving literacy among young parents. As important community health providers, hospital staff are able to offer these programs advice and assistance in targeting appropriate community members and in designing effective referral systems.

Mercy Health System

The other major hospital operating in the area, Mercy Health System, also serves as an important community health resource for Beloit residents. Although its hospital facility is located in the nearby city of Janesville, Mercy operates several primary care clinics in the area, including one clinic located in central Beloit. In addition, the system contains a mental health treatment facility, several outpatient specialty clinics, and a health maintenance organization. Systemwide, ~10% of the patients served are Medicaid beneficiaries, and 8% receive uncompensated care.

Administrators at Mercy report that the organization's involvement in community health issues stem both from its mission as a nonprofit organization and from its growing involvement in managed health care. As part of its community service mission, Mercy operates the county's training program for emergency medical technicians, which previously had been maintained by the county health department. The hospital system also assists in supporting the free health care clinic operated by the Salvation Army and local volunteer physicians. The system donates office equipment and supplies to the clinic and provides all laboratory and imaging work to the clinic at cost.

The hospital system's growing involvement in managed care provides much of the motivation for its activities in community wellness and health promotion. In an effort to promote health and reduce the costs of illness among enrollees in its HMO, Mercy operates a corporate wellness and occupational medicine program in partnership with local employers. Through this program, the system conducts work site health assessments and develops health promotion programs for employee groups. System staff also provides technical assistance to employers in identifying potential work site health risks. These activities assist the community in making progress toward one of the US Department of Health and Human Services Year 2000 health objectives: "to increase to at least 85 percent the proportion of workplaces with 50 or more employees that offer health promotion activities for their employees."[3]

Mercy Health System's managed care plan, MercyCare HMO, currently serves ~8400 enrollees through contracts with local employers. System administrators hope to develop a plan for serving Medicaid beneficiaries once the state's mandatory enrollment program is implemented within the county. Such a plan is anticipated to expand upon the system's current role as a provider of health services to vulnerable and underserved population groups. The system's network of community-based primary care centers are well positioned to serve these groups.

Mercy's administrators indicate that the system currently maintains little regular interaction with the local public health agencies at the county or city level. As the system expands its involvement in community health issues, administrators anticipate developing closer ties with these agencies. Areas identified for possible future collaboration include community health assessment and communitywide planning and priority setting. As the system expands its capacities in providing wellness services and in serving vulnerable population groups, administrators anticipate a need for enhanced coordination with other community organizations, including public health agencies.

Managed Care Plans

In addition to the managed care plans operated by local hospitals, at least four other HMOs serve residents of Beloit and Rock County. All of these plans are located in the surrounding metropolitan areas of Madison and Milwaukee, and none of them maintain regular interaction with the local health department. These network-model and independent practice association-model HMOs maintain contracts with local physician practices for managing the care of their enrollees. Rather than establishing direct relationships with the area's two local health departments, HMO administrators indicate that they depend on their contracted physician practices to maintain these relationships. HMOs pay these practices on a capitated basis to manage the health needs of their enrollees, including establishing linkages with public health agencies where such arrangements might be appropriate and effective. The majority of HMO contracts are managed by two local physician practices—the Beloit Clinic in Beloit and the Riverview Clinic in nearby Janesville—plus the network of primary care clinics operated by Mercy Health System. As described earlier, Mercy's clinics operate independently of the local public health agencies serving the area; however, both the Beloit and Riverview clinics maintain relatively strong working relationships with these agencies.

Private Physicians

The Beloit Clinic serves as the city's primary source for private medical care, as very few solo practitioners remain active within the area. A long history of collaboration exists between the clinic and the Beloit health department. Long-standing informal agreements between the clinic and the health department regarding indigent care have largely eliminated a need for the department to engage in comprehensive primary care delivery. Clinic physicians readily accept Medicaid beneficiaries, and participate in the state's voucher program for providing health services to uninsured beneficiaries of Wisconsin's general relief public assistance program. Moreover, health department and clinic staff routinely work together on a case-by-case basis to identify member physicians who are able to provide pro bono care to uninsured residents.

The clinic has proven instrumental in helping to build the health department's capacity and expertise for providing clinical public health services such as sexually transmitted disease diagnosis and treatment, well child health services, and preventive health screenings and assessments. The clinic provides medical oversight for maternal and child health services delivered through the Fourth Street Center, as well as the health screenings and assessments performed through the community health nurse program. One of the clinic's pediatricians, Dr. Donald Burant, serves as health officer within the Beloit health department and oversees all of the agency's clinical programs.

The Beloit Clinic also serves as an important collaborator with the health department in supporting community health initiatives. Clinic physicians are kept informed of the social support programs maintained by the health department and other community organizations, so that physicians are able to make informed referrals to programs addressing such issues as parenting skills and domestic violence prevention. In cooperation with the local health department, the also clinic maintains Beloit's only communitywide childhood immunization registry. Through this system, the clinic tracks all immunizations given through health department clinics and through visits to local pediatricians—all of whom are members of the clinic. This system allows the health department's public health nurses to identify cases of underimmunization and to provide follow-up through telephone reminders and home visits. Finally, members of the Beloit Clinic serve as important contributors to the community health assessment processes underway within the area. Through these processes, physicians and staff from the clinic are able to offer first-hand accounts of outstanding health needs among community members and to assist in devising plans to address these needs.

Currently, ~15% of the Beloit Clinic's patients are HMO enrollees. Clinic administrators indicate that many physicians are still adjusting to the characteristics of managed care medicine, such as the constraints imposed by capitated payment, the imperatives of efficient practice, and the implications of provider feedback and profiling systems. None of the HMOs that contract with the clinic are currently certified to enroll Medicaid beneficiaries; however, several of these plans anticipate entering the Medicaid market in the near future. The clinic's early experience with managed care, its substantial expertise in serving Medicaid beneficiaries, and its strong linkages with the local health department suggest that the clinic could effectively function within these impending Medicaid managed care systems.

The other major physician practice in the area, the Riverview Clinic, contains ~60 physicians and is based in Janesville. This clinic maintains relatively few linkages with the Beloit health department but does interact regularly with the Rock County's health department. Most of this interaction occurs through the free health clinic which is operated collaboratively by the local Salvation Army, the county health department, and other community agencies. Riverview donates equipment and supplies to the clinic, and many of its physicians provide pro bono care through the clinic.

Riverview is by far the largest provider for managed care plans in the area, serving more than 15,000 enrollees of DeanCare, a for-profit, network-model HMO based in Madison. DeanCare also anticipates developing a Medicaid managed care plan in the near future, through its contracts with Riverview. Riverview has some experience in serving vulnerable populations through its work with the local free clinic, but its location in relatively affluent Janesville may limit its ability to provide adequate access to care for low-income, underserved residents of the county. For this reason,

DeanCare is also exploring the potential for expanding its relationship with the Beloit Clinic.

Other Community Agencies

A wide range of other community-based organizations support and expand upon the community health efforts of Beloit's local health department. The nonprofit Nutrition and Health Services agency serves as the area's provider of nutritional services under the federal Special Supplemental Food Program for Women, Infants, and Children (WIC). This agency is also an important partner with the local health department in providing maternal and child health services through the Fourth Street Clinic. The local chapter of the YMCA operates numerous youth programs in the community and collaborates with the local health department in operating many of its programs aimed at teen self-sufficiency and violence prevention. Also involved in providing health and human services to area youth is the newly formed Beloit Youth Services, a nonprofit organization formed by the consolidation of several local organizations involved in youth issues. The local school system also participates in the planning and management of many area youth services, such as the after school drop-in program operated by the local health department.

The local chapter of the United Way is active in providing financial support to many of the community health programs maintained by the local health department and other organizations. The United Way is also instrumental in implementing the countywide health and human services needs assessment process. A local philanthropic organization, the Beloit Foundation, provides financial assistance for many local community health programs and services. The Rock County Department of Human Services also exists as an important funding source for local community health services. Faculty and staff at the local Beloit College provide the health department with expertise in evaluating local community health programs and services.

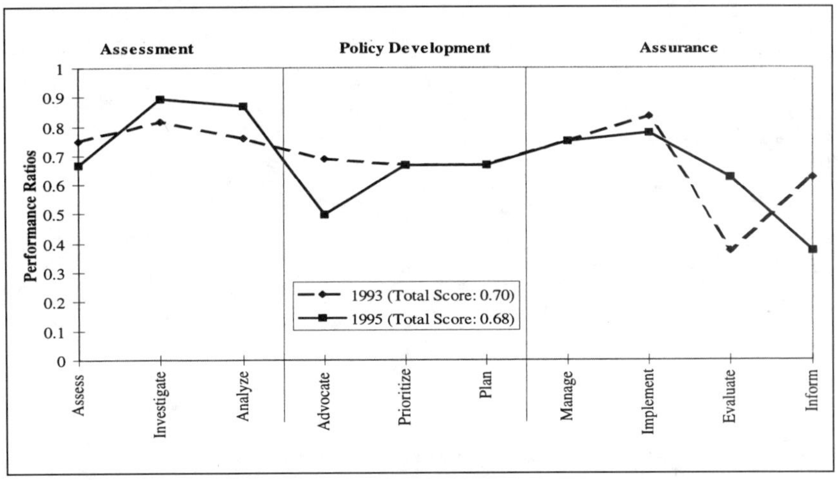

Figure 1. Community public health performance, Beloit, Wisconsin, 1993 and 1995.

Measures of Public Health System Performance

Performance Assessment Results: 1993 and 1995

Responses from Beloit's local health department director to the *Local Public Health Assessment Survey*[4] in 1993 and 1995 suggest that, overall, community performance of core public health functions has remained steadily above average during this period (see Chapter 8 for details on the survey and its measures). Overall, community performance was rated at 68% of the maximum possible score in 1995, compared with 70% in 1993 (**Figure 1**). By comparison, surveys conducted during 1992 and 1993 with a diverse collection of 63 local public health jurisdictions in 15 states indicated that the average jurisdiction reached only 51% of the maximum possible score. Beloit results suggest that community performance increased somewhat during the 1993-1995 period for the core public health practices of investigating health threats in the community, analyzing the determinants of community health needs, and evaluating the effects of health programs and services. Over this same period, community performance appeared to decrease somewhat for the practices of assessing health needs in the community, advocating for public health issues, implementing public health programs and policies, and informing and educating the public about pressing health issues. The largest decreases in performance appeared to occur for the practices of advocacy and evaluation.

When we examine only those public health activities performed by the local health department, total performance levels appear to decrease substantially from 51% of the maximum in 1993 to 39% of the maximum in 1995 (**Figure 2**). This drop in health department performance, when taken together with the stable levels of community performance, suggests that a greater share of the total public health effort is being performed by organizations other than the local health department. Health department performance appears to have increased only for the practices of managing public health resources and evaluating public health

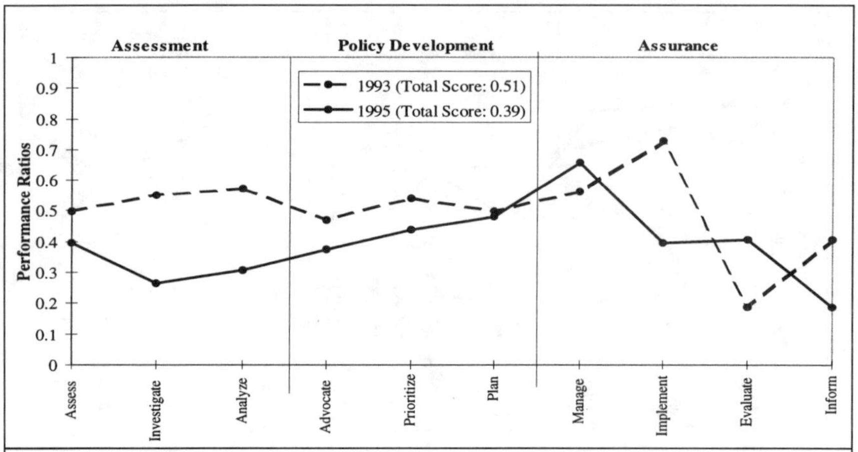

Health department performance score as a percentage of community score

	Assess	Investigate	Analyze	Advocate	Prioritize	Plan	Manage	Implement	Evaluate	Inform
1993:	67%	68%	76%	68%	81%	75%	75%	88%	50%	65%
1995:	59%	29%	35%	75%	66%	72%	88%	51%	65%	50%
Chg:	-11%	-57%	-53%	+10%	-19%	-04%	+17%	-42%	+30%	-23%

Figure 2. Local health department performance scores, Beloit, Wisconsin, 1993 and 1995.

programs and policies. The largest decreases in health department performance appear to occur for the practices of investigating health threats, analyzing the determinants of health threats, and implementing public health programs and policies.

When we examine the participation of organizations other than the local health department in public health functions, the health director's responses in 1993 and 1995 suggest that many types of organizations have increased their involvement in policy development activities (**Figure 3**). Hospitals, nonprofit agencies, state government agencies, and private physicians show the largest increases in policy development participation during this period. At the same time, most organizations appear to have decreased their participation in assurance activities. The largest decreases in assurance activities appear to occur among local government agencies, private physicians, and state government agencies. Participation in assessment activities appears to have remained relatively stable for most types of organizations—except for local government agencies, whose participation has substantially declined.

Interpretation of Performance Assessment Results

Results from the performance assessment surveys in 1992 and 1995 suggest that public health roles and responsibilities are changing within the community but that overall levels of performance are being maintained. The local health department appears to be shedding some of its responsibilities in directly performing public health practices, while other community organizations are stepping in to assume them. These trends may stem in part from the numerous pilot projects and demonstration initiatives that have been launched by the local health department in recent years. As the outside funds supporting these initiatives have waned, the local health department has achieved notable success in continuing many of them through assistance from other community organizations. Notable examples include the health and human service centers that were started with funds from the Robert Wood Johnson Foundation and the maternal and child health "one-stop shopping" center that was initiated with funding from the state health agency. In each of these cases, the health department provided the leadership and expertise necessary for funding, designing, and implementing these initiatives. Once successfully underway, the local health department has sustained these initiatives through growing collaboration with other community organizations—a strategy that has often entailed transitioning the responsibilities of program maintenance and growth to these other stakeholders. Through these types of activities, the local health department appears to be cultivating the community's capacity for public health performance.

Despite the jurisdiction's success in maintaining overall levels of community performance, several trends warrant attention regarding the public health contributions made by community organizations. Community organizations appear to be increasing their involvement in public health functions primarily through policy development activities such as communitywide planning, advocacy, and priority setting. These activities are often important first steps in interorganizational collaboration, as they allow organizations to identify common interests and concerns and to develop coordinated plans for action. Unfortunately, involvement in the vital assurance function appears to be declining for many types of organizations. Assurance activities often entail greater commitments of time, effort, and resources than other public health practices, because they typically involve the "front-line" tasks of providing services and managing resources. As a result, these activities may be the most vulnerable when funding sources change and responsibilities are shifted among community organizations. Results from the performance assessment surveys in 1993 and 1995 suggest that Beloit's public health agencies need to examine and encourage continued organizational contributions to assurance activities, as changes occur within their public health system. These

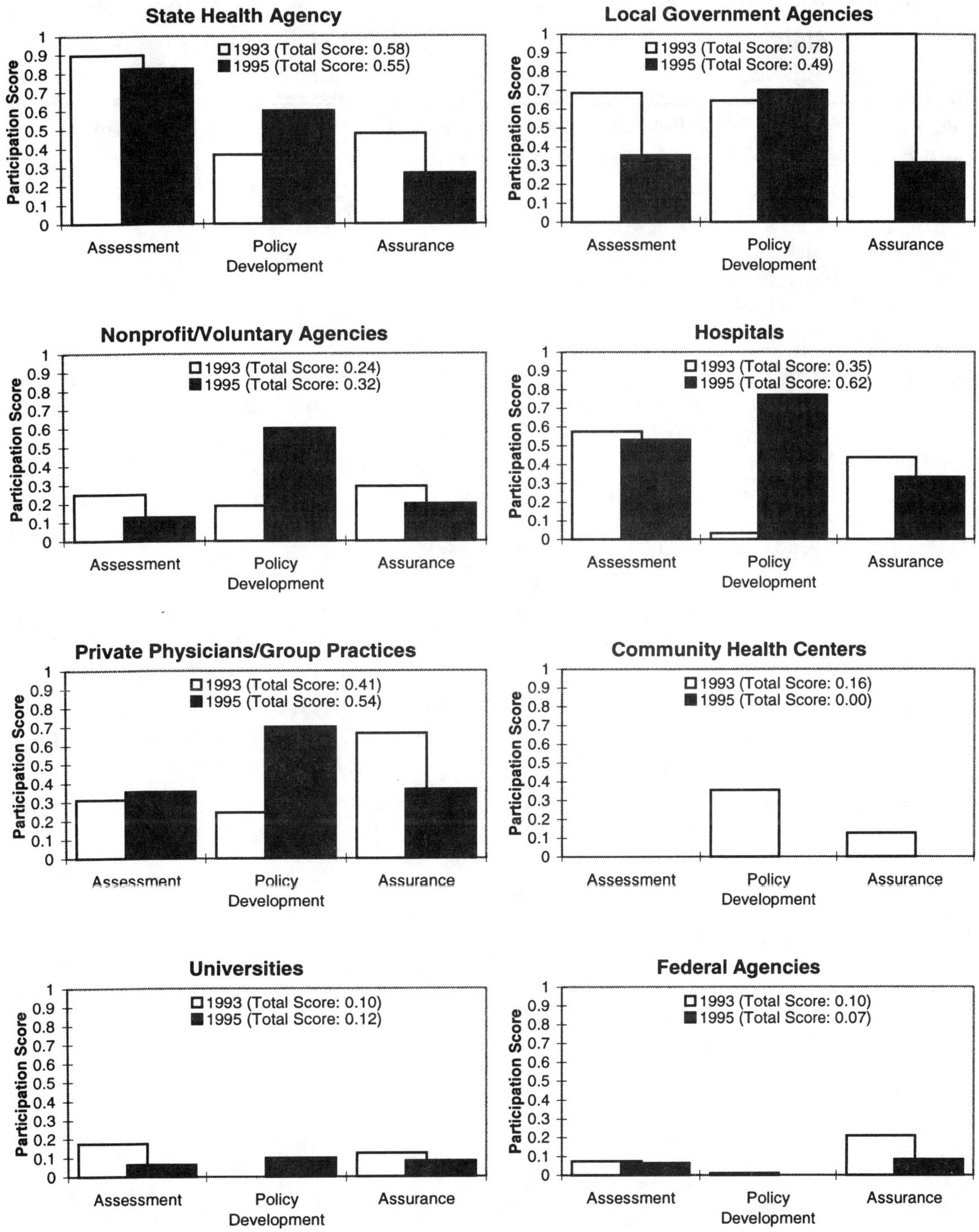

Figure 3. Participation in local public health acitivites by other organizations, 1993 and 1997 (as reported by the local health director).

contributions are difficult but essential components of the task of achieving improvements in community health status.

Future Prospects and Projections

A continuing strength of Beloit's local public health system lies in the close working relationships among the major service providers in the community. These relationships are surviving, and even strengthening, in the face of mounting external pressures created by such trends as local hospital competition, managed care growth, and political pressures for local health department consolidation. In maintaining and strengthening these relationships, Beloit's public health organizations need to guard against the tendency toward insularity, which could greatly diminish the public health system's ability to adapt to and capitalize upon these larger changes. As managed care continues to grow within the public and private health care sectors, the constellation of organizations contributing to health in Beloit is likely to grow in size and complexity. Similarly, competition among hospitals and other health care organizations is likely to bring Beloit's population within the service areas of numerous service providers. To be optimally effective in assuring health within its jurisdiction, Beloit's local health department needs the ability to interface with the full extent of organizations contributing to the health and health care of its residents.

This task will undoubtedly require the health department to move beyond the geographic boundaries of its jurisdiction in interacting with health care organizations. Additionally, this task will require the department to remain detached from, but cognizant of, the competitive pressures that inevitably consume health care providers in an increasingly market-based health system. Finally, this task may require the local health department to work in tandem with the county health department and other local public health agencies in order to achieve the necessary leverage, coverage, and visibility to interact effectively with other health care organizations—whose scale and scope of operations may far surpass those of the department. Beloit Health Department's skills in interorganizational collaboration and coalition-building are highly developed and should leave the organization well positioned to achieve these emerging objectives. Future success will likely hinge upon the department's ability to realize the strengths of the department's long-standing relationships with other community providers, while rising above the inherent trappings of these relationships.

References

1. US Centers for Disease Control and Prevention. State and national vaccination coverage levels among children aged 19-35 months—United States, April-December 1994. *MMWR Morb Mortal Wkly Rep.* 1995;44(33):613,619-623.
2. American Medical Association. *Physician Data by County, 1992.* Chicago, Ill: American Medical Association; 1992.
3. US Department of Health and Human Services (DHHS). *Healthy People 2000: National Health Promotion and Disease Prevention Objectives.* Washington, DC: DHHS; 1991.
4. Miller CA, Moore KS, Richards TB, Monk JD. A proposed method for assessing the performance of local public health functions and practices. *Am J Public Health.* 1994;84(11):1743-1749.

Chapter 10

Case Study of Denver, Colorado

Key Attributes

- Integrated organizational structure encompassing a local health department, hospital, network of community health centers, and a managed care plan.
- Strong collaborative activities among the public and nonprofit health organizations serving the community.
- Competitive relationships within the growing for-profit health care sector.
- Active involvement of managed care plans in community health activities.

Community Characteristics

Demographic and Socioeconomic Characteristics

Metropolitan Denver comprises a five-county area containing a population of almost 2 million residents. Approximately 500,000 of these residents live within the city and county of Denver, the urban core of the area (**Table 1**). The area continues to grow rapidly with an expanding local economy fueled by technology firms and service industries. This recent growth stands in stark contrast to the stagnant local economy that emerged after the oil industry faltered during the 1980s.

Denver's population contains a diversity of ethnicities and cultures. Census data indicate that residents of Hispanic origin comprise 23% of the county's total population, and almost 12% of the population speak Spanish at home. African Americans comprise 12% of the county population. Educational attainment and income appears higher in Denver than in many similar urban counties. Almost 80% of Denver residents are high school graduates, and 30% hold Bachelor's degrees. The median family income of $32,038 is only slightly below the national average, and less than 18% of residents live below the federal poverty threshold.

Denver's population appears generally younger and healthier than many comparable urban areas. Less than 14% of the county's population has reached age 65. Infant mortality stands at 8.1 for Whites and 10.4 for non-Whites (per 1000 live births) based on 1995 data. Leading causes of death include heart disease (351 per 100,000 population), cancer (193 per 100,000), and stroke (54 per 100,000) (**Table 2**).

Parts of this chapter are reprinted, with permission, from: Mays GP. Integrated public and private health care systems in Denver, Colorado. In: Halverson PK, Kaluzny AD, McLaughlin CP (eds). *Managed Care and Public Health.* Gaithersburg, MD: Aspen Publishers; 1998:201–221.

Local Health Resources and Manpower

The city and county of Denver benefit from a wide array of public and private health resources. Access to health services remains a concern in low-income neighborhoods and some communities with large minority populations. In these areas, private providers are less

Table 1
Demographic Characteristics: Denver, Colorado

Population (1996)	496,470
Percent of metropolitan area population	23.4
Median age in years (1996)	34.3
Percent 65 years and older (1991)	13.8
Percent non-White (1991)	30.3
Percent speaking Spanish at home (1991)	11.9
Percent completing high school degree (1991)	79.2
Percent below federal poverty level (1989)	17.1
Median household income (1989)	$25,106
Average percent unemployed (1996 metropolitan area)	3.8

Data from US Department of Commerce, Bureau of the Census.

Table 2
Health Status Indicators: Denver, Colorado, 1995

Infant mortality rate per 1000 live births	8.2
Percent of births to mothers age 10-17	7.1
Percent of infants with low birth weight	10.5
Percent of births with prenatal care later than first trimester	27.7
Deaths per 100,000 population, age-adjusted	597.6
Cancer, all types	128.5
Lung cancer	31.7
Female breast cancer	21.7
Heart disease	124.6
Other cardiovascular diseases	168.2
Cerebrovascular diseases	28.3
Chronic obstructive pulmonary diseases	27.4
Motor vehicle accidents	15.3
Suicide	20.6
Work-related injury	2.6
Percent of deaths due to pneumonia and influenza	3.6
HIV/AIDS	4.3
Diabetes mellitus	1.9
Injury by firearms	2.3
Alcohol-induced deaths	2.3

Data from Colorado Department of Public Health and Environment (unpublished data, 1997).

abundant, health insurance coverage is low, and language and cultural differences pose barriers to care. An estimated 12.5% of the population did not have health care coverage in 1994.[1] A total of 3204 active nonfederal physicians practiced in city and county of Denver during 1994, yielding a comparatively high ratio of 661 physicians per 100,000 population (**Table 3**).[2] A relatively low proportion of these physicians practice in primary care disciplines, with only 21% practicing in the specialties of family medicine, general medicine, pediatrics, and obstetrics/gynecology.

Ten community hospitals serve the city and county of Denver and the surrounding metropolitan area, with a total inpatient capacity of 2889 beds, or 596 beds per 100,000 population.[1] Consolidation continues to occur rapidly in the local hospital market, as evidenced by a recent hospital closure (1995) and several nonprofit hospital acquisitions by the for-profit corporation Columbia/HCA. Most of the Denver area hospitals are now affiliated with one of four multihospital systems. Two public hospitals—the local Denver Health authority and the state-affiliated University hospital—provide the bulk of charity care in the area.

A network of 11 community health centers operates as part of the Denver Health authority.[7] These federally funded centers provide primary care services to uninsured and underinsured populations, as well as Medicaid and Medicare beneficiaries. The centers also receive federal funding to provide specialized human immunodeficiency virus (HIV) services under the Ryan White program as well as substance abuse services under the federal block grant program. A federally funded homeless health clinic also operates in Denver's downtown area, under the management of a private nonprofit corporation.

Managed care has become a dominant form of local health services delivery and financing for commercially insured individuals as well as Medicaid and Medicare beneficiaries in Denver. Almost 50% of the total population in the Denver metropolitan area receive health services through health maintenance organizations (HMOs).[8] At least 10 commercial HMOs report operating in the city and county of Denver.[5] Two of these HMOs enroll Medicaid beneficiaries, five hold federal contracts for serving Medicare beneficiaries on a capitated basis, and one plan serves Medicare beneficiaries under cost-based reimbursement. Three of Denver's private multihospital systems also operate HMO products that serve primarily employee groups. Additionally, the Denver Health authority operates an HMO that serves municipal employees and maintains part ownership in another HMO that serves Medicaid beneficiaries.

Table 3
Health Resources: Denver, Colorado

Number of nonfederal physicians (Number per 100,000 population) 1992[a]	3204 (661)
Family practice	177 (37)
General practice	46 (9)
Internal medicine	587 (121)
Obstetrics/gynecology	174 (36)
Pediatrics	271 (56)
Number of community hospital beds (FY1995)[b]	2,889
Beds per 100,000 population	596
Number of community hospitals (FY1995)[b]	10
Number of HMOs (1994)[c]	11
Number of federally qualified health centers (1994)[d]	18
Total number of clinic sites	7
Local public health expenditures (1997)	$8,613,783
Percent from direct federal sources	14%
Percent from state sources (including federal pass-throughs)	52%
Percent from local sources	18%
Percent from Medicaid	0%
Percent from Medicare	0%
Total federal funding for community health centers (1996)[e]	$8,967,188
Total federal funding for migrant health centers (1996)[e]	$1,378,617
Total federal block grant funds for preventive health services (1996)[e]	$2,215,454
Total federal block grant funds for maternal and child health services (1996)[e]	$7,509,545
Total federal block grant funds for substance abuse services (1996)[e]	$4,415,098
Total federal funding for homeless health services (1996)[e]	$983,485
Total federal funding for National Health Service Corporation (1996)[e]	$146,549

[a]*Data from American Medical Association Physician Masterfile.*[3]
[b]*Data from American Hospital Association.*[4]
[c]*Data from Group Health Association of America.*[5]
[d]*Data from US Bureau of Primary Health Care (unpublished data, 1994).*
[e]*Data from US Department of Commerce.*[6]

The Local Health Department

Organizational Structure

The local public health department for the city and county of Denver resides within the consolidated Denver Health authority . This authority also encompasses a general acute-care hospital, a network of community health centers, and a managed care plan serving county employees. The public hospital and health department have operated under a consolidated organizational structure since 1912, when a state home rule amendment took effect that separated the city of Denver from its surrounding county jurisdiction and designated Denver as a combined city and county government. Under this amendment, the public hospital and health department were combined with the local public assistance program into a single agency of local government, under the authority of Denver's elected mayor and city council. An amendment to the city charter in 1951 moved the hospital and health department into a separate agency named Denver Health and Hospitals and created a seven-member board of health and hospitals to govern the institution.

Several important organizational components have been added to the Denver Health system over the past 30 years. In 1966, Denver Health expanded to include a community health center funded through the US Office of Economic Opportunity's Neighborhood Health Center program. In subsequent years, Denver Health expanded this center into a network of 10 community health clinics for providing ambulatory health services to low-income population groups within the city. In 1988, Denver Health established a network of school-based health clinics through a collaborative effort with the Denver school system, the University of Colorado, the private not-for-profit Children's Hospital, and several mental health and substance abuse providers. Denver Health's foray into managed care began in 1991 with the formation of City Care, an HMO serving employees of the city and county of Denver. Three years later, the agency began operating a prepaid health plan serving Medicaid beneficiaries. Soon after, in 1995, the agency joined with University Hospital, Children's Hospital, and a network of community health centers to form Colorado Access, a not-for-profit HMO designed to serve Medicaid beneficiaries. With its capacities in inpatient care, ambulatory services, public health, and managed care, Denver Health evolved into one of the earliest and most complete examples of a public sector integrated health care delivery system.

The organizational structure of Denver Health changed markedly on January 1997, when the system converted from an agency of the city and county of Denver to an independent health services authority. Denver Health leaders worked for several years to develop a legal and political framework that would allow the system to operate more efficiently by escaping restrictive municipal requirements in areas such as purchasing products and services, hiring and firing personnel, and entering into contracts and agreements with other public and private organizations. In 1994, state legislation passed that authorized the creation of an independent political subdivision within the state for Denver Health, which would be free of both state and local administrative control.[9] This legislation authorized a nine-member governing board for the authority to be appointed by the mayor and approved by the city council of Denver. Members of the Board of Health and Hospitals authorized under Denver city charter were designated to serve as ex officio nonvoting members of the authority's governing board. During 1996, Denver's city council approved an agreement to transfer the city's health system assets and authority to the independent authority, effective January 1, 1997. Under this agreement, the city has taken steps to (1) transfer its health care facilities, equipment, and assets to the authority, (2) transfer responsibility for management and operation of the health system to the authority, and (3) establish contracts with the authority for the provision of health services that the city remains responsible for under its charter, including indigent care at both inpatient and ambulatory levels and specified public health functions. Existing Denver Health staff were given the choice to remain employees of the city and be leased to the authority or to become employees of the authority. New staff for the Denver Health system has been hired as employees of the authority.

The current organizational structure of the Denver Health system consists of eight general service areas, supported by a range of administrative and operational divisions. The eight service areas include hospital operations, community health services, public health services, managed care operations, school-based services, substance abuse services, emergency medical services and the 911 system, and poison control services. Denver Health administrators emphasize that, while an identifiable public health department exists within the organizational structure of the authority, public health functions and activities are tightly integrated with other components of the organization. Public health functions are therefore carried out within and across the full range of departments that comprise Denver Health. Environmental health services, however, are no longer carried out within the agency. When Denver Health moved from a city agency to an independent authority in 1997, environmental health functions were separated from the agency and organized under a new city department of environmental health.

A range of cross-functional divisions support the core service areas within Denver Health. A finance division handles the billing, medical records, and contract management functions for the system. A quality review and improvement division houses continuous quality improvement initiatives, infection control, and medical staff review activities. Physicians practicing in inpatient, outpatient, and community settings within Denver Health are all salaried employees of the system and are organized into a single, multispecialty group. Similarly, all nursing and ancillary services provided within the system are administered through a consolidated division.

Governance

Management and governance structures for the Denver Health system begin with the nine-member governing board for the Denver Health authority, established by the 1994 state enabling legislation. This body, which is appointed by Denver's mayor and approved by its city council, holds broad authority for the administration of the Denver Health system. As one of its powers, the governing board is responsible for hiring and evaluating a chief executive officer for the system.

Two other municipality-appointed boards provide governance and oversight for categorical activities within the Denver Health system. The Neighborhood Health Program board oversees programs and services provided through the network of community health centers, and the Rocky Mountain Poison Center Foundation Board serves in an advisory capacity to the poison and drug centers operated under Denver Health's public health department. The mayor appoints members of both boards, subject to the city council's approval.

Health Officer and Staff

Patricia Gabow, MD, serves as the organization's chief executive officer and medical director. A 24-year veteran of Denver Health, Dr. Gabow began her tenure as a staff physician within the hospital and progressed through the positions of Chief of Medicine and Deputy Manager of Medical Affairs. Denver's Mayor Wellington Webb appointed Dr. Gabow as co-manager of the Denver Health system in 1991, along side the municipality's former budget director Thomas Moe. Mr. Moe's retirement in 1995 left Dr. Gabow as the sole administrator of the system, a position she retained when the organization converted from a municipal agency to an independent authority in early 1997. As Denver Health's chief administrator, Dr. Gabow holds primary responsibility for balancing and integrating the public health and medical care components of the system.

Frank Judson, MD, serves as the Director of the Public Health Department within Denver Health and as the Chief of Infectious Diseases within Denver Health's hospital. Dr. Judson's position as Public Health Officer holds statutory authority under state and municipal law for issuing health orders related to communicable disease control and public health and safety. Correspondingly, the public health department within Denver Health maintains primary responsibility for services and activities in the areas of disease control, health promotion, disease prevention, community health assessment, and public health policy development and enforcement. In carrying out these activities, Dr. Judson and his office work closely with staff in the other Denver Health divisions.

Richard Wright, MD, heads the Division of Community Health Services, which encompasses the network of 11 federally qualified community health centers. These centers provide primary care services to uninsured and underinsured residents and to Medicaid and Medicare beneficiaries in the city and county of Denver. These centers originally operated as neighborhood health centers under the federal Office of Economic Opportunity program. Currently, the network of centers receives federal funding under the Section 330 Community Health Centers program and exists as one of the largest programs of its type in the country. The centers also provide HIV/AIDS outpatient services with funding from the federal Ryan White Act program and substance abuse treatment services through the federal substance abuse prevention and treatment block grant. One of the clinics operates as an outpatient center within the Denver Health hospital.

Douglas Clingscales serves as the chief administrator of the managed care division within Denver Health. Mr. Clingscales' responsibilities center around the two managed care products offered within Denver Health: the City Care plan, which operates as an HMO for municipal employees, and Denver Health's component of the Colorado Access HMO. Approximately 3300 municipal employees (25%) receive their health care through City Care, and more than 16,000 Medicaid beneficiaries are enrolled Denver Health's component of Colorado Access. Mr. Clingscales works in tandem with a senior staff composed of an administrator and a medical director for managed care operations.

Several administrative structures exist within Denver Health to facilitate integration and coordination among the divisions. An executive committee, comprised of the chief administrators and medical directors in each of the divisions of public health, community health, and quality assurance, serves as the principal forum for managerial communication and coordination across the divisions. Other cross-division working groups and advisory committees provide opportunities for integration at operational levels. A managed care advisory committee comprises clinical staff from the hospital, community health, and public health divisions and provides guidance on operational and policy issues for the authority's two HMO products. Similarly, a services committee comprised of the directors of all departments providing health services within Denver Health meets every 2 weeks to address issues of service coordination, duplication, and shared resources. The organization also makes use of cross-division appointments to achieve coordination and integration within Denver Health. Dr. Judson, for example, serves not only as the director of the public health division but also as Chief of Infectious Diseases within the hospital division.

Program and Service Areas

Public Health Department

The Denver Health system provides for a wide range of public health programs and services through its integrated structure. The public health division that exists within this structure directly performs some of these public health activities, while other activities are provided through other components of the Denver

Health system. The public health division serves as the focal point for programs related to disease control, health promotion, community health assessment, and public health policy development.

Within its disease control section, the public health department provides personal health services as well as surveillance, investigation, and research activities related to communicable disease prevention and control. The department's sexually transmitted disease clinic offers free diagnostic and therapeutic services to area residents 5 days and 2 nights per week, providing more than 20,000 patient visits per year. A separate teen clinic offers sexually transmitted disease screening as well as birth control services, pregnancy testing, and counseling and referral for area residents 19 years of age and under. Staffing and funding shortages have limited the department's ability to expand service volume in this clinic beyond the roughly 500 patient visits provided annually.

A tuberculosis clinic provides free education, screening, treatment, and follow-up for residents who have contracted or are at risk of contracting the disease. This clinic provided more than 50,000 patient visits during 1993, including active treatment sessions, preventive therapy visits, and refugee screening. The outreach program component of this clinic now extends to jails, homeless shelters, and boarding homes.

The public health department conducts childhood immunization activities in coordination with the Denver Health community health services division, which oversees the network of community health centers and school-based health clinics. Routine childhood immunizations are administered to sixth- and seventh-graders through school-based clinics, and underimmunized children less than 2 years of age are targeted through outreach programs in the community health centers. In addition, the department provides immunization injections for individuals exposed to hepatitis A and active surveillance for cases and contacts of hepatitis A, B, and C.

Denver Health's public health department also maintains extensive programs and services for the prevention, diagnosis, and treatment of HIV and AIDS. An infectious disease / AIDS clinic operated by the department manages the care of more than 500 patients who have developed AIDS, other manifestations of HIV, or other infectious diseases. This clinic provides intensive diagnostic and therapeutic services such as chemotherapy sessions and pharmaceutical counseling. Additionally, the department administers a storefront outreach and education program targeting IV drug users, an HIV counseling and testing program that is operational in multiple community sites, and an extensive battery of clinical research efforts related to HIV prevention and control.

Several other components of the public health department's disease control section reinforce its achievements in clinical service provision and surveillance. The department operates a full-service laboratory to process its large volume of screening and diagnostic tests. Additionally, the department operates a Sexually Transmitted Disease Prevention and Control Training Center in partnership with the Colorado Department of Health and the University of Colorado Health Sciences Center. This center is one of 11 federally funded centers across the nation that offer health care providers education and training in the clinical management of sexually transmitted disease and HIV infection.

Community Health Services

The community health services division within Denver Health provides extensive primary care and preventive health services to area residents through its network of community health clinics and school-based health clinics. The system includes 11 health clinics located in Denver neighborhoods where access to private health care has traditionally been limited. Eight of the centers are staffed by nurse practitioners and family practitioners, and three centers are staffed by teams of nurse practitioners, general internists, pediatricians, and obstetricians. The clinic system is designated as a federally qualified health center and receives Section 330 funds for the provision of care to low-income uninsured and underinsured residents. The system also receives funds under the federal Ryan White Act for the provision of outpatient services to HIV patients and under the Substance Abuse Services Block Grant for delivering treatment and counseling services for patients with addictions to alcohol and other drugs. State and city funding for the provision of indigent care services complete the system's revenue sources. More than 90,000 ambulatory care visits were provided by Denver Health during 1996.

Denver Health also operates a network of school-based health clinics, in partnership with Denver's school system, the University of Colorado, Denver Children's Hospital, and several mental health and substance abuse providers. Clinics currently operate in five Denver high schools and in all of the grade and middle schools that are located within a specific medically underserved area in Denver's urban core (a total of 11 school-based clinics). All of the clinics are staffed by nurse practitioners or nurses receiving nurse practitioner training, with physician support provided by pediatricians within the Denver Health system.

Also included in the community health system is a hospital-based ambulatory care center that provides both primary and subspecialty care on an outpatient basis. A dental clinic and a pharmacy services division complete the range of ambulatory health services provided through the system.

As a whole, the community health system appears to function effectively within the larger Denver Health delivery system. In total, the community health system provides ~433,000 patient visits per year. Administrators report the following statistics for the system's 100,000 regular users who access clinics at least 3 times in a 2-year period ending in 1996: 66% of pregnant women enter prenatal care during the first trimester; 88% of children ages 2 to 5 are immunized with the basic series; 75% of patients diagnosed with hypertension are treated for this disorder; 86% of women over age 18 have had pap smears at appropriate intervals; and 73% of women between ages 50 and 75 have had mammography at appropriate intervals.

Managed Care Division

Managed care has become a key component of the Denver Health system during the past decade. The system began its foray into managed care when it jointly developed an HMO for serving city employees through a partnership with FHP, a large for-profit HMO with a strong local presence in Denver. After several years of joint operation, Denver Health chose to end its agreement with FHP and operate the employee plan on its own. Currently, the City Care plan serves ~3300 municipal employees, or almost one quarter of the city's work force. Administrators of the managed care division emphasize that, because the City Care plan is now wholly owned and financed by the Denver Health system, it permits the system to use revenues from this program to support the delivery of nonrevenue generating services in other areas of the system. Income generated through operation of the City Care plan therefore helps finance the delivery of public health services and personal health care to the uninsured.

In 1994, the Denver Health system initiated a managed care plan for serving Medicaid beneficiaries. Colorado's Section 1915b Medicaid waiver demonstration program began that year, creating a mandatory enrollment requirement for beneficiaries eligible for the Aid to Families with Dependent Children (AFDC) public assistance program who reside in the state's metropolitan counties. Choice Care, as Denver Health's Medicaid plan was called, was one of four HMOs that contract with the state Medicaid agency for serving Medicaid beneficiaries. This plan was later consolidated with the Colorado Access HMO that Denver Health launched with its partnering organizations in 1995. Colorado Access now exists as the state's largest Medicaid HMO, with the Denver Health component alone serving almost 18,000 enrollees. Colorado Access also is the only HMO in the state that serves all types of Medicaid beneficiaries—not only AFDC beneficiaries—on a voluntary basis. The decision to serve non-AFDC beneficiaries under the same capitation rate as AFDC clients is notable, given the difficulties and financial risks entailed in efficiently managing the often complex service needs of Medicaid eligibility groups such as supplemental security income beneficiaries and the aged, blind, and disabled.

The Denver Health component of Colorado Access functions as a staff-model HMO in that all physicians within the Denver Health system are salaried employees. Enrollees choose a primary care physician operating in one of the system's community health clinics, and beneficiaries failing to make this choice are assigned a clinic and physician nearest to their residence. Clinic physicians serve as case managers for enrollees by insuring that routine primary care and preventive services are utilized appropriately and by providing referral authorizations for specialist services.

Colorado Access operates an extensive quality assurance program to insure that its Medicaid enrollees receive appropriate, accessible, and timely health care. Through this system, plan administrators track indicators of preventive services utilization, prenatal care delivery, birth outcomes, service accessibility, and enrollee satisfaction. Denver Health reports a subset of these indicators to the state Medicaid agency in response to contract requirements and to the National Commission for Quality Assurance as a step toward accreditation by this body.

Hospital Services

Denver Health Medical Center (formerly Denver General Hospital) serves as the system's inpatient care facility and as the region's level one trauma center. The facility is centrally located in Denver's urban core and contains a total of 349 licensed beds of which 313 are currently staffed. The facility serves as the primary provider of hospital services to the uninsured and Medicaid-eligible residents of the city and county of Denver. Among Denver area hospitals, Denver Health Medical Center serves a larger proportion of minority and low-income patients (Colorado Hospital Association, unpublished data, 1995).

A referral agreement with the nearby University of Colorado Hospital transfers responsibility for meeting the indigent care needs of nonresidents to this state-affiliated hospital. Nonetheless, the Denver Health system provides nearly 40% of the charity care that is delivered in the state. Medicare beneficiaries make up a comparatively small proportion of the medical center's patient mix, despite a unique reimbursement arrangement the hospital holds with the Health Care Financing Administration for bundling physician and hospital costs into a single reimbursement rate. The hospital handled 18,369 inpatient admissions during 1996 and maintained an average daily census of 219 patients (69% of capacity). An active obstetrics program managed 2617 births during this period. Despite the high acuity level of patients served by the medical center, admitted patients spend an average of only 4.8 days in the hospital.

Other Programs and Services

The Denver Health system includes several other programs and services that complete its integrated service continuum. The emergency medical services division operates the area's paramedic and ambulance service and the area's 911 emergency access network. Denver Health's poison control section administers two information and consultation centers for both consumers and health professionals. The Denver Health poison center provides toxicological information and treatment recommendations by telephone on a 24-hour basis. Additionally, the agency operates the Rocky Mountain Drug Information Center, which provides information regarding the proper use of both prescription and nonprescription medications. This center also serves as Denver Health's central reporting vehicle for adverse drug events that occur among patients in the system.

Denver Health also maintains an array of behavioral health programs. The agency operates a 90-bed alcohol treatment center, which provides transportation, detoxification, and treatment services to over 7000 patients on an inpatient basis and 96,000 patients on an outpatient basis. As an outgrowth of its behavioral health care activities, in 1996, Denver Health joined with the University of Colorado Health Sciences Center and several mental health and substance abuse providers to create a managed behavioral health plan known as Signal Behavioral Health Network. This plan provided more than 20,000 detoxification episodes and 18,000 substance abuse treatment episodes during fiscal year 1997. Denver Health also recently joined with several partners—including a local community mental health center, a psychiatric hospital, and its collaborators in the Colorado Access HMO—to form Access Behavioral Care, a managed behavioral health care plan designed to serve Medicaid beneficiaries in Colorado's Mental Health Capitation and Managed Care Program.

Until its reorganization as an independent authority in 1997, Denver Health also maintained responsibilities in environmental health, consumer protection, and animal control. These functions are now carried out by the city and county of Denver and housed in a new department of environmental health. Environmental protection activities fall into three categories: pollution control, pollution prevention, and industrial and occupational health. Within the pollution control arena, the department oversees the regulation of air and water pollutant emissions from both residential and commercial sources. The department serves in an advisory capacity for pollution-prevention programs that target consumer and commercial adoption of low-emissions technologies in transportation and industrial production. Industrial and occupational health programs include asbestos abatement inspections, indoor air quality investigations (including environmental tobacco smoke investigations), and complaint-driven noise exposure inspections. The consumer protection division provides food safety inspections, housing code investigations, health facilities licensing, and childcare licensing. The animal control division operates the municipal animal shelter and enforces the city's animal control ordinances.

Infrastructure and Resources

Physical infrastructure for the Denver Health system consists of an acute care hospital, 11 community-based health clinics, 11 school-based clinics, a hospital-based ambulatory care center, an alcohol treatment facility, and several specialty centers for public health services. All centers providing personal health services are linked through a single medical record that is maintained for each patient seeking care within the system. Development of a computer-based information system is currently underway to reduce duplication and transport costs associated with medical records and to better link the operations of multiple system components. Major components of this system are already in place, including billing, laboratory, imaging, and radiology. Within 3 years, the system will include the full patient record, as well as components for pharmacy, personnel, and management.

Financial resources for the Denver Health system derive from a broad base of federal, state, and local support combined with payments from private insurers and patients. The system receives funding from the city and county of Denver through three contractual agreements: a service agreement for providing public health services mandated by city charter, a service agreement for providing uncompensated care, and capitated contract for providing specified health services to city employees enrolled in the Denver Health Municipal Plan HMO. The first two sources of local funding amount to ~16% of the system's total budget, while HMO premiums account for ~3% of this budget.

Medicaid payments for patient services represent the largest single share of the system's budget. Combined revenue from fee-for-service payments and from capitated payments for enrollees in the Choice Care HMO total ~26% of the budget (more than $38 million). This revenue is generated from personal health services delivered in the community health clinics, HIV / AIDS clinics, and the hospital. An additional 9% of the system's budget derives from an annual Medicaid disproportionate share hospital payment the system qualifies for as a major provider of uncompensated hospital care. These payments, which increased substantially when the state Medicaid plan was revised in 1993, played a major role in helping the system to retire a $39 million deficit and to build its current $40 million revenue surplus. Currently, administrators rely on disproportionate share hospital payments to finance the computerized information network that is being phased in across the Denver Health system. Denver Health receives one additional revenue source linked to the provision of uncompensated care through the state's Medically Indigent Fund. This fund specifically covers the provision of ambulatory and hospital services to populations without health insurance who are ineligible for Medicaid coverage. Revenue from this fund accounts for an additional 9% of the system's financial resources.

Medicare payments for services provided to beneficiaries in the hospital and community health clinics total ~8% of the system's budget. This proportion is substantially lower than other hospitals operating in the area, suggesting that the system does not attract a preponderance of Medicare beneficiaries residing in the area. Because all physicians practicing within Denver Health are salaried employees of the system, Medicare uses a combined fee schedule to cover the hospital and physician services for beneficiaries admitted to the hospital.

The Denver Health system serves a moderate number of commercially insured individuals, primarily through its hospital inpatient departments, emergency department, and ambulatory care center. Commercial insurance payments for patient services amount to 14% of the system's annual budget. Other funding sources for the system include federal and state grants for research and special programs (6%) and self-pay patient revenue (3%).

Other Contributors to Local Public Health Practice

State Health Agencies

Public health and medical care programs for the state of Colorado are administered through separate agencies. A reorganization effort in 1994 created a separate state agency for administering medical care programs, named the Department of Health Care Policy and Financing. This agency serves as the state's single agency for administering medical care programs and services. The Department of Public Health and Environment administers public health and environmental programs within the state. Finally, the Department of Human Services houses programs related to mental health, social services, and alcohol and drug abuse.

A Health Division within the Department of Public Health and Environment administers programs and services related to disease control and epidemiology, health promotion and disease prevention, family and community health, emergency medical services, and health facilities licensing and inspection. These programs serve as important sources of funding and technical assistance for services provided by Denver Health and other county public health agencies. A decentralized administrative relationship exists between county public health agencies and the state Department of Public Health and Environment. The state department provides little direct governance or oversight in county public health functions outside of its responsibilities in contract enforcement and administration of state public health codes. Denver Health administrators characterize their relationship with this department as strong and supportive, noting that the department operates mainly as a resource to Denver Health in carrying out its public health functions.

The Department of Health Care Policy and Financing administers the state's $1.4 billion Medicaid program and $71 million Colorado Indigent Care Program. More than 280,000 individuals are served through the Medicaid program. Almost 70% of these beneficiaries are enrolled in one of the state's two Medicaid-waiver managed care programs: a fee-for-service case management program that operates in most Colorado counties and a capitated managed care program that operates in Denver and other urbanized counties within the state. Both programs operate with a 1915(b) demonstration waiver from the US Health Care Financing Administration, which provides for mandatory enrollment of AFDC program beneficiaries in the managed care programs. Under the capitated program, approved

HMOs may choose to enroll supplemental security income beneficiaries on a voluntary basis. The department holds primary responsibility for developing and administering contracts with Medicaid providers, including HMOs participating in the capitated managed care program underway in Denver and other urbanized counties. This responsibility includes insuring compliance with HMO enrollment and marketing procedures and reviewing quarterly reports of utilization and outcome data reported by HMOs. HMO data reported and reviewed by the agency include the following: enrollee utilization of preventive and screening services, family planning services, and prenatal care; low birth weight rates; cesarean section rates; emergency services utilization; disenrollments and member grievances; and annual enrollee satisfaction survey results. All HMOs participating in the capitated Medicaid waiver program must also meet state Department of Insurance licensing requirements regarding levels of capitalization and financial reserves.

Denver Health maintains a strong working relationship with the Department of Health Care Policy and Financing, which provides funding for a substantial portion of the medical services delivered through the organization's hospital, managed care plan, and community health center network. Denver Health officials note that their organization operates not only as a contractor but also as a partner with this state agency. Denver Health serves as a pilot for many of the innovations that the agency explores for its health care financing programs. For example, the department modeled its Medicaid HMO quality assurance reporting system after a system developed by Denver Health for its Medicaid managed care plan. Additionally, the department has used Denver Health as a model in establishing policies for Medicaid disproportionate share hospital payments, which are designed to compensate facilities that serve large proportions of uninsured individuals.

Along side Denver Health's integrated public health and medical care system, a constellation of other public and private organizations contribute to public health in Denver. Some of these organizations engage in public health activities through partnerships and alliances with Denver Health. Many other organizations support public health initiatives that are independent of the "official" public health system, either alone or in partnership with other organizations. Denver Health administrators report that they do not pursue an "all-inclusive" strategy of convening health care organizations to work on public health issues. Rather, the authority places emphasis on working through the components of its own integrated system and through the limited network of local organizations that maintain an explicit mission of community health. This network includes the local medical center operated by the University of Colorado and the nonprofit Children's Hospital. Perhaps as a consequence of this approach, many of the other local health care organizations report disengagement from the formal public health system in Denver. The sections that follow describe the major types of organizations contributing to public health in Denver and the relationships that they maintain with Denver Health as the local public health authority.

Hospitals

In addition to Denver Health's facility, Denver's local hospital market consists of a state university medical center, four private hospital systems, a children's hospital, and several specialty facilities such as the National Jewish Center for Immunology and Respiratory Medicine and a veterans affairs medical center. The pressures of managed care and cost containment continue to drive mergers, consolidations, closures, and acquisitions in Denver's hospital market as in many other areas of the country. Over the past 3 years, two major nonprofit hospital systems have merged, one independent hospital closed, and Denver's largest system converted from nonprofit to for-profit status under a merger with a facility owned by the national Columbia/HCA hospital corporation. These market dynamics appear to affect the roles and responsibilities that hospitals undertake regarding public health activities and community health issues and in the interorganizational relationships they establish to accomplish these activities.

University Hospital

University Hospital maintains a close working relationship with Denver Health and is a substantial contributor to the local public health system in Denver. Although formally affiliated with the state-owned University of Colorado Health Sciences Center, University Hospital operates as an independent hospital authority similar to the Denver Health system. The facility includes 316 licensed beds and an extensive outpatient clinic system that handled almost 245,000 patient visits in 1994. University Hospital stands as the second largest provider of uncompensated care in Colorado and maintains a formal agreement with Denver Health to meet the primary care needs of the medically indigent who reside within the Denver metropolitan area but outside the city and county of Denver. University Hospital also maintains responsibility under state law for providing specialty care to all medically indigent residents of Colorado. As a consequence, most of the indigent care provided by University Hospital involves specialized medical diagnosis and treatment rather than primary care. Hospital administrators report that ~25% of the hospital's patient care expenditures are for uncompensated care, with expenditures for Medicaid and Medicare beneficiaries accounting for another 25% each, and expenditures for commercially insured individuals accounting for the remaining 25%.

University Hospital and Denver Health interact through a diversity of both formal and informal relationships. Both University Hospital and Denver Health serve as teaching facilities for the University of Colorado Health Sciences Center. The medical staffs of both institutions interact frequently through their appointments as faculty of the university. On an operational level, the two institutions engage in several joint ventures and partnerships for providing public health by the University of Colorado Health Sciences Center, Children's Hospital, Denver Health, and the Denver school department operate school health clinics in eleven public high schools, middle schools, and grade schools in Denver. Under this arrangement, University Hospital provides staff and training for nurses who staff the clinics. All contributing organizations provide oversight and governance for the initiative through representation on an executive council.

University Hospital and Denver Health also interact frequently in programs and services for HIV and AIDS patients. University Hospital maintains a respected clinical research program for HIV / AIDS and related diseases, while Denver Health provides an extensive array of prevention, control, and treatment services—as well as clinical research—through its public health department. The organizations maintain joint referral arrangements for service delivery and recruitment for clinical trials and sponsor several collaborative research efforts. Additionally, both organizations serve on a statewide AIDS advisory panel. University Hospital's administrator reports that the extensive involvement of both organizations in AIDS services and research has created some tension over funding issues and service responsibilities, but most often the organizations have found collaborative solutions to their conflicts.

Building on the success of previous joint initiatives, University Hospital and Denver Health joined with Denver Children's Hospital and a statewide consortium of federally funded health centers in 1995 to form Colorado Access, an HMO for serving Medicaid beneficiaries. The new, jointly owned HMO provides coverage to beneficiaries in all of the counties included in the state's Medicaid waiver program. Ownership of the venture is equally shared among the four participating organizations. Colorado Access provides a mechanism for pooling the capacities and skills of the four institutions in serving vulnerable population groups. The venture also represents a strategic effort among the affiliated public and nonprofit institutions to remain viable service providers for the Medicaid population under a state waiver program that creates opportunities for private managed care plans to serve these populations. Under the joint venture, Denver Health provides all health services to enrollees who reside within the city and county of Denver, University Hospital provides specialty care for all enrollees within the plan, and Children's Hospital provides primary pediatric care in geographic areas outside the city, as well as specialized pediatric services to all plan enrollees. The network of federally funded health centers completes the plan's primary care base in areas outside Denver. By collaborating rather than competing in the Medicaid managed care market, the four organizations hope to develop a level of expertise in managing the care of vulnerable population groups that will serve as a benchmark for other plans participating in the waiver program.

University Hospital and Denver Health also interact through a network of Colorado-based not-for-profit hospitals formed in 1996 to facilitate collaboration in activities such as managed care contracting, outcomes research, and health education interventions. A total of 11 hospitals currently participate in the network, named Healthcare Colorado, including one other Denver-based hospital (St. Joseph's Hospital). Most recently, the network sponsored a community campaign to train residents in CPR techniques. The participating organizations launched a mass media advertising campaign followed by a series of low-cost training classes held at the Colorado Convention Center. Other collaborators in this initiative included local chapters of the American Red Cross and the American Heart Association.

Denver Children's Hospital

As a partner in the school health clinic program and the statewide Medicaid HMO, Denver Children's Hospital stands as a major contributor to the public health system in Denver. Children's Hospital operates as an independent, not-for-profit corporation with a 209-bed inpatient facility and a network of specialty outpatient clinics located throughout the Denver metropolitan area and a larger five-state region. The hospital serves as a regional referral center for pediatric specialty care in this region, and in 1994 handled more than 7700 inpatient admissions and 267,000 outpatient visits. Approximately 40% of the hospital's revenue derive from patient care services to Medicaid beneficiaries. The hospital plays an active role in primary care as well as specialty care through the physician-hospital organization it maintains with both hospital-based and community-based pediatricians in Denver. This physician-hospital organization, called Kidsmart, serves as the primary vehicle for delivering physician services to enrollees of Colorado Access, the jointly sponsored HMO for Medicaid enrollees.

Children's Hospital engages in a wide range of public health initiatives for the Denver community. The hospital operates a primary care clinic that provided over 25,000 patient visits during 1994, including care to Medicaid beneficiaries, uninsured children, and other vulnerable and underserved populations. This clinic helps to alleviate demands on the hospital's emergency department by providing routine and preventive services to families without other sources of care. Additionally, the hospital provides leadership for the Colorado Immunization Coalition, a statewide collaborative of health services providers and community organizations aimed at improving childhood immunization rates. Through this coalition, the hospital facilitates the development of community-wide strategies for improving the delivery and uptake of childhood vaccines. With the participation of Denver Health, the state health department, and community service organizations such as Rotary International, the coalition is currently engaged in efforts to develop a community-wide immunization registry for monitoring the vaccination status of all children in Denver.

Children's Hospital maintains several other school health initiatives in addition to the jointly sponsored clinics it operates with Denver Health and the University Health Sciences Center. First, the hospital maintains an active community health nursing program that holds agreements with several public school systems in the state for providing school nurse services. Additionally, the hospital operates a medical day treatment program in partnership with Denver public schools for providing education and medical treatment to special needs children with serious illnesses. Under this program, children with serious chronic or acute illnesses receive instruction from Denver public school teachers in treatment settings maintained by the hospital. The hospital's administrator reports that this program has reduced rehospitalizations in this population by 75% and has increased the high school graduation rate in this population by 400%.

Administrators at Children's Hospital report a strong and effective relationship with Denver Health and the formal public health system in Denver. The multiple collaborative projects that the hospital maintains with Denver Health offer clear evidence of this relationship. The hospital's chief executive anticipates that Denver Health's reorganization as an independent health care authority will only improve the effectiveness and efficiency of their collaborative efforts, as "local politics invariably complicate health care relationships from time to time" (Lou Blankenship Jr, Chief Executive Officer of Children's Hospital of Denver, personal communication, 1996). Other efforts such as the Colorado Access program continue drawing together the triumvirate of Children's Hospital, Denver Health, and University Hospital as a coordinated public-private partnership for public health and medical care delivery.

Other Private Health Care Systems

Denver Health, together with its partners at University Hospital and Children's Hospital, maintain an extensive multi-institutional system for providing public health and medical care services to the Denver community. Outside this system, private health care organizations serve most of the area's privately insured and Medicare beneficiaries, as well as substantial numbers of Medicaid recipients. Interaction between these private health care organizations and Denver's formal public health system is relatively limited. Denver Health administrators view the two hospital systems that share their mission in indigent care and community health services as their primary partners. Together, these systems serve as the safety-net providers for the Denver community. Extensive collaboration with other private health care organizations appears unlikely given the divergent missions and capacities of these institutions. Denver's private health care organizations are examined in detail elsewhere.[10] Below we summarize the major organizations that contribute to local public health practice in Denver.

The largest of the private health care organizations in Denver, HealthOne, is an integrated delivery system owned in part by the for-profit hospital corporation Columbia-HCA. Comprised of six acute care hospitals, four rehabilitation and psychiatric hospitals, and 60 clinics for outpatient and community-based care, HealthOne is the dominant medical care provider in the region but a relatively minor contributor to public health activities. The corporation maintains periodic outreach efforts such as child safety campaigns and school health screenings, and operates several ambulatory care clinics that serve large numbers of Medicaid recipients in addition to privately-insured patients.

HealthOne administrators indicate a desire to expand the system's involvement in preventive health and wellness services, especially for its growing HMO population. To date its activities in health promotion and disease prevention services have been sporadic and limited primarily to personal health services delivery.

Kaiser Foundation's Colorado health plan is one of the two largest commercial HMOs operating in the Denver metropolitan area, with more than 300,000 enrollees or ~15% of the total metropolitan population. Kaiser Colorado is a regional affiliate of the nation's largest nonprofit HMO corporation. Kaiser does not operate its own inpatient facilities in Denver; rather, it maintains a contract with the nonprofit St. Joseph Hospital for providing hospital services to members. Kaiser is one of several private managed care organizations that enroll Medicaid beneficiaries in Denver.

Kaiser is an important contributor to public health efforts in Denver. Community-based initiatives maintained by the HMO include an educational theater program that tours schools and community organizations year-round with information about child health and safety; adolescent health; HIV and AIDS; and issues of aging. Kaiser also operates a "Tele-Health" initiative in partnership with a local telecommunications company that provides local residents with free telephone access to a variety of prerecorded messages on issues related to health and parenting. With support from a Robert Wood Johnson Foundation grant, Kaiser is working with Denver Health and the local public school system to study the utilization of school health centers in Denver. Results from this study will inform the health care delivery strategies employed by the participating organizations. Kaiser also contributes to several community health planning efforts that seek solutions to pressing health issues in the community. These efforts include task forces on influenza and smoking cessation led by the Colorado Lung Association and a childhood immunization initiative led by Denver Children's Hospital.

In addition to these community-based efforts, Kaiser provides an array of health promotion and disease prevention interventions that target enrolled members of Kaiser. These efforts include an outreach program for mammography screening that uses direct mailings to age-appropriate enrollees and a computerized tracking system to monitor compliance. Kaiser maintains a similar outreach and tracking system for influenza immunizations among the elderly and those with chronic diseases. Outreach programs are also targeted at members for smoking cessation and dietary modification among enrollees identified as hypercholesterolemic. The organization recently completed development of a health risk appraisal protocol that will be administered to all members and used for planning health promotion and disease prevention programs and for targeting interventions to high-risk groups. Kaiser also offers its members 40 different health education classes on a variety of health promotion topics.

Kaiser's collaborating hospital, St. Joseph's Hospital, maintains additional public health activities. The hospital operates a community health clinic in a low-income Denver neighborhood that serves Medicaid beneficiaries and the uninsured. The hospital also provides free monthly health education classes on topics such as diabetes management, hypertension, teen pregnancy, AIDS and sexually transmitted diseases, and parenting skills. Other community health activities provided by St. Joseph include a mobile dental clinic for serving homeless individuals and a free childhood immunization clinic conducted every 6 weeks.

Two other hospital-based health care systems operate in Denver, the Provenant/St. Anthony health care system and the Adventist health system, both of which are nonprofit institutions affiliated with religious organizations. These institutions contribute to local public health activities primarily through the provision of charity care services and the sponsorship of periodic health fairs and health education initiatives. The Adventist health care system maintains a strong historical emphasis on health education and health behavior programs, and continues to offer the community a range of seminars and support groups in areas such as smoking cessation, diet, and chronic disease management. Adventist also administers a free health information telephone line staffed by trained nurses, who provide community residents with advice on a variety of health and wellness issues.

The numerous managed care organizations operating in Denver play relatively limited roles in the local public health system, beyond maintaining health promotion and disease prevention interventions for their members. Several of these plans, such as MetraHealth, have become active in marketing worksite wellness programs to large employers in the Denver area. Other plans such as PacifiCare and QualChoice make substantial investments in public education campaigns around topics such as mammography, immunization, and child injury prevention that also serve as marketing opportunities for the HMOs. Additionally, many of the local HMOs are participating in a regional effort to develop standardized clinical practice guidelines in areas such as cancer screening, immunization, and child wellness screenings. This effort, which is maintained by the local HMO association, promises to improve medical practice at the community level while also improving HMO operations.

Other Community Organizations

A wide range of other organizations makes important contributions to Denver's public health system. Local chapters of voluntary associations such as the American Heart Association, American Lung Association, the American Cancer Society, the American Red Cross, and the United Way provide leadership for a wide range of community health initiatives. Additionally, a variety of nonprofit organizations contribute to the public health system through the direct provision of health-related services and through community-wide planning agenda-setting activities. Voluntary and nonprofit agency efforts include the following activities:

- Both the Red Cross and the American Heart Association sponsor work site health programs that provide screening, health education, and counseling services to employees, in partnership with local businesses.
- The American Cancer Society maintains a statewide task force on smoking cessation in partnership with the Colorado Department of Public Health and Environment.
- The local United Way chapter is responsible for conducting Denver's only comprehensive community health assessment, which was completed during 1996 as part of a larger evaluation of the human services system in Denver.
- The National Jewish Center for Immunology and Respiratory Medicine operates a nurse-staffed telephone information and advice line to field questions from community members regarding immune system and lung disorders.
- Several nonprofit coalitions and neighborhood groups in Denver sponsor violence prevention efforts in the community, including efforts targeted at domestic violence and gang activity.
- Several nonprofit agencies, including Planned Parenthood and Alternatives Pregnancy Center, provide services related to family planning, teen pregnancy prevention, and parenting.
- A range of nonprofit foundations provide advocacy, counseling, and prevention and treatment services regarding a variety of specialized health issues, such as the Brain Injury Foundation, the Arthritis Foundation, the Colorado Coalition for the Protection of Children, the Safe Kids Coalition, the Colorado SIDS program, and the Denver Indian Health and Family Education program.

Some of the efforts underway by voluntary and nonprofit organizations appear to occur independently of the local public health system in Denver and entail little if any collaboration with Denver Health. The state public health agency maintains involvement in many of the activities undertaken by these organizations. The prevalence of state rather than local public health involvement in nonprofit and voluntary agency may stem from two interrelated factors: (1) many of the activities underway target statewide populations and health issues, and (2) the Colorado Department of Public Health and Environment offers funding and technical assistance to many of these agencies through the federal and state grants it administers.

Measures of Public Health System Performance

Health Department Perceptions of Performance

The local public health performance assessment protocol was administered to Denver Health administrators in April 1992 and again in June 1995. The assessment protocol asks health department directors to indicate the availability of 84 public health services and practices in the community, rate the adequacy of these activities in meeting community needs, and indicate the relative proportion of the activity that is performed by the local health department (see Chapter 8 for detailed description of the methodology). These ratings are used to produce performance scores for each of 10 core public health practices, as well as overall performance scores.

In 1992, Denver Health's total community performance score of 0.61 ranked the agency well above the median score of 0.51 for all 63 health departments surveyed during 1992 and 1993 (**Figure 1**). In 1995, this community performance score is somewhat lower (0.53) but still above the 1992-1993 median score. Much of the difference in scores between 1992 and 1995 appears to be in the functional areas of *assessment* and *assurance*. Results from the 1992 survey suggest that community public health performance in Denver was highest for assessment activities (score of 0.71) and substantially lower for policy development and assurance activities (0.57 and 0.54, respectively). The 1995 survey shows a reversal of this trend, with assessment activities being the lowest area of community performance (0.49) and activities in policy development and assurance being highest (0.58 and 0.67, respectively). These results suggest that activities related to the as-

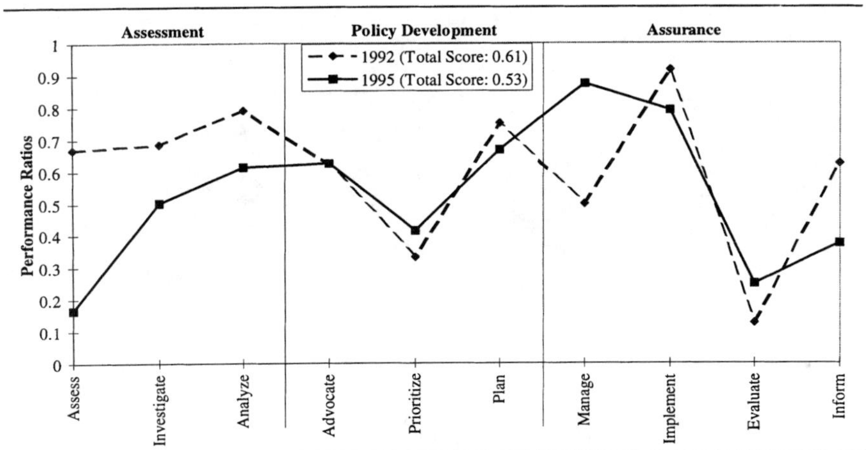

Figure 1. Community performance scores for Denver, Colorado: 1992 and 1995.

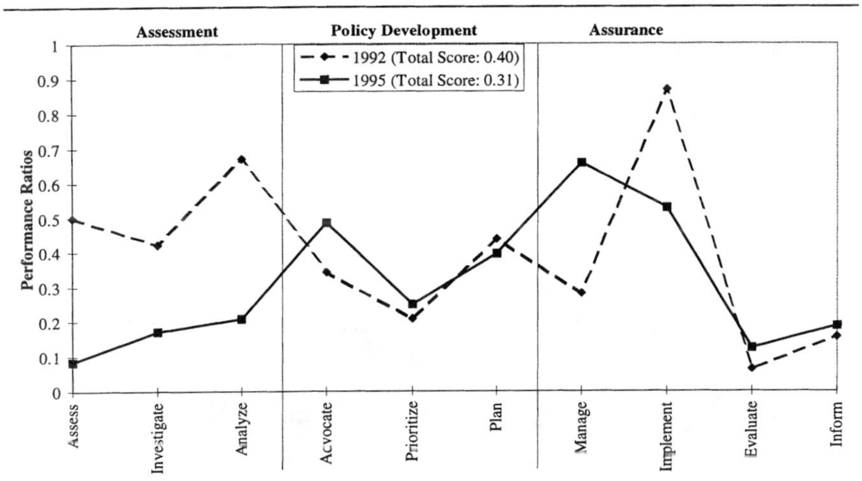

Health department performance score as a percentage of community score

	Assess	Investigate	Analyze	Advocate	Prioritize	Plan	Manage	Implement	Evaluate	Inform
1992:	75%	62%	85%	55%	62%	58%	56%	95%	50%	25%
1995:	50%	34%	34%	78%	60%	59%	75%	67%	50%	50%
% Chng:	-33%	-44%	-60%	41%	-04%	02%	33%	-30%	00%	100%

Figure 2. Health Department performance scores for Denver, Colorado: 1992 and 1995.

surance function may have improved in their availability and adequacy in the community, whereas assessment activities may have declined during this 3-year period.

The local health department's contributions to public health performance mirrors the trends noted in the community performance scores (**Figure 2**). Denver Health's effort in assessment activities appears to have declined somewhat between 1992 and 1995, whereas efforts in assurance activities have increased for three of the four practices. Denver Health's effort in policy development activities also appears to have increased in two of the three areas of performance. When local health department effort is measured as a percent of total community performance, it appears that Denver Health's share of total community performance has declined during 1992-1995 for the practices of *assess, investigate, analyze,* and *implement* (Figure 2). Denver Health's share of total community performance increases over this time period in the practices of *advocate, manage,* and *inform*. These results suggest that Denver Health's operations may have undergone a change in emphasis from assessment activities to assurance activities during 1992 to 1995. Denver Health's efforts to develop a Medicaid managed care plan to expand its network of community and school-based health clinics exemplify the organization's growing role in assurance activities. The decline in assessment activities may signal an area in need of renewed attention for Denver Health and other contributors to the local public health system.

The range of organizations contributing to public health practices in Denver appears to have expanded for certain public health practices while diminishing for others (**Figure 3**). Overall, local government agencies are reported to participate in more activities in 1995 than in 1992, and nonprofit agencies are reported to participate in fewer activities. State agency participation in most activities has remained strong during the 3-year period, with decreases noted only for the function of assurance. Community health centers and federal agencies are reported to have increased their involvement in public health activities during the period, particularly in the area of policy development.

Perceptions of Other Providers Regarding Public Health Performance

The performance measurements described above are based on reports from Denver Health administrators, who are assumed to be among the most informed community representatives regarding the availability and adequacy of public health services. Nonetheless, the perspectives of other individuals and organizations in the community may reveal important additional attributes of the local public health system. Using only reports about the availability of public health services in the community (and not perceptions about the adequacy of these services), we find that administrators of the health department, hospitals, and HMOs in

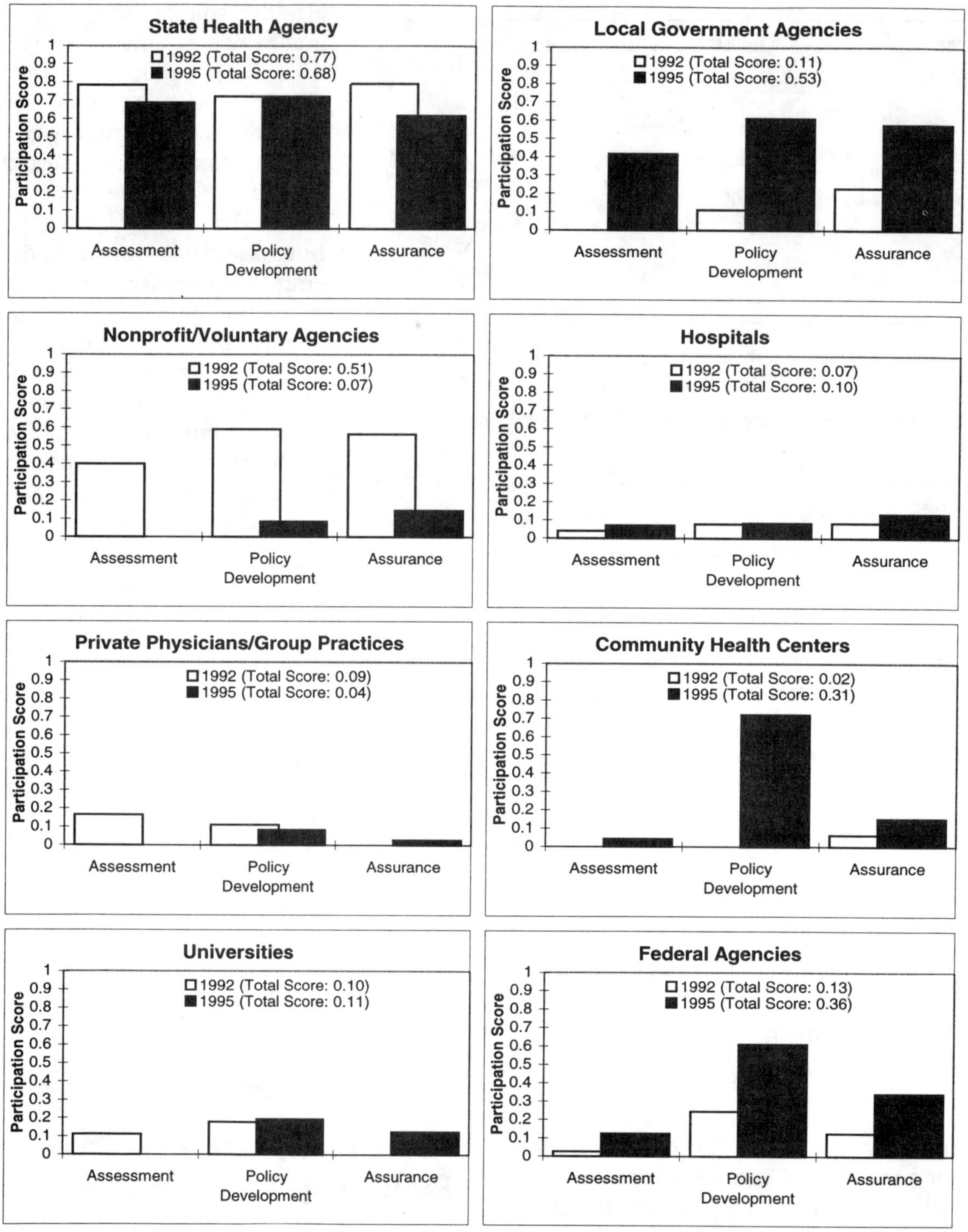

Figure 3. Participation in local public health activities by other organizations, 1992 and 1995 (as reported by the local health department director).

Denver differ substantially in their awareness about public health services in the community (**Table 4**). The health department administrator reports that approximately two thirds of the services involving *assessment of health needs* are available in the community. By comparison, hospital administrators report that all of these services are available, and administrators at two of Denver's largest HMOs report that they have no knowledge about assessment activities in the community. The administrators of hospitals and HMOs indicate that all of the public health activities relating to *analyzing the determinants of health needs* are available, but the health department administrator reports that only half of these activities are performed in the com-

Table 4

Proportion of Public Health Practices Performed in Denver, as Reported by Administrators of the Local Health Department, Hospitals, and HMOs

Practice	Health Department (N=1)	Hospitals (N=8)	HMOs (N=2)
Assess	0.67	1.00	*
Investigate	1.00	1.00	*
Analyze	0.50	1.00	1.00
Advocate	0.75	0.83	0.50
Prioritize	0.67	0.63	*
Plan	1.00	0.54	0.25
Manage	1.00	*	*
Implement	1.00	1.00	1.00
Evaluate	0.50	0.00	0.01
Inform	0.50	1.00	1.00

**One or more activities in this category were reported as "unknown."*

munity. By contrast, the health department reports that activities for *developing community health plans and policies* are fully available, while hospital and HMO administrators report that many of these activities are not available. All of the administrators agree that activities involving the *implementation of programs and services* are fully available in the community.

These differences in the reported availability of public health services in Denver suggest that local health care organizations may not be fully aware of the programs and services provided by other organizations in the community. These findings further suggest that communication and collaboration among health care organizations may be limited for many activities. That the organizations reach consensus about the availability of *implementation* activities may indicate that interorganizational communication and collaboration is greater in this area than in many others. This finding appears consistent with changes taking place in Denver's local health care system. Colorado's Medicaid managed care initiatives appear to be driving many of the alliances among local health care organizations, and these initiatives most often center around the implementation of delivery systems for personal health services.

Future Prospects And Projections

Denver's integrated public health and medical care system demonstrates notable success in serving the health care needs of broad segments of the community population. The recent restructuring of this organization as an independent health care authority holds potential for strengthening the organization by creating greater flexibility in its management and operation. Nonetheless, our analysis of Denver's public health system reveals two basic challenges that the system faces as it moves into the future: maintaining and expanding linkages with private health care organizations and retaining adequate capacity and expertise for assessment activities in public health. These challenges also create opportunities for Denver Health and other contributors to public health within Denver's evolving health care system. Many of Denver's public and private organizations note the need for greater levels of interorganizational collaboration around community health issues, particularly under the state's expanding Medicaid managed care initiatives. This organizational climate appears ideal for forging new partnerships between the public and private service providers operating in Denver, provided that competitive issues among organizations can be held at bay.

The need for greater levels of involvement in public health assessment activities emerges at a time when Denver Health and other health care organizations are intensively focusing on the implementation of programs and structures for service delivery. Pressures for service delivery are likely to increase under federal and state welfare reform initiatives that threaten to reduce the number of individuals who receive access to health services through the Medicaid program. Nevertheless, opportunities for enhancing assessment activities in the community may exist among the host of public and private organizations currently expressing concern about the demise of Colorado's Health Data Commission. Clearly, this concern indicates growing levels of interest within both the public and private sectors for reliable and accurate information on the health risks, health care needs, and utilization patterns of community residents. Given this level of interest, collaborative efforts to expand public health assessment activities in the community appear at once appropriate and feasible.

References

1. American Hospital Association (AHA). *AHA Guide to the Health Care Field, 1995*. Chicago, Ill: AHA; 1996:A68.
2. American Medical Association (AMA). *Physician Data by County, 1994*. Chicago, IL: AMA; 1996.
3. American Medical Association. *Physician Data by County*. Chicago, Ill: AMA; 1992.

4. American Hospital Association. *AHA 1997 Guide to the Health Care Field*. Chicago, Ill: AHA; 1997.
5. Group Health Association of America. *1995 Directory of HMOs*. Washington, DC: GHAA; 1995.
6. US Department of Commerce. 1995 Consolidated Federal Funds Report. Washington, DC: Census Bureau; 1997.
7. US Health Resources and Services Administration, Bureau of Primary Health Care (BPHC). *1995 Directory of Primary Health Care Programs*. Bethesda, Md: BPHC; 1995.
8. Group Health Association of America (GHAA). *1995 Trends in Managed Care*. Washington, DC: GHAA; 1995.
9. Colorado Revised Statutes, Denver Health and Hospitals Authority, 25 USC, Article 29 (1994).
10. Mays GP. Integrated public and private health care systems in Denver, Colorado. In: Halverson PK, Kaluzny AD, McLaughlin CP, eds. *Managed Care and Public Health*. Gaithersburg, Md: Aspen Publishers; 1998;201-221.

Chapter 11

Case Study of Genesee County, Michigan

Key Attributes

- Strong public health leadership from government and community-based organizations.
- Substantial interaction between the local health department and local hospitals.
- Growing interaction between the local health department and area managed care plans.
- Growing involvement of employers and business leaders in community health issues.
- Successful responses to diminishing public health grant funds.
- Successful development of formal, multiorganizational coalitions to address community health issues.

Community Characteristics

Demographic and Socioeconomic Characteristics

Genesee County lies in the eastern half of Michigan ~60 miles northwest of Detroit. Flint, the county's largest city, maintains a long history as an industrial and manufacturing hub, including foundry operations in the early 19th century, carriage manufacturing during the mid-1800s through early 1900s, and automobile manufacturing during most of the 20th century. Currently, Flint serves as home to General Motors' largest automobile manufacturing operation. The automotive industry is by far the largest employer within the county.

US census data from 1990 indicate that a population of 430,459 individuals resides within the county, representing a 4% decline from 1980 (**Table 1**). Approximately 141,000 of these individuals reside within the city of Flint. Similar to state and national trends, 10% of the county population are 65 years of age or older, and 28% are under 18 years of age. The county population reflects a greater degree of racial and ethnic diversity than state or national populations, with Whites comprising 78% of the population, African Americans comprising 19%, and Hispanics comprising 2%. Although the county population as a whole has declined over the last decade, minority populations have substantially grown. Between 1980 and 1990, the African American population grew by 7%, the Hispanic population grew 16%, and other minorities grew by 41%. Racial diversity is even more pronounced in the city of Flint, with 50% of the population being White and 48% being African American.

Residents of Genesee County appear to experience greater levels of socioeconomic need than state and national populations. Growth in per capita income over the past 25 years has been slower in Genesee County than in the state and national populations, reaching $16, 808 in 1995. Approximately 31% of Flint residents and 17% of Genesee County residents subsist below

Table 1
Demographic Characteristics: Genesee County, Michigan

Population (1990)	430,459
Median age in years	29.7
Percent 65 years and older (1990)	10.2
Percent non-White (1990)	21.8
Percent speaking a language other than English at home (1990)	4.6
Percent completing high school degree (1990)	76.8
Percent of individuals below federal poverty level (1989)	16.5
Median household income (1989)	$31,030
Average percent unemployed (1991)	12.6

Data from US Department of Commerce, Bureau of the Census.

Table 2
Health Status Indicators: Genesee County, Michigan, 1996

Infant mortality rate per 1000 live births	12.1
Percent of births to mothers age 10-17	6.6
Percent of infants with low birth weight	9.7
Percent of births with prenatal care later than first trimester	12.3
Deaths per 100,000 population, age adjusted	942.4
Cancer, all types	204.9
Lung cancer	61.8
Female breast cancer	26.1
Heart disease	326.3
Cerebrovascular diseases	63.3
Chronic obstructive pulmonary diseases	51.6
Suicide	13.5
Pneumonia and influenza	24.7
HIV/AIDS	4.3
Diabetes mellitus	31.9
Motor vehicle accidents	20.8
Homicide	12.2

Data from Michigan Department of Community Health, 1997.

the federal poverty level, compared with 13% of the state and national populations. Moreover, unemployment rates in Flint and Genesee County have remained higher than state and national averages during the last decade. High school educational attainment appears substantially lower among Flint residents (31%) in comparison to county, state, and national averages. Moreover, residents of Flint and Genesee County are less likely to obtain college or graduate degrees than state and national populations.

Community Health Status Indicators

Mortality data suggest that chronic diseases pose substantial health threats to Genesee County residents (**Table 2**). Age-adjusted death rates in Genesee County (972 per 100,000) are 11% higher than state and national averages. When deaths are expressed as years of potential life lost before age 65, Genesee County residents lose 12% more years of life than the state average. Similar to state and national trends, cardiovascular diseases are the leading cause of death within the county (44% of deaths), followed by cancer (24%). Nonetheless, death rates from leading chronic diseases—including heart disease, cerebrovascular disease, chronic obstructive pulmonary disease, cancer, and diabetes mellitus—are higher among Genesee County populations than among state or national populations. County residents die at younger ages from these chronic diseases than state or national averages, resulting in higher years of potential life lost.

The performance of disease prevention efforts in Genesee County appears mixed. A 1991 study by the Greater Flint Area Hospital Assembly suggests that Genesee County residents are somewhat more likely to have prostate cancer diagnosed at its earliest stage but somewhat less likely to have breast cancer diagnosed at its earliest stage, compared with state averages. Rates of cholesterol screening among county residents (69) appear lower than Healthy People 2000 objectives, but rates of mammography screening among women 40 years and older (71%) exceed state trends and Healthy People 2000 objectives.

Maternal and child health issues also pose substantial threats to the health of Genesee County residents, especially those who reside in the city of Flint. During the 1991-1993 period, infant mortality stood at 15.3 per 1000 live births among Flint residents and 10.8 per 1000 births among Genesee County residents, both exceeding state and national averages. The infant mortality rate among African Americans in Genesee County exceeds the rate among White residents by more than 150%. Low birth weight infants are also more common among Genesee County residents (9.2% of births) than among state and national populations (6.7% and 7.1%, respectively). As a likely contributor to the area's adverse birth outcomes, births to teenagers appear more prevalent among Flint and Genesee County residents than among state and national populations. A birth rate of ~426 per 1000 population was observed among Flint residents age 15-19 during 1990-1992, compared with a county rate of 76, a state rate of 59, and a national rate of 62. Genesee County performs better than state and national trends in the proportion of pregnant women who receive prenatal care during the first trimester (80% compared with 74 and 78%, respectively). Nevertheless, the county still falls short of the Healthy People 2000 goal of a 90% prenatal care rate. Hospital data from 1993 suggest that Genesee County infants are substantially more likely to be delivered by cesarean section (29%) than state and national trends (22 and 24%, respectively). The cesarean section rate also substantially exceeds the Healthy People 2000 goal of 15%.

Communicable diseases appear to pose fewer problems for Genesee County residents than for other populations. Case rates for tuberculosis, syphilis, and AIDS/HIV are substantially lower in Genesee County than in state and national populations. Death rates for pneumonia and influenza are also lower in Genesee County. The case rate for gonorrhea, however, substantially exceeds state and national trends. The county population appears relatively well protected against infectious childhood diseases. The vaccination coverage rate for the basic series (4:3:3:1) stands at 74% among children under 2 years old, which does not yet meet the Healthy People 2000 objective of 90%. Immunization rates for children in licensed day care facilities and for newly enrolled school children stand at 95%.

Local Health Resources and Manpower

Three major hospital systems serve residents of Genesee County, providing a combined capacity of 1016 staffed beds or 236 beds per 100,000 population (**Table 3**). The largest of these systems, Genesys Health System, grew from the consolidation of four separate nonprofit hospitals during the past two decades. Until early 1997, Genesys provided services through four separate hospital campuses containing a total of 613 staffed beds. Three of these facilities were located in Flint, and one was located in an outlying area of the county. During the spring of 1997, Genesys opened a new, 379-bed hospital campus in southern Genesee County and began closing its other four facilities. McLaren Health Care Corporation exists as one of two remaining hospital systems within the city of Flint. Located in the western half of the city, this private, nonprofit system operates a 387-bed hospital facility that provided services to 16,733 inpatients and 349,720 outpatients during calendar year 1994. Flint's other hospital, Hurley Medical Center, is owned and operated by the city of Flint and located in the heart of the city. Hurley served more than 20,000 inpatients and almost 286,000 outpatients through its 324-bed hospital facility. Hurley serves as the area's level one trauma center and operates the region's only burn center, neonatal and pediatric intensive care units, and kidney transplant center. Genesee County patients may also be referred to the larger tertiary care centers in Ann Arbor and Detroit for specialized medical services. Among the three area hospitals, Hurley Medical Center provides the majority of care to Medicaid beneficiaries and the uninsured.

A total of 912 physicians operate within Genesee County, yielding a physician-to-population ratio of 210 physicians per 100,000 population. Fifty-four percent of these physicians practice in the primary care disciplines of family practice, general practice, internal medicine, obstetrics/gynecology, and pediatrics. Adjusting for population size, the county has somewhat fewer total physicians but somewhat more primary care physicians than the nation as a whole. Doctors of osteopathy and medical residents account for substantial shares of the county's physician work force (17 and 29%, respectively).

Despite a relatively healthy supply of physicians, several geographic areas of the county remain underserved by medical professionals owing to the uneven distribution of the work force. One federally qualified community health center, the Hamilton Family Health Center, operates two clinics in underserved areas of Flint that provide primary care services for uninsured and underinsured populations as well as Medicaid beneficiaries. A federally qualified dental health center also operates in an underserved Flint neighborhood. Other primary care resources for underserved populations include the following: an ambulatory care center operated by the Hurley Medical Center in a low-income, underserved neighborhood within Flint; three public health clinics operated by the local health department that provide categorical public health services in underserved areas; and a free medical clinic operated several days per week through a partnership among local hospitals, the local medical society, and the local health department.

An estimated 90% of Genesee County residents have health insurance coverage of some type. Approximately 60% of the population has employer-based coverage, 11 has coverage through Medicare, 10% has coverage under Medicaid, 8% maintain self-purchased health care insurance, and 1% has coverage through the federal CHAMPUS program for family members

Table 3
Health Resources: Genesee County, Michigan

Number of nonfederal physicians (Number per 100,000 population) 1992[a]	912 (210)
Family practice	100 (23)
General practice	29 (7)
Internal medicine	159 (37)
Obstetrics/gynecology	40 (9)
Pediatrics	62 (14)
Number of community hospital beds (FY1995)[b]	1016
Beds per 100,000 population	354
Number of community hospitals (FY1995)[b]	3
Number of HMOs (1995)[c]	9
Number of federally qualified health centers (1994)[d]	2
Total number of clinic sites	3
Local public health expenditures (1992)	N/A
Percent from direct federal sources	N/A
Percent from state sources (including federal pass-throughs)	N/A
Percent from local sources	N/A
Percent from Medicaid	N/A
Percent from Medicare	N/A
Total federal funding for community health centers (1996)[e]	$609,615
Total federal funding for migrant health centers (1996)[e]	0
Total federal block grant funds for preventive health services (1996)[e]	0
Total federal block grant funds for maternal and child health services (1996)[e]	0
Total federal block grant funds for substance abuse services (1996)[e]	0
Total federal funding for homeless health services (1996)[e]	$202,766
Total federal funding for National Health Service Corporation (1996)[e]	0

[a]*Data from American Medical Association Physician Masterfile, 1992. American Medical Association. Physician Data by County. Chicago, IL: AMA; 1992.*
[b]*Data from American Hospital Association, 1997. American Hospital Association. AHA 1997 Guide to the Health Care Field. Chicago, IL: AHA; 1997.*
[c]*Data from Healthcare Blue Book, 1996.*
[d]*Data from US Bureau of Primary Health Care, 1994. Unpublished data, Bureau of Primary Health Care, US Health Resources and Services Administration, 1994.*
[e]*Data from US Department of Commerce, 1997. US Department of Commerce. 1995 Consolidated Federal Funds Report. Washington, DC: Census Bureau; 1997.*

of active-duty military personnel. Approximately 21% of the county population are enrolled in health maintenance organizations (HMOs), according to enrollment data from 1994.[1] Ten different HMOs report operating within Genesee County, seven of which are now certified to enroll Medicaid beneficiaries and three of which actually enroll these beneficiaries.

Medicaid beneficiaries have been served through managed care plans in Genesee County since 1988, when a special demonstration program began with funding from the Robert Wood Johnson Foundation to offer managed care options to Medicaid beneficiaries and the uninsured. This program allowed Medicaid beneficiaries either to enroll in an HMO or to sign up with participating physicians as part of a primary care case management program. Beginning in the spring of 1997, a new state program was implemented requiring all Medicaid beneficiaries in Genesee County to enroll in one of the seven approved HMOs. These HMOs are now competing to enroll beneficiaries who have traditionally been predominantly served through the primary care case management program. Over 90% of Genesee County's Medicaid beneficiaries now participate in some form of managed care.

The Local Health Department

Genesee County maintains a thriving local health department that strives to protect and improve health within the community by supporting a wide range of personal health services, environmental health services, and community-level interventions within the county. In shaping the organizational structure and operations of the agency, local health department officials draw heavily on principles established in an influential report by the National Association of County and City Health Officials, entitled *Blueprint for a Healthy Community*.[2] The department's primary organizational objectives are based on the ten essential elements of a community health system that are identified in this report. In keeping with these essential elements, health department officials place emphasis on performing core public health activities in collaboration with other community organizations that can offer needed resources and expertise.

Organizational Structure

The Genesee County Health Department operates as a unit of county government under the direction of a nine-member elected board of county commissioners. The department is headed by a full-time health officer who is appointed by and reports to the board of commissioners. A seven-member board of health serves in an advisory capacity to the board of commissioners. The board of health comprises three county commissioners, and two community representatives who are appointed by the board of commissioners. Robert M. Pestronk, MPH, maintains a 12-year tenure as the department's health officer.

A full-time medical director reports to the health officer and oversees the department's programs for quality assurance, epidemiology, and laboratory services. As a physician, the medical director also serves as the county's medical examiner and acts as the primary liaison between the health department and the local medical community. Dr. Gary Johnson, MD, a board-certified pediatrician, serves as the department's medical director and also spends 30% of his time as a practicing physician in the department's pediatric clinics. In addition, Dr. Johnson serves on the board of directors of the county medical society and chairs its community health committee.

The department's public health programs and services are organized within four functional divisions. A *division of personal health* administers services for maternal and child health, family planning, pediatric and adult primary care, and nutrition support services under the federal Special Supplemental Food Program for Women, Infants, and Children (WIC). These services are delivered through three public health clinics located in geographically dispersed, underserved areas within the county.

A *division of community health* administers health department programs for health promotion and disease prevention, early detection of chronic diseases, and infectious disease prevention, detection, and treatment. These services are performed by teams of community health nurses during scheduled programs held at the department's three public health clinics and, for immunization services, at church-based sites. A *division of behavioral health* manages the department's programs for sexually transmitted disease prevention and control, family planning, HIV/AIDS counseling and testing, tobacco use prevention and control, and substance abuse prevention and treatment. Finally, a *division of environmental health* houses departmental programs for water quality protection and management, food safety inspection, solid waste management, vector control, and air quality monitoring.

Administrative support for the department's four functional divisions is provided through a central services division, which houses the department's systems for management information, accounting, billing, payroll, and personnel. Responsibilities in strategic planning, program development, and grant processing are shared by the central services division, the medical director's office, and the health officer.

Overview of Programs and Services

Personal, Community, and Behavioral Health Services

Maternal and Child Health Services. The health department offers a wide range of personal health services through its three public health clinics. Maternal and child health programs figure prominently among these services. Pediatric examinations are provided to children who do not have access to private providers, by a team comprising the medical director and nurses who staff the health department clinics. For infants and children eligible for Medicaid, the local health department provides outreach and support services to insure that these beneficiaries receive the necessary screening services from their managed care providers. In collaboration with the public and private school systems operating within the county, the local health department conducts hearing, vision, and lead poisoning screenings for elementary and middle school children. The health department also provides special developmental screening services to at-risk school-age children in Flint's public school district, as part of a larger program to enhance family literacy under the US Department of Education's "Even Start" grant program. The department provides nutritional assistance and counseling to all eligible clients under the WIC program at each of its public health clinics.

The maternal and child health services offered by the health department have been scaled back over the last 5 years as the community's capacity to provide personal health services to this population has grown. Expansions in Medicaid eligibility and the increased participation of private providers in the county's Medicaid primary care case management program have allowed the local health department to discontinue its involvement in the direct provision of prenatal care and maternity support services. As the health department has transitioned these responsibilities to private physicians and hospital systems, it has developed enhanced capacities in the areas of assessment and data collection, outreach, and educational services to assure the accessibility and effectiveness of privately provided care.

The health department developed a community health nurse program using resources that were previously committed to the department's maternity and infant support services programs. Through this program, the department provides education and referral services to community members regarding available maternity and infant health services. The community health nurse program also conducts community education campaigns around topics such as sudden infant death syndrome awareness and prevention, family planning, adolescent pregnancy prevention, prenatal care, and substance abuse during pregnancy. Most of these projects are carried out in collaboration with other community organizations such as churches, schools, neighborhood associations, and other health and social service providers.

Immunization Services. The department maintains active programs for both child and adult immunization services. Infant and child immunization services are available daily through the department's three public health clinics. Additionally, immunization clinics are held one day per month at each of nine area churches and one shopping mall, which are geographically dispersed throughout the county. Teams of public health nurses provide immunization services through these clinics and offer advice and referral for other public health services that may be needed. Evening and weekend hours are offered to provide enhanced access to immunization services. Adult vaccinations for pneumonia and influenza are offered by the health department each fall at churches and senior centers located throughout the county.

As part of a statewide program, Genesee County Health Department serves as the hub for a newly developed, regional childhood immunization registry. The health department collects and processes information from public and private providers in a nine-county region that includes Genesee County. All managed care organizations that serve Medicaid beneficiaries are required to submit immunization information for their enrollees. Additionally, state and local medical societies work to insure the participation of other private providers in the community. Immunization data are stored on a central computer server maintained at the health department. Providers can submit and retrieve information from the registry in one of three ways: using a personal computer and modem which run special software developed for the registry, using telephone or fax transmissions, and using specially developed vaccination encounter forms that were designed to be completed and sent to the health department. Before the development of this regional registry system, the health department had developed plans for a countywide registry in collaboration with the county medical society, local hospitals, and a local children's health center. This early work greatly facilitated the process of implementing a larger, regional registry and insured the full participation of Genesee County health care providers.

Communicable Disease Services. The health department offers testing, treatment, and counseling for sexually transmitted diseases through its two public health clinics. These services include HIV antibody testing and counseling services. Contact tracing and partner notification services are also performed as part of these services. Additionally, the department operates a weekly tuberculosis clinic that offers testing for exposed and high-risk individuals and treatment and follow-up for all confirmed tuberculosis cases. The department provides directly observed therapy for all noncompliant cases.

Family Planning Services. The health department offers a comprehensive range of family planning services two of its public health clinics. These services include pregnancy testing and counseling, sex education, and contraceptive services. The department also provides broad-based access to family planning education and counseling services through its community health nurse program. Through this program, a team of six nurses implements a wide range of outreach and community education interventions throughout the county on topics such as adolescent pregnancy prevention, parenting skills, and decision-making skills for family planning. The community health nurses also offer information and referral to residents regarding other available family planning services in the community. Most of these interventions are carried out in collaboration with other community organizations, such as schools, churches, and neighborhood associations.

Health Promotion and Disease Prevention Services. The health department maintains a breast and cervical cancer screening program for low-income, uninsured women age 40 to 65 years. Screenings are provided through one health department clinic and two community clinics (Hamilton Family Health Center and Women to Women P.P.C.), with funding received through a state program supported by the US Centers for Disease Control and Prevention. Because this program only provides funding for screening services—and not for the definitive diagnosis and treatment services that may be needed after diseases are detected—the health department maintains an additional program for covering some of the costs incurred in providing these services for low-income uninsured and underinsured women. All three of the area hospitals contribute funds to support this program. Contracts are maintained with area physicians to deliver many of the diagnostic services, and community physicians also donate services to this program.

The local health department also operates an active work site wellness program that provides consultation and grants to local small employers (less than 500 employees) to assist them in developing health promotion programs for their employees. Through this program, health department staff assist eligible employers in designing programs that may include on-site employee health assessments, exercise and diet programs, smoking cessation programs, and projects to reduce the risk of illness and injury on work sites. An annual grant from the state health agency provides funding for this program.

The health department maintains a diabetes outreach and referral project in collaboration with area hospitals. High-risk individuals who receive care through the department's public health clinics are screened for diabetes, and indicated clients are referred to the diabetes management programs maintained by the three area hospitals. The department's community health nurse program also contributes to this program by implementing community educational campaigns about diabetes awareness and disease management strategies. Hurley Medical Center remains the program's largest referral source.

The local health department also operates a heart health promotion campaign in collaboration with area hospitals. This project sponsors community presentations on heart disease risk reduction strategies and holds periodic cholesterol testing campaigns within the community. The organizations collaborating in this program also conduct joint planning and priority-setting efforts aimed at developing new community interventions to address high-risk behaviors and populations within the community.

Substance Abuse Services. The local health department serves as the county's substance abuse coordinating agency for uninsured and underinsured residents of Genesee County. Health department staff identifies individuals in need of substance abuse services through client contacts in the department's public health clinics and community health nursing program or through referrals from other community agencies. Individuals who do not have access to substance abuse services through public or private health insurance coverage are referred to local prevention and treatment providers, who maintain contracts with the local health department for providing these services. Health department staff monitor and audit the programs to ensure that residents receive appropriate and coordinated services.

Other Community Health Services. The health department is involved in providing a range of other community health services that endeavor to promote health and assure access to health services within Genesee County communities. Most of these activities are implemented in collaboration with other community-based organizations, in an effort to pool the diverse resources and skills of multiple organizations and to ensure that public health interventions are targeted at priority issues in the community. Many of these initiatives have their origins in a unique initiative sponsored by the W. K. Kellogg Foundation, the Community-Based Public Health Initiative (CBPHI). A regional public health consortium—comprising local health departments, community organizations, and health professions schools located in Genesee County and the cities of Detroit and Ann Arbor—was one of seven grantees nationwide to receive funding under Kellogg's CBPHI initiative in January 1993 (see Chapter 5 for more details on the program).

Environmental Health Services

The local health department's environmental health division maintains a comprehensive range of programs and services designed to insure the safety and quality of environmental conditions in Genesee County. The division's water quality programs include licensing, monitoring, and inspection systems for public and private water systems, as well pollution detection and control programs for both ground water and surface water within the county. The division's waste management staff inspects and monitors solid waste disposal sites, hazardous waste transportation and disposal systems, and on-site sewage disposal systems within the county. A new program within this office is investigating and mapping unauthorized and undocumented solid waste disposal sites within the county, in order to inform waste management and clean-up efforts. The health department also conducts routine food safety inspections of temporary and permanent food service establishments, mobile units, and vending machines. Air quality monitoring is a growing area of activity for the health department, with new programs being launched to monitor indoor radon and carbon monoxide levels and inspect indoor air handling systems in schools and other public institutions. Staff performs outdoor air quality inspections on an ad hoc basis. The environmental health division also operates programs for insect and rat control and for conducting safety and health inspections of campgrounds, trailer parks, and swimming pools.

The health department's environmental health division works in tandem with the community health division to operate both primary and secondary prevention programs for lead poisoning. Under the primary prevention program, the health department conducts lead inspections and lead abatement procedures in a high-risk region of Flint, which has a high proportion of aging housing stock. The department also conducts training sessions with area residents and builders regarding proper maintenance and clean-up practices in homes likely to have lead exposure problems. The health department conducts these activities in collaboration with several community organizations that participated with the health department in the community-based public health program funded by the W. K. Kellogg Foundation. These activities are also supported through a primary lead poisoning prevention grant from the US Centers for Disease Control and Prevention.

Secondary lead poisoning prevention activities involve health department inspections of the housing and recreation areas of children who have been identified to have elevated blood lead levels. The department initiates lead abatement activities once the source of lead exposure is identified. These activities are triggered when health department staff identify cases of elevated blood lead levels in children screened through the department's clinic-based and school-based screening programs. Private physicians are also informed to report cases of elevated blood lead levels to the health department in order to initiate secondary prevention activities.

As a final environmental health activity, the health department operates several successful tobacco control programs through its behavioral health division. An enforcement section within the department monitors and licenses tobacco retailers to insure sales are not made to minors. This section also inspects public buildings on a periodic basis to insure that local smoking regulations are enforced. Additionally, the health department maintains a tobacco prevention coalition in collaboration with the local medical society and other community organizations. This group conducts planning and advocacy activities regarding potential new regulations to restrict environmental exposure to tobacco smoke and works with local businesses to encourage the adoption of policies that limit exposure to tobacco smoke among their employees and customers.

Infrastructure and Resources

The health department maintains a central office located in downtown Flint, which houses the department's administrative offices as well as one of its public health clinics. The department operates two other public health clinics within the county: one located in the northern end of Flint, and another located in the southern region of Genesee County. All three public health clinics are open 5 days per week, and one includes some evening hours.

A total staff of ~150 full-time equivalent positions work within the health department. A total operating budget of approximately $13.5 million supports these staff and the programs and services they administer. This budget produces an annual public health expenditure of approximately $31 per resident in Genesee County, which exceeds the median local health department expenditure of $20 per capita identified through a national survey of departments in 1992.[3] The health officer reports that the health department's funding and staffing levels have remained relatively even during the past 5 years, even though the department's programs and services have continually evolved and, in many cases, expanded over this period.

In keeping with the county government's desire to contain local expenditures for public services, the health department has pursued a strategy of "expansion through collaboration" in maintaining necessary resources for public health. Through this strategy, the health department has identified ways to use existing resources in the community—such as those maintained by local hospitals, physicians, and other community organizations—to launch new programs and services. Given relatively constrained funding from state and local sources, the department has also been successful in attracting outside grant funding from federal and private sources to develop and pilot test new public health programs and services. The health officer reports that, because of their transitory nature, these types of grant funds are often used to develop capacities in the community for performing public health functions, rather than for supporting ongoing health department activities.

For example, the health department participated in collaborative project funded by the Robert Wood Johnson Foundation beginning in 1988 to develop a managed care program for serving uninsured residents. This project helped private physicians and hospitals to develop the skills and capacities necessary for serving vulnerable populations and assisted the health department in developing strategies to support and encourage the capacities of these private providers. More recently, the health department participated in a project funded by the W. K. Kellogg Foundation to develop community-based strategies for public health improvement in collaboration with nearby universities and local community-based organizations. This project allowed the department to develop a structure and process for information-sharing, coordination, and collaboration with these organizations on a broad range of health and social interventions. Although the outside funding streams that supported both of these projects have now terminated, the community capacities that were developed through these projects continue to serve the department and the community's public health system.

Other Contributors to Local Public Health Activities

A wide array of other organizations and individuals make important contributions to local public health activities in Genesee County. Genesee County appears somewhat unique among local public health jurisdictions in that many of these contributions are made through formalized, multiorganizational initiatives rather than through independent, individualized efforts. One of the largest and most visible interorganizational initiatives, the Greater Flint Health Care Coalition, maintains membership from local and state government agencies, local hospitals, managed care plans, physicians, the local health department, and employers. Originally formed by a collection of local agencies, this effort is now largely sustained with resources from General Motors, the United Auto Workers union, and local hospitals. The work of the coalition is gradually expanding from an initial focus on medical care quality and efficiency to broader concerns of health promotion, disease prevention, and community-wide access to health care.

A second multiorganizational initiative is maintained through a partnership between the local health department, a network of community-based health and human service organizations, and two university-based health professions schools. This initiative, originally launched with funding from the W. K. Kellogg Foundation under its Community-Based Public Health Initiative, focuses on developing collaborative strategies for implementing public health practice, training, and research opportunities that are optimally responsive to community needs and priorities. Activities conducted through this initiative, which is known as the Genesee Team (and locally as the Broome Team after a local community leader), originate from low-income, vulnerable neighborhoods and populations within the Genesee County.

These types of multiorganizational efforts, along with the independent efforts of numerous community organizations and individuals, complement the range of activities directly performed by the local health department. The sections that follow examine both the independent and collective contributions to public health made by specific types of organizations operating within Genesee County.

State Health Agency

Michigan's state public health agency resides in the newly consolidated Department of Community Health. This agency, which is the largest of the 18 state government departments, maintains responsibility for all of the state's publicly funded, health-related programs and services. Michigan's Governor John Engler created the department by executive order in January 1996 by consolidating the state's existing Department of Public Health, Department of Mental Health, Medical Services Administration (the state's Medicaid agency), Office of Drug Control Policy, and Office of Services to the Aging. During this reorganization process, responsibility for environmental health programs was moved from the Department of Public Health to three other state health departments: the Department of Environmental Quality, the Department of Agriculture, and the Department of Consumer and Industrial Affairs. The combined Department of Community Health operates with more than $7 billion in appropriations and 6500 employees.

Genesee County Health Department maintains a decentralized administrative relationship with the state health agency, in which the county government retains overall responsibility for operating and managing public health programs and services. The state agency serves primarily as a source of funding and technical assistance for Genesee's local health department. Under this arrangement, the county health department establishes a comprehensive contract with the state health agency that covers all of the local public health programs and services that are funded in whole or part by the state health agency. For each local public health program and service, this contract specifies the level of service to be performed by the health department, and the amount of funding to be contributed by the state health agency and by the county. In establishing this contract, the local health department works with the state health agency and state legislature in determining the range of programs and services that should be supported by the state agency and the appropriate funding levels for these activities. As part of this process, the department must be able to determine and report the costs of specific public health services and activities, as well as to demonstrate community need and program impact.

Genesee County's local health officer indicates that his department's relationship with the state health agency is still evolving in response to its recent reorganization. To some extent, the state reorganization effort appears to have deemphasized public health issues and activities and collapsed them within the larger health care delivery and financing issues faced by the state. Local health department staff are now working to reestablish relationships with new staff and new divisions within the reorganized state agency and to help these officials understand the unique roles and responsibilities of local public health agencies. Genesee County staff suggest that the state agency has shown a tendency to regard local health departments as simply another contractor for service provision, without sufficiently appreciating the vital but somewhat intangible roles these agencies play in health care leadership, service coordination, coalition-building, advocacy, oversight, and policy development. Local officials express hope that over time, the state health agency will develop an enhanced understanding and appreciation for local public health functions.

Local health department officials note that Michigan's expanding Medicaid managed care program represents a policy arena that is especially in need of improved state-local relationships. These officials indicate that, to date, local health departments have not been involved in the state health agency's efforts to develop and enforce appropriate contract provisions with managed care plans. The state health agency maintains the exclusive responsibility for designing and implementing these provisions. Moreover, a newly appointed managed care advisory panel recently created by the agency does not include representation from local health departments. The agency's approach to Medicaid managed care delivery does not appear to fully recognize the strong and effective roles that local departments can play in monitoring and encouraging health plan performance of key public health services. Officials in Genesee County are particularly eager to assume larger roles in assuring health plan performance of childhood immunizations and maternal and child health visits—services they view as having a high public health impact and a high risk of underservice within managed care delivery systems. Currently, the state health agency requires health plans to develop and report a strategy for interfacing with local health departments, as part of their application for participation in the Medicaid managed care program. Genesee County officials indicate that stronger provisions are needed to assure that health plans give emphasis to local, state, and national public health goals. There appears to be room for enhanced collaboration between the local and state health department in assuring the quality and accessibility of care under the state's growing Medicaid managed care initiative.

Hospitals

Local hospitals are important contributors to the public health system in Genesee County, and their roles within this system appear to have grown somewhat over the last decade through collaboration with the local health department. Genesee County's health officer indicates that, beginning in the early 1990s, the health department began to actively recruit assistance from the area's hospitals in addressing the growing unmet needs for personal health services among the county's underserved population groups. Rather than seeking resources to expand the health department's capacity to provide personal health services, the health officer and staff sought to establish collaborative arrangements with the hospitals to increase the community's capacity through shared staff, equipment, and services. Currently, the health department and three local hospitals are developing an arrangement whereby each hospital sponsors one of the health department's three public health clinics. Through this sponsorship, a hospital contributes a team of clinical staff to provide services through a public health clinic on a part-time basis or in some cases provide financial support for construction. One hospital also makes annual financial contributions to a fund maintained by the health department to pay for specialty medical services that may be needed by uninsured patients treated in the health department's public health clinics. Beyond their involvement in providing personal health services, hospitals have collaborated with the health department on a broad range of other multiorganizational initiatives aimed at assessing community health needs and developing coordinated strategies for addressing pressing health issues.

All three of Genesee County's hospitals are assuming growing roles in providing population-based services through programs for health education, health promotion, disease prevention, and occupational health. These activities mirror national trends among hospitals and appear to be a response to growing demands for these services on the part of health care consumers, employers, and payers—particularly managed care organizations. Whether their motivations are altruistic or economic, Genesee County's hospitals are making important contributions to the local public health system by expanding access to health promotion and disease prevention services. While all three of the local hospital systems make notable contributions to public health, important differences exist across the organizations in the extent and nature of their contributions.

Hurley Medical Center

Hurley Medical Center, the area's only public hospital, is a substantial contributor to local community health activities. As a city-owned hospital, Hurley maintains a long tradition of providing medical care to uninsured and underinsured residents of Flint and surrounding communities. Hospital data from 1991 suggest that Hurley serves a larger proportion of Medicaid beneficiaries and uninsured patients than the other two hospital systems in Genesee County. Approximately one third of the hospital's patients are covered by Medicaid, and almost 40% of the hospital's annual charges are for uncompensated indigent care services. These services totaled almost $55 million in 1991, including both charity care services and unpaid medical bills. The hospital's disproportionate share of vulnerable and underserved patients can be explained in part by its location in central Flint and its stature as the area's only source for high-risk obstetrical services and neonatal and pediatric intensive care services.

Recently, the hospital has expanded its role in serving these populations by opening a primary care and urgent care clinic in an underserved community in northern Flint. The clinic, which opened in mid-1996, contains 30 examination rooms and 4 treatment rooms, operates 6 days per week from 9:00 AM to 11:00 PM. Two of Hurley's board-certified family practice physicians staff the clinic, along with nurse practitioners and registered nurses. The clinic also provides a wide range of health education services in the community, such as programs for diabetes self-management, cardiovascular health, and smoking cessation.

Hurley's involvement in providing primary care services to underserved populations is motivated partly by financial and strategic issues and partly through its mission of public service as a government-owned corporation. Although owned by the city of Flint, Hurley does not receive financial support from the City. Hurley's administrator during the past 5 years, Glenn Fosdick, reports that this arrangement creates an imperative for the hospital to operate as efficiently as possible in order to support its mission of community service. Hurley's expansion into primary care delivery represents a strategy to improve operating efficiency by curbing the demand for more costly care delivered through its emergency room. Mr. Fosdick indicates that before the opening of its primary care clinic, almost 60% of its emergency room patients came from two zip code areas in the northern Flint area. The hospital's involvement in primary care delivery for underserved populations is intended to reduce overall costs for indigent care by encouraging the utilization of routine primary care and preventive services among underserved populations.

The hospital's growing involvement in primary care for underserved populations also exists as a strategic response to the growth of managed care in the community, especially for Medicaid beneficiaries. By developing the capacity to provide primary care services, Hurley seeks to retain its role as the dominant Medicaid provider in a market that has recently moved to mandatory HMO enrollment for Medicaid beneficiaries. HMOs participating in the Medicaid program view Hurley Medical Center as a preferred contractor, given its experience in serving vulnerable populations and its ability to provide beneficiaries with easy geographic access to a comprehensive range of health services.

Currently, Hurley is planning for the construction of another primary care facility in southern Genesee County, which it hopes to operate jointly with the Genesee County Health Department. The clinic would be staffed by personnel from the hospital and health department and would serve to replace the aging and cramped Burton Health Center which the health department currently operates in this area. Clearly, this project promises to expand the primary care capacity of Hurley Medical Center. Moreover, this project is expected to allow the hospital and health department to realize efficiencies through shared staff and equipment, as well as to encourage improvements in program effectiveness and accessibility through colocated and coordinated service delivery.

In addition to its own primary care programs, Hurley Medical Center engages in a broad range of activities to support the clinical services programs maintained by the local health department.[4] For example, the hospital maintains a contract with the health department for operating its tuberculosis clinic. Under this arrangement, a team of physicians and nurses from Hurley provides services for tuberculosis diagnosis, drug therapy, and medical follow-up for health department clients. Through a similar contract, the hospital's pathology department assists in administering the health department's medical examiner program. Hurley also maintains a contract with the local health department for providing a hospital pediatrician to work in one of the department's public health clinics. Clinical staff from Hurley also assists the department in conducting breast and cervical cancer screenings at the department's clinics on a weekly basis.

Staff from the health department's program for children with special health care needs works closely with Hurley's pediatric intensive care unit to insure that appropriate hospital patients are targeted for the health department's program. The health department's children with special health care needs staff works with Hurley's nursing and social work staff to conduct assessments of patient needs during their stay in the hospital and with Hurley's home health care staff to jointly manage the delivery of services to these patients once they are discharged. For children eligible for early intervention services under Part H of the federal Individuals with Disabilities Education Act, an arrangement between the hospital and the health department allows for automatic referrals from the hospital to the health department's children with special health care needs program.

Hurley Medical Center and the local health department maintain several additional collaborative arrangements for clinical service delivery within the county. Hurley's pediatric clinic performs all of the follow-up medical work for children identified by the health department as having elevated blood lead levels. Additionally, most of the laboratory testing procedures conducted through the health department's HIV testing and counseling program is performed by Hurley's laboratory. Health department staff indicate that this arrangement allows the department to obtain test results much faster than would be possible through other arrangements. Finally, participants in Hurley's infectious disease residency program rotate through the local health department's sexually transmitted disease clinic. This arrangement provides the health department with additional clinical manpower while enhancing Hurley Medical Center's commitment to medical education and increasing physician exposure to and experience with problems of community health.

Hurley Medical Center's contributions to community health issues extend beyond the realm of clinical services delivery. The hospital is an important collaborator in the Greater Flint Health Care Coalition, which is taking steps to assess community health needs and develop community-level interventions to improve health status. Much of the hospital's work on this initiative to date has involved community-wide planning and priority setting regarding strategies to address the community's most pressing health issues. As part of the coalition's work to address issues of service duplication and inefficiency, Hurley has established agreements with the area's two other hospitals to facilitate community-wide service coordination. For example, Hurley recently discontinued its cardiac surgery services and began referring all of its cases to McLaren Health Care Corporation in southwestern Flint. In exchange, McLaren discontinued its pediatric inpatient services and transferred these cases to Hurley. Hurley also agreed to provide the pediatrics training for physicians participating in McLaren's family practice residency program. Additionally, Hurley developed an agreement with Genesys Health System to own and operate jointly a combined oncology center, as an alternative to the institutions' separate programs. A similar agreement established with the Mott Children's Health Center, a local provider of specialized child health services, allows Hurley Medical Center physicians to assume responsibility for providing pediatrics services in the clinics operated by the center. Currently, the three area hospitals are negotiating the possibility of a jointly operated behavioral medicine program to replace the separate programs that currently exist. These types of collaborative efforts between Hurley Medical Center and other providers of specialized medical services endeavor to create efficiencies in service delivery within the community, while also enhancing quality of care for "volume-sensitive" services that may require a sufficient patient volume in order to achieve optimal health outcomes.[5,6]

The hospital also collaborates with the local health department and community mental health center in operating a violence prevention project. Under this project, the hospital provides vehicles, radios, and salary support to a team of social workers who conduct assessments, investigations, and follow-up counseling for every reported case of domestic violence within the county. Currently, the hospital is working to expand the program's operations to 7 days per week, from the current 6 days.

As part of a community-wide childhood immunization initiative, the hospital operates a immunization support program that covers every infant born within the hospital that continues to reside within the surrounding five-county region. Under this program, hospital staff provide periodic telephone follow-up with families to encourage timely immunization delivery, using the newly established community-wide immunization registry to identify cases at risk of underimmunization. For chronically underimmunized children, the hospital sends nurses to the home to administer immunizations. Under this project, Hurley Medical Center staff work closely with the local health department's immunization program staff in developing strategies to encourage immunization utilization and in ensuring coordination between the two organizations' outreach efforts.

Through its individual and collaborative efforts, Hurley Medical Center exists as a vital contributor to community health initiatives within Genesee County. The hospital's strong and enduring relationships with the local health department and other community agencies play a vital role in its operations. Unlike many public hospitals across the country, Hurley appears to be successfully responding to the larger health care trends of managed care growth and increased competition among providers. Perhaps even more notably, the hospital appears to be successfully maintaining and expanding its involvement in community health issues in the wake of these changes.

McLaren Regional Medical Center

McLaren Regional Medical Center exists as the other remaining hospital facility within the city of Flint. This facility is operated by the nonprofit McLaren Health Care Corporation, which also encompasses an extended care facility, several home health agencies, a community hospital located in a neighboring county, and more than 50 ambulatory care centers located in an eight-county region surrounding Flint. The hospital corporation exists as an important source of care for uninsured and underinsured populations by providing approximately $8 million in uncompensated care services during 1996. Services to Medicaid beneficiaries currently comprise only ~5% of the hospital's payer mix, ranking the hospital behind both Hurley and Genesys in service to the area's Medicaid population. Because McLaren's hospital facility has not until recently marketed themselves to Medicaid eligible residents, demand for services from Medicaid beneficiaries remains relatively modest. Hospital administrators report that most of the uncompensated care that is provided by the hospital is received by Flint's substantial employed uninsured population, rather than the area's more severely impoverished population groups.

Several recent developments in the local health care environment promise to increase McLaren's role in serving vulnerable population groups. First, the recent relocation of Genesys' health care facilities from western Flint to southern Genesee County has removed a substantial Medicaid and uncompensated care provider from the city. In fact, Genesys's Flint Osteopathic facility, which had been located across the street from McLaren's hospital, has long served as the area's second largest provider of care to Medicaid beneficiaries and uninsured individuals. The closure of this facility appears likely to increase McLaren's role in serving these population groups. Additionally, McLaren's recent efforts to increase its capacity for providing primary care services within the community also promise to expand the hospital's role in serving vulnerable and underserved population groups. McLaren currently operates several primary care clinics that serve substantial numbers of Medicaid beneficiaries and is considering plans for opening a new clinic within the county that will be designed primarily to serve Medicaid beneficiaries. McLaren administrators report that the hospital system's effort to expand its primary care capacity is a principal component of its strategy to adapt to the growth of managed care within the local health care system. Under the state's new Medicaid initiative, an increasing number of the area's managed care plans are contracting to serve these beneficiaries. To compete effectively in the local managed care market, McLaren's administrators are striving to enhance their organization's capacity to serve the full range of managed care enrollees, including Medicaid beneficiaries.

Many members of McLaren's clinical staff already have substantial experience in serving vulnerable and underserved populations within the community. The hospital and its staff are key supporters of the Genesee County Free Medical Clinic, which is operated jointly by local hospitals, the county medical society, and the local health department. A Gastroenterologist at the hospital, Dr. Marigowda Nagaraju, MD, spearheaded the opening of the clinic in 1991 and currently serves as the clinic's president. Numerous other members of McLaren's clinical staff volunteer their services at the clinic, which now boasts at total of 41 primary care physicians, 65 specialists, 68 nurses, 9 pharmacists and pharmacy technicians, and 27 administrative staff—each of whom volunteer several hours per year.

McLaren maintains several other programs and services that target community health issues. McLaren's child evaluation clinic serves as Genesee County's central resource for evaluating and treating suspected cases of child sexual abuse. Opened by the hospital in 1992, the clinic is staffed by a pediatrician, a family practitioner, and a team of nurses and social workers. Local police officials and social workers make referrals to the clinic when suspected child sexual abuse cases are identified. Since its inception, the clinic has served over 560 children using approximately $175,000 in annual appropriations from McLaren.

McLaren also maintains an expanding range of health promotion and disease prevention programs in the Genesee County area. Through its wellness program, the hospital conducts a wide range of health education classes and seminars on topics such as cardiovascular health, diabetes management, and smoking cessation. During 1996, more than 10,000 individuals were served through these initiatives. As part of this program, the hospital launched a community-based health education project in Genesee County's Fenton community, in partnership with a local chamber of commerce. The project was designed to identify residents at high risk for chronic disease problems using individual health risk appraisals conducted at area community centers and to offer targeted health education interventions aimed at reducing health risks. The hospital is currently considering plans for implementing this project on a broader scale within the county. In another project, the hospital is conducting tobacco cessation programs in a collection of public high schools in three counties (including Genesee), using video conference technology. A national information technology firm, Ameritech, is cosponsoring this health education effort.

McLaren maintains an active and expanding occupational health program that is enhancing access to and utilization of wellness services among the community's employed population. More than 2500 employers in mid-Michigan currently hold contracts with McLaren for providing health assessments, screening services, health education, and counseling to their employees. The hospital currently operates three free-standing occupational health centers across Genesee County to support these activities. The hospital also provides employers with customized computer software for profiling their occupational health programs and identifying high-priority health issues within their workforce. Finally, McLaren's occupational health program maintains an employer advisory council that comprises representatives from local employers who provide the hospital with valuable input regarding emerging occupational health concerns. This council also assists the hospital in disseminating information regarding occupational health issues to the larger community of employers within the area.

Other community health resources maintained by McLaren include the following:

- The local Visiting Nurse Association, which provides skilled home care services to area residents. A grant from the local United Way totaling $102,000 in 1996 allows the association to provide care to indigent clients requiring home care services. The hospital also participates in annual plant sales in order to raise additional revenue to support indigent home care services.
- The local emergency management service, which provides both emergency response services and nonemergency patient transportation services to county residents.
- A hospice program that provided more than $145,000 in absolute charity care and $400,000 in care that exceeded insurance reimbursement for individuals needing end-of-life health and support services during 1996. The program also provided hospice education and grief support services to more than 800 individuals in 1996.
- A telephone "ask-a-nurse" program operated by McLaren's nursing staff, which provides free health care information, advice, and referrals to area residents. The program handled more than 100,000 calls during 1996.
- A partnership with two local elementary schools to provide health and nutritional counseling and to conduct classes on nutrition, hygiene, and physical fitness for students.
- A program to provide unused hospital food items to a local food bank and soup kitchen.

McLaren's relationship with the local health department in Genesee County is cooperative but relatively limited in scope. McLaren makes an annual donation of $75,000 to the health department to help fund physician services to uninsured residents of the county, including follow-up diagnostic and treatment services for women found to be at-risk for breast or cervical cancer through the department's screening program. The hospital also provides financial assistance to support a pediatrician to work part-time in one of the health department's public health clinics. McLaren participates in several community-wide initiatives and coalitions that provide additional opportunities for interacting with the local health department as well as other community agencies. Prime among these activities is the Greater Flint Area Health Coalition, which has primarily served as a forum for the hospital to engage in joint planning and information sharing with the health department and other organizations. McLaren participates in several other community-wide health planning and policy development activities, such as the following:

- a breast and cervical cancer working group that brings together the local hospitals, the county medical society, the local university, and the health department to share information on the range of activities underway within the county to prevent, detect, and treat these diseases;
- a diabetes outreach and referral project, through which the local hospitals agree to serve as disease management referral sites for individuals identified by the health department as being at-risk for diabetes;
- a community-wide heart health coalition, which conducts joint planning to develop community-wide interventions for reducing cardiovascular disease within the county;
- a communicable disease network, through which infectious disease representatives from each of the hospitals meets periodically with the local health department to review policies and procedures for communicable disease testing, reporting, and treatment;
- a tobacco control and reduction coalition, through which local hospitals collaborate with the county medical society and the local health department in developing policies and community-wide interventions to reduce tobacco use within the county;
- a community hospital oncology program that supports the development of joint strategies for collecting data on cancer incidence within the county and serves as a forum for developing coordinated efforts in cancer prevention, detection, and treatment.[4]

Administrators at McLaren anticipate that their relationships with the local health department and with other community-based public health agencies will need to be strengthened as the hospital continues to expand its involvement in primary care and preventive services, especially for Medicaid beneficiaries and other vulnerable and underserved populations. In the past, the hospital's focus on tertiary care and highly specialized medical services appears to have limited the need for stronger relationships with the public health community. McLaren's service population of largely employed and insured community residents also appears to have limited the degree to which the hospital shared common interests with the public health community in serving vulnerable and underserved populations. Recent changes in the hospital's scope of services and in its service population provide motivation for developing stronger linkages with local public health organizations, including the county health department.

Genesys Health System

The county's third and largest hospital system, Genesys Health System, maintains a 70-year history in the community as a nonprofit corporation affiliated with the Sisters of Saint Joseph of Nazareth Catholic order. The current system brings four separate Genesee County hospitals under common ownership and management—St. Joseph Hospital in central Flint, Genesee Memorial Hospital in western Flint, Flint Osteopathic Hospital in western Flint, and Wheelock Memorial Hospital in southeast Genesee County. Historically, both St. Joseph and Flint Osteopathic have served as important sources of care for Medicaid beneficiaries and uninsured and underinsured populations. Hospital records indicate that during 1991, Medicaid comprised 18% of Flint Osteopathic's patient revenues and 10% of St. Joseph's patient revenues. During this same year, Flint Osteopathic provided more than $18 million in services to indigent patients (or 20% of its total charges), while St. Joseph provided a similar amount (representing 15% of its total charges).

In early 1997, Genesys opened a new hospital facility in the city of Grand Blanc, a suburban area ~12 miles southeast of central Flint. Consequently, Genesys is currently in the process of closing its four previously existing hospital facilities, which will reduce its hospital capacity from 683 staffed beds to 379 staffed beds. This action promises to enhance efficiency within the system by eliminating excess service capacity and consolidating operations, but it also imposes substantial changes in the geographic accessibility of medical services within the county. As a result of these changes, Genesys is likely to experience declines in the demand for services from Medicaid beneficiaries and uninsured individuals, because these groups are largely concentrated within the city of Flint and are more likely to experience difficulties in transportation.

Genesys maintains involvement in a broad range of community health activities that should remain largely unaffected by the system's recent consolidation and relocation. Genesys contributes a team of perinatal staff to provide prenatal care and well child examinations through one of the health department's public health clinics 2 days per week. This team includes a board-certified physician and several residents, nurses, and social workers who are employed with Genesys. Genesys also contributes clinical staff on a weekly basis to provide free health screenings for senior citizens at one of the health department's clinics. Additionally, Genesys helps to support the health department's clinical capacity by rotating participants in its family practice residency program through the health department's clinics for sexually transmitted diseases and family planning. Along with other community providers, Genesys is an important collaborator in the Genesee County Free Clinic program, which provides primary care services to uninsured individuals. Genesys staff serve on the clinic's advisory board, and many provide clinical services through the clinic on a voluntary basis.

Genesys maintains substantial involvement in school health programs within Genesee County. Genesys funds a program in one of Flint's public elementary schools that is designed to promote healthy lifestyles and to prevent youth violence, adolescent pregnancy, and other social problems through education and counseling services. The hospital system also funds a competitive minigrant program in Genesee County that is designed to support innovative health programming in area schools.

Genesys also serves as an important source of health promotion and disease prevention services for community residents. An active health education program offers classes and seminars on topics such as nutrition, weight control, physical fitness, diabetes management, and smoking cessation. The hospital also maintains a newborn telephone hotline staffed by nurses who provide free information and advice regarding infant health issues. Finally, an expanding occupational health program offers a broad range of work site health services that are aimed at preventing injury and disease and promoting health in the workplace. Employers may contract with Genesys to receive services such as the following: industrial hygiene consulting, environmental health and safety compliance audits, safety inspections, employee training in health and safety procedures, on-site employee health assessments, and support services for developing work site health promotion, wellness and fitness programs.

Like the other local hospitals, Genesys serves as an important participant in many of the community-wide planning and policy development initiatives that are underway in Genesee County. These initiatives include the Greater Flint Area Health Coalition and the health department's collaborative projects for diabetes management, tobacco control, cardiovascular health, communicable disease control, and breast and cervical cancer prevention and control.

The relationship between Genesys and the local health department appears largely cooperative in that the agencies maintain agreements for joint funding of public health activities, shared staff, referrals for service delivery, and joint planning and policy development activities. The recent relocation of Genesys hospital services from Flint to the new Grand Blanc facility has created some tension between the organizations, however. This tension stems largely from concerns about changes in the accessibility of care and about changes in the roles that public and private health care providers may play in serving vulnerable and underserved residents within the county. Nonetheless, the multiple collaborative efforts maintained by Genesys and the local health department insure that the organizations will be able to monitor changes in health care delivery and pursue collective strategies to address any problems.

Managed Care Plans

Managed care plans are a relatively small but growing component of Genesee County's local health care delivery system. In contrast to many other areas of the nation, nonprofit health plans are the dominant providers of managed care services in Genesee County and statewide. Genesee County's first local HMO formed in 1979, largely through the work of the local medical society. Since this time, a number of other plans have begun operations in Genesee County, many of which are based in Detroit. An innovative demonstration project, spearheaded by the health department and funded in part by the Robert Wood Johnson Foundation during the mid-1980s, helped to encourage the growth of managed care plans in Genesee County, especially among small employers and uninsured populations. Through this program, known nationally as the Health Care for the Uninsured Program, a group of 10,000 low-income, uninsured residents of Genesee County received health care coverage either through a designated HMO or through a primary care case management plan. This same plan was marketed to area small employers who could not afford to offer health insurance benefits to their employees. The program, which operated from 1986 through 1992, was carried out through a collaborative effort between Genesee County's three hospitals, the local medical society, the local health department, and the state department of social services.

In 1992, the state began a mandatory managed care program in Genesee County and five other Michigan counties for all Medicaid beneficiaries who are eligible through the Aid to Families with Dependent Children program (now known as the Temporary Assistance to Needy Families program) and the Supplemental Security Income program. Michigan implemented this initiative under the authority of a 1915(b) waiver from the US Health Care Financing Administration. Under this initiative, which was patterned after the earlier program for the uninsured, Medicaid beneficiaries could choose to enroll either in an HMO or in a primary care case management program operated by local physicians. Until early 1996, only one HMO served Medicaid beneficiaries in Genesee County—the Detroit-based Wellness Plan.

Several other plans began involvement in serving Medicaid beneficiaries during 1996 in anticipation of the state's new policy of mandatory HMO enrollment for Medicaid beneficiaries eligible under the Aid to Families with Dependent Children and Supplemental Security Income programs. The state began phasing in this new policy during 1997 by allowing physicians participating as Medicaid primary care case management providers to "roll over" their Medicaid enrollees into one of the seven HMOs that were approved to enroll Medicaid beneficiaries in Genesee County. Over a period of several months, this policy has allowed several HMOs to assume substantial roles in serving vulnerable and traditionally underserved populations within the county.

The managed care plans operating in Genesee County have maintained relatively limited interaction with the local health department to date. Some of these plans serve on community-wide planning groups with the local health department, such as the Greater Flint Area Health Coalition and the community-wide immunization coalition. Several plans have also engaged in dialogue with the health department regarding collaborative strategies for providing public health services within the community. Despite these efforts, the organizations so far have been unsuccessful in developing strong and productive joint efforts in performing core public health services. To facilitate collaboration under the state's new mandatory HMO enrollment program for Medicaid beneficiaries, the local health department drafted a memorandum of understanding to be established between itself and local Medicaid HMOs. This draft agreement was designed to help the department in delineating service responsibilities and establishing joint referral and information-sharing mechanisms with area health plans. Unfortunately, the department was unable to secure agreements with any of the health plans operating in Genesee County. Nevertheless, several health plans remain optimistic about the potential for future collaboration as the local managed care market and the public health system mature.

HealthPlus of Michigan

HealthPlus was founded in 1979 as Genesee County's first HMO, largely through the efforts of the local medical society to offer an alternative to the traditional Blue Cross Blue Shield indemnity insurance plan that dominated the local insurance market. The HMO has remained a nonprofit, federally qualified plan organized as an independent practice association model. The plan is now licensed to operate in a 13-county area surrounding Flint, and contracts with more than 2100 physicians on a nonexclusive basis. HealthPlus maintains an enrollment of almost 114,000 members, ~80,000 of whom reside in Genesee County. Almost 52% of the HMO's enrollees are enrolled through General Motors Corporation, the area's leading employer.

HealthPlus began participating in the Medicaid managed care program in 1996, in anticipation of the state's move to mandatory HMO enrollment for Medicaid beneficiaries. During the first 3 months of 1997, the HMO has seen its Medicaid membership grow from 2000 enrollees to 15,000 enrollees. HealthPlus administrators anticipate that by the end of the phase-in period in 1998, the HMO will have accrued approximately half of the 130,000 Medicaid beneficiaries who reside in its 13-county service area.

Currently, HealthPlus relies largely on its network of independent physician practices to ensure that this large volume of new and potentially vulnerable enrollees receives appropriate and accessible care. The HMO has placed a priority on establishing contracts with the community physicians that have traditionally served these beneficiaries, in order to take advantage of their knowledge and expertise in serving vulnerable populations. The rapid pace with which HealthPlus has received new Medicaid enrollees has so far prevented the organization from developing specialized services and monitoring systems to insure that these individuals receive access to care. These new enrollees are served through the organization's existing quality assurance systems, which include an immunization tracking system and processes for monitoring emergency room utilization and hospitalizations for ambulatory care sensitive conditions. Medicaid enrollees also have access to the HMO's array of health education programs in areas such as prenatal care and diabetes management.

HealthPlus administrators acknowledge that the local health department could be a valuable partner in helping the organization develop targeted systems of care for its growing Medicaid population. To date, however, the plan has been unable to establish workable service agreements with the department. For example, a dialogue between the two organizations has been ongoing for several months regarding the fact that the health department's immunization clinics serve substantial numbers of HealthPlus enrollees without reimbursement from the HMO. This trend has suggested that some of the HMO's enrollees may prefer to obtain immunization services at the health department and also that some of the HMO's providers may refer their clients to the department for these services. In response, HealthPlus has begun a project to educate its physicians and enrollees about the provision of immunization services. HealthPlus and the health department have also established an agreement to reimburse the department for the cost of any immunization services delivered to HealthPlus enrollees. Ongoing dialogue between the two organizations provides hope that other workable agreements will be developed in the future.

HealthPlus interacts frequently with the local health department and other area health care organizations through the communitywide Greater Flint Area Health Coalition. HealthPlus has made substantial contributions of time and effort to this coalition since its inception. As evidence of its commitment to this effort, the HMO assigned one of its vice presidents to work virtually full time on the coalition activities. HealthPlus administrators remain optimistic that this communitywide effort will eventually lead to tangible, collaborative interventions aimed at improving health status within the community. These administrators report that they have much to gain from such community-wide interventions, because they anticipate having at least one fourth of all Genesee County residents enrolled in their plan by the end of 1998.

Wellness Plan

The Detroit-based Wellness plan maintains the longest history in serving Medicaid beneficiaries of Genesee County. This organization served as the HMO option for the demonstration program that began in Detroit in 1986 for covering uninsured residents and for the original Medicaid managed care program that began in 1992. Wellness Plan has its origins in Detroit's neighborhood health center program, which began in 1969 with funding from the US Office of Economic Opportunity's Model Neighborhood Comprehensive Health Program. When funding for this program ended in the early 1970s, the organization reformed itself as a nonprofit, staff-model HMO with support from the federal Health Maintenance Organization Act of 1973 and secured a state contract to serve Medicaid patients. The organization continued to expand its capacity for serving Medicaid patients by constructing community health centers around the Detroit area and directly employing physicians and other clinical staff to operate these clinics. During the mid-1980s, the organization initiated an independent practice association plan, which enabled the HMO to expand by contracting with existing community health centers and private physician practices. The plan initiated its operations in Genesee County in 1987 by contracting with the Hamilton Community Health Center, a federally qualified health center located in northern Flint.

Currently, Wellness Plan serves ~150,000 enrollees in nine Michigan counties, of which 25,000 reside in Genesee County. Approximately 90% of the plan's membership are Medicaid beneficiaries, with the remainder being Medicare beneficiaries and commercially insured enrollees. Although the HMO is working to expand its involvement in serving Medicare beneficiaries and employer groups, Wellness maintains a primary commitment to serving Medicaid beneficiaries and other vulnerable populations (the plan serves ~18,000 uninsured individuals through a special, locally financed program in Detroit). By expanding its revenue base to include contracts with employers and Medicare beneficiaries, the HMO hopes to secure additional financial stability and resources to enable improved levels of service to vulnerable and underserved populations.

To better serve these populations, Wellness establishes relationships with an array of other community organizations, including community mental health centers, substance abuse treatment programs, county social services departments, schools, churches, and neighborhood groups. In Genesee County, Wellness funds a public health nurse to conduct health screenings in one elementary school. The HMO also provides on-site health screenings to area churches and neighborhood associations on a periodic basis.

Interestingly, Wellness maintains only limited interaction with the local health departments that serve the counties in which it operates. In Genesee County, the HMO serves with the health department on a community-wide immunization coalition that has worked to implement the area's immunization registry. However, the two organizations have not yet developed any formal agreements for joint service delivery, referral, or coordination in serving the county's Medicaid population. Administrators at Wellness indicate that such agreements, especially regarding the sharing of utilization information, would be extremely useful to the HMO in serving its Medicaid population. The ability to track enrollee utilization of health department services such as treatment for sexually transmitted diseases and other communicable diseases would greatly assist the HMO in coordinating and managing the delivery of health services to its enrollee population. To date, however, issues of patient confidentiality have prevented the two organizations from establishing such agreements. The implementation of a community-wide immunization registry has resolved the data-sharing issues surrounding childhood immunizations. However, these issues remain for other communicable disease and public health services.

Somewhat surprisingly, Wellness does not maintain membership on the board of the community-wide health planning and development organization known as the Greater Flint Area Health Coalition. The HMO's administrators indicate that they have not received an invitation to participate on the board, most likely because of their lack of involvement in serving employer groups and because of their image as an out-of-town, Detroit-based plan. Staff from Wellness do participate on several of the coalition's working committees. As the county's largest provider of services to Medicaid beneficiaries, Wellness could undoubtedly make valuable contributions to the coalition's work in identifying outstanding health needs and resources within the community. This coalition could also serve as an important vehicle for Wellness to forge stronger relationships with the local health department and other community organizations, particularly as it attempts to expand its role in the commercial and Medicare markets as well as the Medicaid program.

Wellness has demonstrated clearly its success in serving the complex health needs of vulnerable and underserved populations within Michigan. Nonetheless, within Genesee County, the HMO appears to face some difficulties in forging productive partnerships with the full array of organizations that could potentially assist the organization in serving these populations. Overcoming these difficulties may require considerable effort, but it may also offer the organization valuable opportunities for enhancing its service delivery and expanding its service population within Genesee County.

Blue Care Network

Blue Care Network is Michigan's and Genesee County's largest HMO, with ~86,000 enrollees within the county. Four separate Blue Care Network plans operate within Michigan, each of which is a wholly owned subsidiary of Blue Cross/Blue Shield of Michigan. Together, the four plans serve over 550,000 enrollees statewide. Blue Care Network of East Michigan serves Genesee County and surrounding areas. The nonprofit HMO administers both a staff-model health plan and an independent practice association model. General Motors remains the plan's largest client, contributing ~25% of the plan's total membership. Blue Care also serves several thousand Medicaid beneficiaries as part of the state's mandatory managed care program and is in the process of negotiating a contract for serving Medicare beneficiaries.

Blue Care has engaged in a broad range of activities that are designed to improve health status at the community level. Many of these activities have been implemented in collaboration with other health care organizations in the community—often with other participants in the Greater Flint Area Health Coalition. In an effort to improve screening practices for cardiovascular disease, the HMO recently sponsored a community education program among area physicians. This program, which was jointly sponsored with a competing HMO (HealthPlus), recruited area primary care physicians to participate in educational sessions chaired by leading cardiologists from the University of Michigan. These sessions were designed to promote proper screening and diagnostic practices among local primary care physicians, in order to promote early detection, prevention, and treatment for cardiovascular disease. The HMO is now sponsoring a similar physician education program for area primary care physicians regarding the issue of gastrointestinal disorders. Through this program, the HMO is bringing in prominent gastroenterologists to lead educational sessions in areas such as the proper treatment of ulcers and the elimination of *Helicobacter pylori*. To finance these physician education programs, Blue Care secured grants from a national pharmaceutical company.

As part of another community-wide initiative, Blue Care recently sponsored a community-wide breast cancer awareness program in partnership with area hospitals. The program included community-wide media messages and educational seminars conducted at several community locations. These activities were designed to promote proper self-examination practices as well as to encourage the utilization of routine mammograms and clinical examinations.

In January 1997, Blue Care launched a 2-year project to study the effects of an intervention to encourage shared medical decision-making among community physicians and their patients facing treatment for ischemic heart disease. This project, which includes collaboration from HealthPlus and the county's three hospital systems, is designed to enhance informed decision-making by patients regarding treatment options for one of the community's most prevalent chronic diseases. The intervention under study consists of a video to be administered to appropriate patients regarding alternative treatments, risks, and benefits.

Currently, Blue Care is experimenting with community-wide implementation of a computer-based clinical information system that is designed to provide information to clinical staff on treatment standards and guidelines. The system, known as the Care Management System, is being demonstrated in all three of the county's hospital systems. The system is designed encourage provider adoption and adherence to community-wide treatment guidelines, such as those currently being developed by the Greater Flint Area Health Coalition in the areas of cardiac treatment, cesarean section delivery, and diabetes management.

Virtually all of the community-wide initiatives currently supported by Blue Care are related in some way to the community health assessment activities conducted by the Greater Flint Area Health Coalition. Blue Care, together with its parent corporation Blue Cross/Blue Shield of Michigan, serves as a vital participant in the work of the coalition. Blue Care staff serve on several administrative committees within the coalition and chair the coalition's task forces on cardiovascular disease and pharmacy services. As evidence of its commitment to the coalition's work, Blue Care now employs a full-time community health director who is charged with coordinating the plan's contributions to the coalition.

Blue Care administrators suggest that both altruism and pragmatism provide the motivation for their plan's involvement in community health efforts. As a nonprofit organization with a 20-year history within the community, the plan faces a social obligation to provide a certain level of service to the community the form of health promotion, disease prevention, and quality improvement activities that extend beyond the plan's enrolled membership. Beyond this altruistic motivation, Blue Care faces the reality of serving a large proportion of the total community population in Genesee County and eastern Michigan. For many of the chronic health conditions threatening this population, community-wide initiatives appear to be the most promising strategies for improving health status and therefore reducing financial risk among its enrollees.

Despite its substantial involvement in community health issues, Blue Care maintains only loose affiliations with the local health department in Genesee County. The HMO and health department interact as members of the Greater Flint Area Health Coalition and as members of a community-wide immunization task force but otherwise do not maintain regular contact. Blue Care administrators report that their organization does not currently face the need for stronger affiliations with the health department. The plan receives adequate support and assistance for its community health initiatives through the full membership of the health coalition. Furthermore, Blue Care administrators do not perceive a substantial need for assistance in serving the needs of vulnerable and underserved population groups through the plan's Medicaid contract. Virtually all of Blue Care's Medicaid enrollees in Genesee County are served through the plan's staff-model clinic, located in central Flint. Administrators suggest that the plan is committed to serving those beneficiaries who choose Blue Care as their preferred source of care, but Blue Care is not actively involved in expanding its capacity for serving Medicaid beneficiaries. However, once the mandatory HMO enrollment program for Medicaid beneficiaries has been fully phased in across the state, Blue Cross may begin to compete more aggressively for serving this population across its service area. Such a strategy might motivate the plan to develop stronger affiliations with the local health department and other traditional care providers for this population. In lieu of such a strategy, the relationship between Blue Care and the local health department is likely to remain informal and limited.

Other Managed Care Plans

At least five other health plans operate within Genesee County, but these plans currently serve relatively small numbers of county residents and are based outside the county. None of these plans currently maintain any relationship with the local health department. Many of these plans, however, are new participants in the state's Medicaid managed care program. As these plans seek strategies to enhance their capacity and effectiveness in serving vulnerable and underserved populations, they may begin to seek out the health department as a potential resource. Currently, Wellness and Health Plus exist as the dominant providers of managed care services to the Medicaid population in Genesee County. Many of the other health plans currently entering the Medicaid market have little experience in serving potentially underserved and vulnerable populations. As competition grows within the Medicaid market, the local health department may face a growing need to monitor these developing delivery systems, if not directly participate in them, to ensure that accessibility and quality of care are maintained.

Private Physicians

Genesee County is served by an active medical community that maintains strong relationships with the local health department and other community health organizations. The Genesee County Medical Society continues a long history of involvement in public health issues that dates back to the early part of this century, when the society helped to launch the county health department. More recently, the medical society plays an active and ongoing role in developing policies and plans to address pressing public health issues, in launching community interventions to expand access to care for vulnerable populations, and in establishing mechanisms to monitor and improve health care quality delivered within the community.

For example, the society participates in a community-wide tobacco reduction coalition that recently secured the passage of local ordinances restricting tobacco advertising and tobacco use in public places. The society also serves as a founding and operating member of the Genesee County Free Clinic, which provides free health services to uninsured county residents. A charitable foundation that is owned by the medical society provides revenue to support the free clinic as well as other community health initiatives undertaken by the society. Revenue for the foundation is generated from several physician support services operated by the medical society, including an answering service and an urgent care center. As part of its mission to expand health care accessibility, the society also maintains an active effort to encourage local physician participation in the Medicaid program. This effort proved highly effective in encouraging local physicians to participate in the Medicaid primary care case management program which began in 1992, despite the fact that this program offered only a $3 monthly per member payment for providing case management services to beneficiaries. The medical society also administers a $500,000 grant from the federal Ryan White program to cover the costs of treatment services for patients with HIV and AIDS. Finally, the medical society maintains involvement in community health education initiatives, funded largely through its foundation. These initiatives are carried out largely through public television and newspaper messages, on topics such as violence prevention and adolescent pregnancy prevention.

The medical society conducts many of its public health activities in collaboration with the local health department. The two organizations jointly participate on several community-planning coalitions, including those for adolescent pregnancy prevention, violence prevention, and environmental health protection.

To facilitate interaction and coordination between the health department and the medical society, the two organizations share membership on their respective governing boards. The medical society's executive director serves on the local board of health, while the county medical director serves on the medical society's governing board. Medical society staff indicate that their close relationship with the local health department often provides an effective vehicle for circumventing political issues that might otherwise inhibit public action on divisive public health issues. The medical society assumes the lead role in advocating for public action in cases where the health department may be unable to assume this role owing to political constraints.

The medical society works closely with the health department as well as other community health organizations through participation in the Greater Flint Area Health Coalition. The medical society's executive director serves as a key staff person for the coalition, and several physician leaders within the society serve as members of task forces and committees within the coalition. Currently, the society is actively involved on the coalition's project to develop and implement a community-wide, multi-institutional quality assurance and guideline system. At least 52 of the medical society's member physicians are working with representatives from area hospitals, managed care plans, and the local health department to develop quality-of-care guidelines and protocols that can be implemented on a community-wide basis through this system. A wide array of specialty-specific and site-specific protocols are under development, ranging from primary care and preventive health practices to medical and surgical guidelines for inpatient settings. Blue Care HMO is currently working with area hospitals, physicians, and health plans to evaluate a computer system to be used in supporting community-wide adoption of the guidelines and in monitoring compliance with these guidelines. Initiatives such as this guideline development project provide a true test of the coalition's ability to progress from community assessment and planning activities to meaningful community health interventions.

In general, medical society staff remain optimistic about the ability of the coalition's work to improve health care quality and accessibility within the community. The coalition appears to have strengthened the already-solid relationship between the medical society and the local health department by providing an expanding array of opportunities for communication and collaboration. Moreover, the coalition also appears to have created opportunities for the two organizations to work together in seeking new allies for public health initiatives within the community. Together, the two organizations insure that a strong voice for public health exists within a forum whose membership tends to focus on the more high-profile issues of medical care costs and employer-based health insurance.

Other Community Organizations

A wide range of other organizations and individuals make substantial contributions to Genesee County's public health system. These organizations include local business leaders (including General Motors), the local United Auto Workers union, established voluntary organizations such as Planned Parenthood, local churches, local and regional universities, and an array of neighborhood associations and community groups. To be sure, many other communities are served by these same types of organizations. Genesee County, however, appears unique both in the extent to which these organizations engage in community health efforts and in the mechanisms through which these organizations participate in community health efforts.

Two community-wide, multiorganizational initiatives help to motivate and sustain this involvement. The Greater Flint Area Health Coalition—perhaps the most widely recognized, and the most resource-intensive, of these initiatives—consists largely of organized health care providers, government leaders, community members, insurers, and health care purchasers. Another initiative, which began with funding from the W. K. Kellogg Foundation, brings together a diverse collection of community-based organizations with two area universities and the local health department. The local health department serves as the principal agent for linking the activities of these two multi-organizational initiatives. Currently, these two initiatives are beginning to explore opportunities for joint actions to address pressing health issues within the community.

The Greater Flint Area Health Coalition, which began operating in early 1995, represents a reincarnation of an earlier coalition of business leaders, government officials, health care providers, and community organizations which began in 1992. This earlier initiative had conducted a community health needs assessment and had initiated joint planning and priority-setting activities but had begun to unravel after several years of operation. In 1995, General Motors and the United Auto Workers union expressed interest in a community-level initiative to address issues in health care cost and quality within Flint and Genesee County. This interest was motivated by a nation-wide review of health care utilization and outcomes data for the corporation's active and retired employees, which indicated that some of the corporation's highest costs and poorest outcomes occurred within Flint and Genesee County. Rather than initiate a new community effort, the corporation and union chose to invest in the existing community coalition and to restructure it for improved decision-making ability.

After extensive negotiations with the coalition participants, the coalition was restructured in early 1996 and incorporated as a nonprofit corporation. A board of directors was appointed that includes representatives from General Motors and the United Auto Workers union, state and local government representatives, the area's hospitals and managed care plans, the local medical society, and the local health department. General Motors and the United Auto Workers union each appointed a full-time employee to staff the coalition. Many of the other participating organizations also dedicated staff members to work almost exclusively on the coalition's activities. The coalition has now hired a director and core staff members.

Even before the coalition's organizational structure was complete, General Motors and the United Auto Workers union commissioned a community health assessment study to be performed, in an effort to identify the area's most pressing health issues and resource needs. The results of this study were released in June 1996. On the basis of these results, the coalition formed a series of task forces to develop action plans for addressing high-impact health issues. Task forces were formed around the issues of cardiac disease, pharmacy services, cesarean section services, diabetes management, wellness services, oncology services, and maternal and child health issues.

Currently, the coalition's task forces are working to develop community-level interventions to address the identified health issues, with each organizational participant assuming responsibility for specific tasks. For example, the Blue Care Network of East Michigan is leading a community-wide study of cardiac catheterizations to examine the appropriateness and quality of these procedures. The medical society is leading a multidisciplinary effort to develop of care guidelines and protocols suitable for community-wide adoption. Organizational members of the pharmacy task force are implementing a direct mail campaign to community residents who have sought repeated treatments for gastrointestinal problems, in order to encourage participation in an intervention to eradicate the *H. pylori* bacteria, which often cause these chronic problems.

It remains to be seen whether these interventions will be sustainable over the long term and effective in improving health within the community. Nevertheless, it appears clear that the coalition has motivated enhanced levels of involvement in community health issues among local organizations and individuals.

Genesee County's second multiorganizational initiative in community health improvement began formally in 1993 with the support of a grant from the W. K. Kellogg Foundation under its Community-Based Public Health Initiative. This grant provided funding for two "teams" of public health organizations—one based in Genesee County and the other based in Wayne County (Detroit)—to develop collaborative approaches for improving public health practice, education, and training. Each team contained a local health department, a university-based school for health or human services professions, and a collection of community-based organizations.

The Genesee Team grew out of an earlier effort undertaken by the health department to identify potential partners for improving health within an impoverished area within the city of Flint. In an effort to improve health within this region, the health department established a community health clinic within the area and then implemented an active surveillance process to identify organizations, individuals, and groups within the community to collaborate with in designing meaningful community health interventions. Numerous organizations were identified through this process—including schools, churches, and neighborhood associations—and a subset of six organizations ultimately agreed to collaborate with the health department. This group of community-based organizations began working with the local health department, the University of Michigan at Ann Arbor School of Public Health, and the University of Michigan at Flint's health professions program to develop proposals for community-based public health initiatives in the vulnerable Flint neighborhoods. These proposals were assembled in a grant application to the Kellogg Foundation and were funded in early 1993.

During the 3-year grant period, the Genesee Team developed an interorganizational structure to support effective communication, coordination, and joint planning among the participating organizations. This structure included a regular meeting schedule and a consensus-driven approach for identifying public health issues and developing plans to address these issues. A wide range of successful public health initiatives have been launched through this forum, including the following:

- An African American male mentoring program in an elementary school, which sponsors male adult "role models" to provide counseling and advice to minority male students in areas such as educational and career goals, violence prevention, sexuality, and safety issues.
- A church-based program to provide community members with transportation to area health care providers to receive preventive and screening services. The Genesee Team has also initiated an effort with the county's public transportation agency and the University of Michigan's Transportation Research Institute to conduct a comprehensive study of transportation needs within the county.
- A housing improvement program that trained area community groups and individuals on topics such as home renovation, plumbing, tenant's rights, and strategies for discouraging crime and vandalism.
- A health careers program designed to provide students at the secondary-education level with information and on-site training opportunities regarding local career opportunities in health and health education.
- A lead poisoning prevention and abatement project that includes efforts to educate and screen residents of vulnerable neighborhoods, to assist in the development of state lead abatement regulations, and to study the effects of a newly constructed wood-burning incinerator on lead exposure within a high-risk area of the county.
- A church-based health information program, which supports the operation of "church health teams" in five local churches. During scheduled weekly office hours, these teams provide information to community members regarding such issues as smoking cessation, nutrition, chronic disease prevention and treatment, prenatal care, housing concerns, family planning issues, and substance abuse issues. Team members receive training as lay health educators through a program operated jointly by the local health department and the University of Michigan School of Public Health.
- The formation of a countywide violence prevention coalition that conducts joint planning and priority-setting regarding collaborative strategies for violence reduction within the community. The coalition secured the participation of more than 30 community agencies, received external funding for planning and program development activities, and applied for status as a nonprofit corporation.

Although funding from the W. K. Kellogg Foundation has now expired, the Genesee Team continues to function effectively as an interorganizational coalition in supporting and expanding community-based public health initiatives. Many of the programs initiated during the grant cycle continue to operate successfully through alternative funding sources that have been secured from local foundations and state and federal grant-in-aid programs. Additionally, the Genesee Team continues its work in developing new public health initiatives and securing the necessary organizational and financial support to implement them.

The local health department suggests that its relationships with community-based organizations such as those in the Genesee Team serve as powerful political forces for supporting local public health initiatives within the jurisdiction. By working with these organizations, the health department is often able to mobilize community support for public health issues that can then be effectively communicated to local government officials. In this way, community-based organizations play a role that in some other jurisdictions might be played by a local elected official or some other political ally.

Efforts are now in progress to develop linkages between the work of the Genesee Team and the tasks being undertaken by the county's other interorganizational initiative: the Greater Flint Area Health Coalition. These recent efforts reflect a growing recognition by members of the coalition about the problems created by poor access to care and poor health care outcomes among low-income and minority residents. To begin to address these issues, the coalition is undertaking efforts to expand its involvement with community-based organizations. As part of these efforts, a representative from the Genesee Team recently received membership on the coalition. Additionally, several of the coalition's participants have begun participating in community-based projects maintained by members of the Genesee Team. Nevertheless, the extent to which these two multiorganizational efforts will be able to work together effectively remains uncertain. Clear differences exist in the types of organizations that serve on these two initiatives, their organizational missions, and their human and financial resources. The local health department plays a vital role in attempting to link the activities and memberships of these two initiatives. Such linkages offer opportunities to introduce an enhanced focus on community health among the activities underway within the Greater Flint Health Coalition. These linkages may also offer opportunities for the Genesee Team in expanding the resource base for community-based public health initiatives.

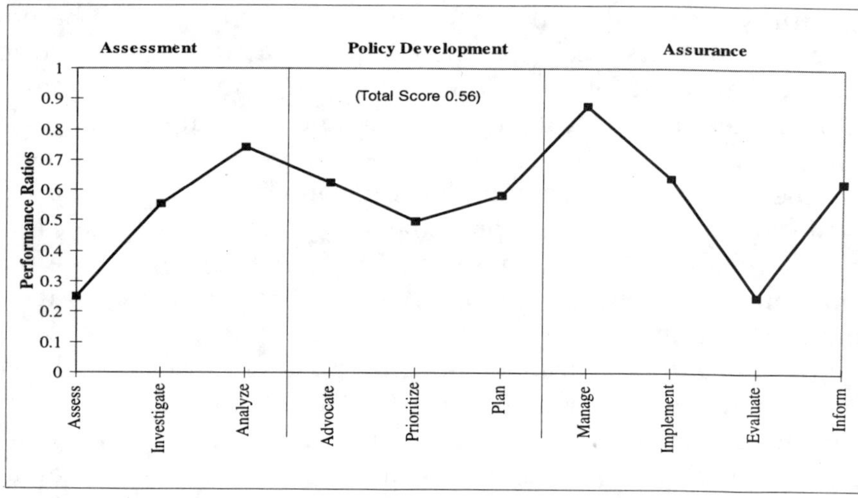

Figure 1. Community public health performance scores for Genesee County, Michigan, 1997.

Measures of Public Health System Performance

Performance Survey Results

On the basis of responses by Genesee County's health officer in 1997, the local public health system serving Genesee County appears to be functioning effectively in carrying out core public health functions. The overall public health performance score for the jurisdiction is rated at 56% of the maximum possible score, which exceeds the median score of 51% that was found in a survey of 63 local public health jurisdictions during 1992-1993 (**Figure 1**). The community's highest performance scores occur for the practices of *managing* health programs and resources, and *analyzing* the determinants of health threats. The community's lowest performance scores occur for the practices of *assessing* health needs and *evaluating* public health programs and services—both of which are below the median scores found during the 1992-1993 survey of public health jurisdictions.

When we examine public health activities specifically performed by the local health department, health department performance scores also appear to exceed the median scores found previously (**Figure 2**). Overall, the local health department's public health performance is rated at 39% of the maximum possible effort, which exceeds the median score of 37% found in the 1992-1993 survey of public health jurisdictions. Health

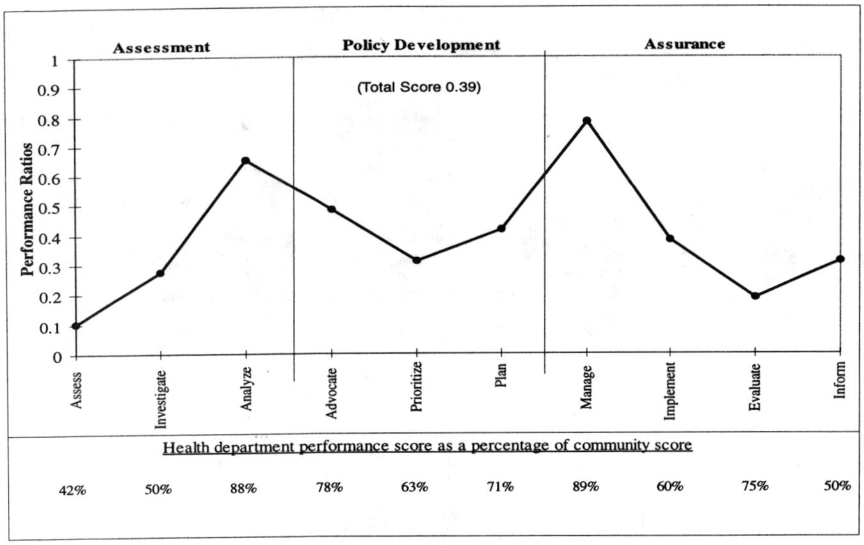

Figure 2. Health department performance scores for Genesee County, Michigan, 1997.

department performance appears highest for the practices of *managing* health programs and resources and *analyzing* the determinants of health threats—a pattern that mirrors the community performance results. Health department performance appears lowest for the practices of *assessing* health needs and *evaluating* health programs and services. Health department performance falls below the median performance scores found previously for these two practices, as well as for the practices of *investigating* health threats and *implementing* programs and services.

When health department performance is expressed as a proportion of total community effort, we find that ~70% of the community's total public health performance is contributed by the local health department. This number is somewhat smaller than the median value of 75% found among the 63 jurisdictions studied in 1992-1993. This result indicates that organizations other than the local health department contribute substantially to local public health performance in Genesee County—~30% of the community's total public health effort can be attributed to these "outside" organizations. The local health department's contributions to community performance are highest for the public health practices of *managing* health programs and resources, *analyzing* the determinants of public health threats, *advocating* for public health issues, and *evaluating* public health programs and services (Figure 2). Conversely, the contributions of outside organizations are highest for the practices of *assessing* health needs, *investigating* public health threats, and *informing and educating* the public.

Among the various types of outside agencies contributing to public health in Genesee County, local government agencies appear to participate in the greatest proportion of local public health activities (**Figure 3**). Nonprofit agencies, state government agencies, hospitals, and private physicians also appear to participate in substantial proportions of public health activities. Most of these outside organizations participate in a greater proportion of *policy development* activities than in *assessment* or *assurance* activities. State agencies and community health centers are the exceptions, as they participate more commonly in *assessment* activities than other types of public health practices.

Interpretation of Performance Survey Results

Results from the 1997 public health performance survey suggest that the local public health system in Genesee County is producing above-average results in performing core public health functions within the community. Nonetheless, the survey responses confirm that, like most other jurisdictions across the nation, Genesee County still has much progress to make in assuring that the community's public health needs are fully met. Public health practices that appear least adequately performed within the community are those involving public health assessment and program evaluation. Interestingly, both of these practices appear to be accruing the involvement of growing numbers of community organizations through the community's two multiorganizational health care initiatives. The work that is now underway within these two initiatives—the Greater Flint Health Care Coalition and the Genesee Team for community-based public health—may ultimately lead to improved community performance in these areas. The local health department must play a critical role in assuring that the activities carried out through these multiorganizational efforts address existing performance gaps in the local health system.

Local health department officials reveal that one of their key strategies for achieving public health improvement involves "expansion through collaboration." Responses to the performance survey appear to reflect this strategy, indicating that ~30% of the community's total public health effort is contributed by organizations other than the local health department. Participation scores for these organizations suggest that most types of organizations are involved more in policy development activities than in assurance and assessment activities. Often, policy development ac-

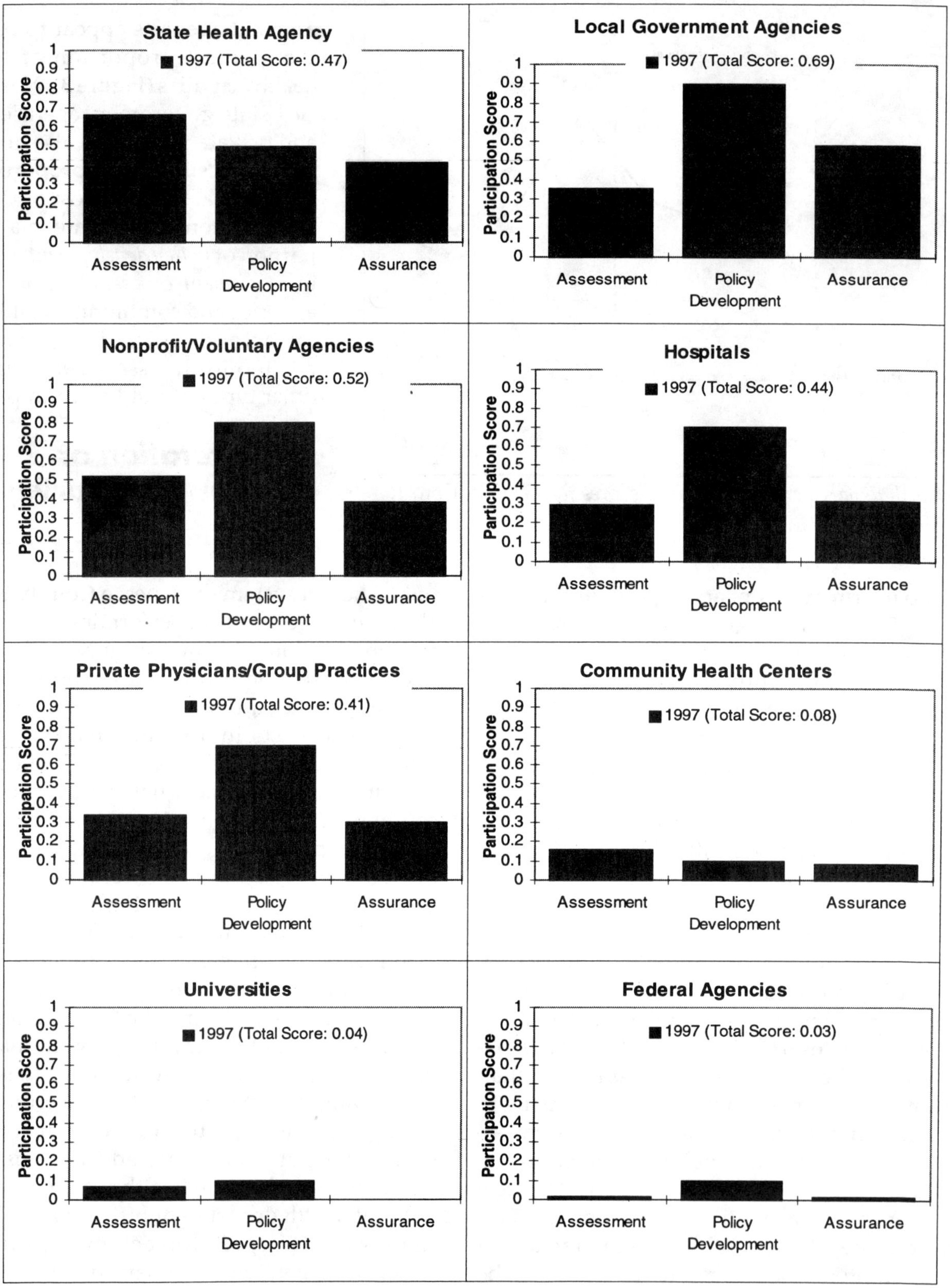

Figure 3. Participation in local public health activities by community organizations, 1997.

tivities such as joint planning and priority-setting efforts offer relatively simple and low-risk ways for organizations to begin working together on public health issues. Assessment and assurance activities, however, may require greater commitments of time and resources and therefore may prove more difficult to initiate through collaborative, interorganizational processes.

The multiorganizational initiatives currently underway within Genesee County are beginning to move beyond policy development activities and address outstanding public health needs in the areas of assessment and assurance. The ability of these initiatives to successfully address outstanding needs in these areas largely remains to be seen. The community faces an expanding need for systems that can assess public health problems and assure access to needed public health services—especially in light of recent health care trends such as the new state policy requiring mandatory HMO enrollment for Medicaid beneficiaries and the relocation of the community's largest hospital system. Keeping pace with the community's growing needs in public health assessment and assurance remains a pressing challenge for the local health department and its allies.

Future Prospects and Projections

Genesee County's local public health system depends heavily on the relationships maintained between the local health department and other community organizations. A somewhat unique feature of this jurisdiction is that many of these relationships are maintained through formal, multiorganizational coalitions. The health department and many community organizations are investing heavily in initiatives such as the Greater Flint Health Care Coalition and the Genesee Team, as measured by commitments of staff time and financial and other resources. The relatively high degree of formalization within these initiatives—both of which have spawned nonprofit corporations, governing committees, and task forces—may give them the organizational structure necessary to weather future conflicts and remain important sources of public health practice for the long term. The ability of these initiatives to produce meaningful, long-term changes in community health status largely remains to be seen. Nonetheless, these multiorganizational coalitions appear to have achieved a degree of permanence within the community that should afford opportunities for affecting community health status over the long term.

The local public health system faces a number of challenges in the near future due to recent health policy and market changes. The mandatory Medicaid managed care program now being phased in within the jurisdiction promises to substantially change the local systems of care for serving this vulnerable and often underserved population group. The local health department has so far been unsuccessful in establishing mutually acceptable service agreements with the health plans that are enrolling Medicaid beneficiaries. Recognizing limitations in the state health agency's quality assessment systems for these plans, the local health department also faces the need to become more involved in monitoring the quality of care provided to Medicaid beneficiaries through these plans and in encouraging adequate levels of service delivery by the plans. In pursuing these objectives, the health department may need to develop stronger working relationships with these plans.

The public health system also faces challenges created by the recent relocation of one of the area's large hospital systems. The burdens of providing services to the uninsured and other vulnerable populations are likely to be redistributed among local health care providers as a result of this change. The local health department must play a major role in assuring that adequate systems of care for these population groups remain available and accessible. The Greater Flint Health Care Coalition may prove to be an effective forum for developing long-term, multi-institutional strategies for addressing any unmet needs that result from this change.

Throughout its history, Genesee County's public health system has proven to be a dynamic constellation of organizations and individuals that has adapted to the changing community health needs and resources within the jurisdiction. The local health department has played a major role in guiding this adaptation. In light of this history, the system's prospects for addressing current and future public health challenges appear promising.

References

1. US Health Resources and Services Administration. *Area Resource File 1994*. Washington, DC: US Department of Health and Human Services; 1996.
2. National Association of County Health Officials. *Blueprint for a Healthy Community: A Guide for Local Health Departments*. Washington, DC: National Association of County Health Officials; 1994.
3. Gordon RL, Gerzoff RB, Richards TB. Determinants of local health department expenditures, 1992 through 1993. *Am J Public Health*. 1997; 7(1):91-95.
4. Pestronk RM. Local health department/hospital collaboration. *Michigan Association of Local Public Health Officials Annual Conference*. Lansing, MI: August 4, 1993.
5. Hannan EL, Racz M, Ryan TJ, et al. Coronary angioplasty volume-outcome relationships for hospitals and cardiologists. *JAMA*. 1997:277(11): 892-898.
6. Jarhult J. The importance of volume for outcome in cancer surgery—an overview. *Eur J Surg Oncol*. 1996;22(3):205-210.

Chapter 12

Case Study of Memphis and Shelby County, Tennessee

Key Attributes

- Continued involvement in comprehensive primary care delivery by local public health department clinics.
- Contractual agreements between the local health department and managed care plans for serving Medicaid beneficiaries.
- Collaborative and competitive relationships with local hospitals.
- Growing capacities in community health assessment, planning, and policy development.

Community Characteristics

Demographic and Socioeconomic Characteristics

Memphis and Shelby County encompass a population of more than 800,000 residents along Tennessee's western border with the Mississippi River. The densely-populated area is racially diverse, with African Americans comprising 44% of the population.[1] Despite steady economic improvements over the last 5 years, many residents of Memphis' urban core remain in poverty. More than 18% of the total population live below the federal poverty threshold. Educational attainment is low among some population groups, with nearly one-quarter of the total adult population having completed less than 12 years of school. Less than 25% of the adult population in Memphis and Shelby County have completed at least four years of college (**Table 1**).

Community Health Status Indicators

The dominant community health problems facing Memphis and Shelby County largely reflect the economic and social conditions of poverty. Out of wedlock births have begun to decline in the community, but they still comprised 50% of all births and 73% of births to minority women during 1995.[1] More than 19% of births to Memphis residents were to women age 10-17 years. Approximately 10.5% of all resident births were low birth weight, and infant mortality stood at 14.4 per 1000 live births. Like many communities, heart disease, cancer, and cerebrovascular disease top the list of leading causes of death. Other leading causes of death include accidents (fifth), homicides (eighth), and HIV / AIDS (tenth) (**Table 2**).

Local Health Resources and Manpower

A diverse collection of public and private health resources exists across Memphis and Shelby County (**Table 3**). Local hospital resources include six general acute-care facilities, two children's hospitals (one general acute-care facility and one specialty

Table 1
Demographic Characteristics: Shelby County, Tennessee

Population (1990)	826,330
Median age in years	31.5
Percent 65 years and older (1990)	6.1
Percent non-White (1990)	44.9
Percent speaking a language other than English at home (1990)	3.9
Percent completing high school degree (1990)	75.1
Percent of individuals below federal poverty level (1989)	18.3
Median household income (1989)	$27,132
Average percent unemployed (1991)	5.4

Data from US Department of Commerce, Bureau of the Census.

Table 2
Health Status Indicators: Shelby County, Tennessee

Infant mortality rate per 1000 live births (1996)	12.3
Percent of births to mothers age 10-17	7.9
Percent of infants with low birth weight	10.7
Percent of births with prenatal care later than first trimester	20,8
Deaths per 100,000 population, age-adjusted (1996)	633
Cancer, all types	147
Lung cancer	45
Female breast cancer	23
Heart disease	179
Cerebrovascular diseases	44
Chronic obstructive pulmonary diseases	21
Motor vehicle accidents	23
Suicide	10
Pneumonia and influenza	21
HIV/AIDS	4
Diabetes mellitus	16
Homicide	23

Data from Tennessee Department of Health (unpublished data), 1997.

facility), and a Veteran's Affairs medical center. The county-affiliated hospital, Regional Medical Center, provides the majority of indigent care in the community. Two private nonprofit hospitals, Methodist Hospital and Baptist Hospital, dominate the commercial market for inpatient and specialty services. St. Francis Hospital, a facility formerly affiliated with the Catholic Church and currently owned by the one of the nation's largest for-profit hospital systems, stands as the area's fourth largest hospital in terms of market share. St. Joseph Hospital exists as the single remaining Catholic hospital in the area and primarily serves the elderly population in inner-city Memphis.

The managed care market in Memphis and Shelby County has grown rapidly in recent years, spurred by the 1994 implementation of TennCare, the statewide managed care program for Medicaid beneficiaries and the uninsured. The commercial managed care market is dominated by health plans operated by established insurance corporations such as CIGNA, Prudential, and the state's two Blue Cross and Blue Shield associations. The Medicaid market created by TennCare, however, consists largely of a collection of newly formed plans and small affiliates of out-of-state plans. Only lately have plans such as Prudential and Blue Cross begun to participate in this market. Currently a total of seven plans serve the almost 300,000 TennCare beneficiaries in Memphis, including one sponsored jointly by the county hospital and a faculty practice plan of the University of Tennessee at Memphis medical school.

A total of 2841 nonfederal physicians practice in Shelby County, creating ratio of 337 physicians per 100,000 population. Approximately 40% of these physicians practice in the primary care disciplines of general practice, family practice, general internal medicine, obstetrics/gynecology, and pediatrics. Nevertheless, many low-income and minority neighborhoods lack sufficient access to primary care providers due to the mal-distribution of physicians within Memphis. Three federally funded health centers and two additional, locally supported centers help to fill the gaps in access by providing services to uninsured and underinsured populations of Memphis. In addition, the Memphis-Shelby County Health Department operates six full-time primary health care centers and eight part-time specialty clinics at various community locations. Services provided through these clinics include well child care, sick child care, prenatal care, acute and chronic disease care for adults, dental care for children, nutritional education and counseling, and family planning services.

The Local Health Department

The Memphis and Shelby County Health Department maintains a long history as a comprehensive

Table 3
Health Resources: Shelby County, Tennessee

Number of nonfederal physicians (Number per 100,000 population) 1992[a]	2841 (337)
Family practice	149 (18)
General practice	56 (7)
Internal medicine	511 (61)
Obstetrics/gynecology	184 (22)
Pediatrics	239 (28)
Number of community hospital beds (FY1995)[b]	4650
Beds per 100,000 population	552
Number of community hospitals (FY1995)[b]	8
Number of HMOs (1994)[c]	8
Number of federally qualified health centers (1994)[e]	3
Total number of clinic sites	4
Local public health expenditures (FY1992)[d]	$29,000,000
Percent from direct federal sources	1%
Percent from state sources (including federal pass-throughs)	27%
Percent from local sources	40%
Percent from Medicaid	13%
Percent from Medicare	1%
Total federal funding for community health centers (1996)[f]	$2,551,260
Total federal funding for migrant health centers (1996)[f]	0
Total federal block grant funds for preventive health services (1996)[f]	0
Total federal block grant funds for maternal and child health services (1996)[f]	0
Total federal block grant funds for substance abuse services (1996)[f]	$3,459,138
Total federal funding for homeless health services (1996)[f]	0
Total federal funding for National Health Service Corporation (1996)[f]	0

[a]*Data from American Medical Association Physician Masterfile.*[2]
[b]*Data from American Hospital Association.*[3]
[c]*Data from Group Health Association of America.*[4]
[d]*Data from Bureau of Primary Health Care (unpublished data, 1994).*
[e]*Data from National Association of County and City Health Officials.*[5]
[f]*Data from US Department of Commerce.*[6]

provider of both clinical and population-based public health services. Rather than scaling down its involvement in clinical services provision under the TennCare program, the department chose to remain an active primary care provider by developing contracts with the managed care plans participating in this program. This strategy, which has been examined in detail elsewhere,[7] enabled the department to retain a leading role in assuring access to health care for vulnerable and underserved populations, while also performing a continuum of population-based public health activities for the community at large. The department has relied heavily on this strategy in pursuing its stated mission of "providing an effective and efficient health care system that offers available, accessible, and affordable health care to all citizens of Shelby County."[8]

Organizational Structure

The local health department receives its funding and administration jointly from the City of Memphis and the County of Shelby. The county government assumes direct responsibility for overseeing the activities of the health department and approving its budget. A full-time health director serves as the administrative head of the health department and is appointed by the county mayor and approved by the 13-member board of county commissioners. The department does not operate under a separate board of health; rather, a five-member committee of the board of county commissioners provides oversight for the department. In keeping with Tennessee state law, the department is also served by a physician-trained medical officer who is appointed by the mayor and reports directly to the health director. The health department also maintains regular contact with the city mayor and city council, although these officials typically do not exercise direct administrative control over the health department.

Yvonne S. Madlock began her tenure as the health director in 1997, after serving almost 4 years as director of the department's division of personal health services. Ms. Madlock assumed the directorship from Hugh Barnes, a popular 12-year veteran of the department who managed the organization through the early years of the state's Medicaid managed care program. Ms. Madlock acquired an extensive knowledge of Memphis' public health issues through her work in managing several local community health centers before joining the health department in 1993.

John D. Kirkley, MD, has served as the health department's health officer on an interim basis since 1995. Dr. Kirkley's 14-year history with the health department began soon after he discontinued work as a private practice obstetrician / gynecologist in 1980. Dr. Kirkley worked in several of the local community health centers over the past two decades and developed a strong working relationship with health director Ms. Madlock even before her tenure began at the health department. Dr. Kirkley has served as interim health officer since Dr. Sherman Kahn, another popular public health practitioner, departed the health officer position to assume a local health directorship in a neighboring state. The local health department has experienced substantial difficulty in finding a suitable permanent replacement for Drs. Kahn and Kirkley, given their unique knowledge and skills in public health practice within Shelby County.

The health department is organized into four basic operational units. The largest of these units in terms of staffing and budget is the bureau of personal health services, which administers all clinic-based and community-based clinical services. Within this bureau, an office of clinical services manages the operations of the department's six full-service primary care clinics and eight specialty clinics. An office of community health services administers community health nursing and health promotion programs, as well as the department's two school-based health clinics. An infectious disease office operates programs that target tuberculosis control, sexually transmitted disease and HIV prevention and control, and epidemiological investigation. A second major operational unit within the health department houses environmental health activities. This division includes offices for environmental sanitation and inspection, vector control, and pollution control. A third division headed by the health officer administers professional and technical support activities involving the department's pharmacy, laboratory, and physician services. The health officer provides clinical oversight and quality assurance for these professional services. Finally, an administrative services division houses the department's activities in vital records collection and management, billing, and contract and grant processing. This division also maintains the department's clinical and administrative information systems. Additionally, the health department maintains a regional forensics center, a public relations office, and a human resources office that stand independent of these four operational divisions.

Overview of Programs and Services

Clinic-based Services

The health department operates a comprehensive array of personal health services that ranges from routine primary care to specialized disease control services. Comprehensive primary care services are delivered through the department's network of six full-time and eight part-time health clinics located in medically underserved areas of the jurisdiction. Clinics provide well and sick child care, prenatal care, dental care for children, adult health services for the treatment of acute and chronic diseases, nutrition education and counseling services, and family planning services. One of the part-time clinics operates as an after-hours pediatric clinic. Clinics are staffed by teams of pediatricians and family practice physicians, nurse practitioners, public health nurses, social workers, and nutritionists. During calendar year 1994 the full-time clinics provided 153,000 patient visits, and part-time clinics provided an additional 142,000 visits.

In addition to these comprehensive clinics, the department operates several additional clinics that provide targeted personal health services. A sexually transmitted disease clinic located within one of the comprehensive clinics provides confidential testing, diagnosis, treatment, education, and partner notification services. The department also operates four community-based clinics for confidential HIV testing and counseling services. Tennessee state law no longer provides for anonymous testing services.

The department's two full-time school-based health centers provide routine primary care as well as family planning and health education services to students in two public junior high schools. These clinics, which are staffed by teams of public health nurses, nurse practitioners, and social workers, provide more than 6000 visits annually to 1100 adolescents and 160 of their children. Additionally, the health department maintains a staff of 11 part-time school health nurses to serve in 40 public schools on a rotating basis, providing health education services as well as a limited range of screening and primary care services.

The health department operates three targeted childhood immunization clinics in addition to the services provided through the comprehensive primary care clinics. These clinics administer more than 15,000 immunizations annually. Additionally, the department operates seasonal clinics for pneumonia and influenza vaccinations, as well as a part-time vaccination clinic that administers vaccines required for international travel.

Other specialty clinics operated by the health department include the following: a tuberculosis control clinic that provides screening, diagnosis, and treatment services for the disease; an employee health clinic designed to address occupational health and general health issues among city and county employees; and several clinics offering nutritional counseling and support services under the federal Special Supplemental Nutrition Program for Women, Infants, and Children. The health department also administers a program for providing medical care services to disabled and chronically ill children through its existing network of health clinics. Clinic physicians and nurses provide all primary care services and arrange for any specialty services, drugs, medical equipment, and hospital services that may be required. Approximately 2500 children are served through this program annually.

Community-based Services

The health department provides an array of home and community-based services through its community health nursing and health promotion programs. The department's community health nursing program provides in-home outreach, education, case management, and clinical follow-up to high-risk pregnant women, infants, children, and adults. This program also provides outreach to homeless individuals, families experiencing sudden infant death syndrome, and participants in the health department's program for disabled and chronically ill children. The program receives referrals from area hospitals, clinics, private providers, and other community agencies. More than 3000 home visits are provided through this program annually.

The health department's health promotion program sponsors public awareness campaigns, workshops, and seminars on a variety of wellness and disease prevention topics. Smoking cessation classes, mammography awareness campaigns, physical activity classes, and blood pressure screening fairs are some of the most common interventions implemented through this program. An active child car seat loan program is also operated through this office.

Environmental Health Services

The local health department's environmental health division maintains responsibility for assuring the safety of food service establishments, hotels and motels, swimming pools, personal care homes, day care centers, public institutions, rural sewage disposal facilities, barber shops, and mobile home parks. The division conducts periodic inspections of these facilities, provides education and training to their owners and operators, and carries out enforcement activities. This division also has responsibility for investigating and resolving lead hazards, rodent infestations, food-borne illness outbreaks, and vector and animal control problems. Finally, the environmental health division operates a pollution control program with monitoring and enforcement activities for both air and groundwater protection. Through this program, the division monitors ambient air quality, investigates complaints of air pollution and dust, inspects industries that emit regulated air and water pollutants, and monitors asbestos removal projects and open burning sites.

Infrastructure and Resources

The department maintains a central office and clinic in downtown Memphis that serves as the administrative hub for its public health programs and services. In addition, the department maintains a network of five full time satellite clinic sites, eight part-time clinic sites, and two additional school-based clinic sites. Other major capital resources include a full-service public health laboratory, and an environmental health field office.

Human resources for the department total almost 800 employees, representing 753 full-time equivalent positions. These staff include 11 physicians, 15 nurse practitioners, 90 public health nurses, two dentists, nine social workers, and two epidemiologists.

An annual budget of approximately $29 million sustains the programs and services operated by the Memphis-Shelby County health department. The largest share of these funds are derived from local sources, with the county contributing 23% of the funds and the city contributing 17%. State funding sources are also important, accounting for ~27% of the department's annual revenue when federal pass-through grants are included. Direct federal grants amount to only 1% of the department's budget. Medicaid payments comprise ~13% of the department's revenue, while Medicare payments account for 1% of revenue. The remaining 19% of funds are derived from private grants and fees.

Tennessee's move to mandatory managed care enrollment for Medicaid beneficiaries in 1994 does not appear to have substantially affected the patient care revenues received by the health department. The health department has successfully developed service contracts with most of the managed care plans that serve Medicaid beneficiaries in Shelby County and thereby retained much of its Medicaid revenue. These contracts have actually created opportunities for the health department to expand its patient care revenue under the capitated payment arrangements used by managed care plans. These arrangements allow the department to assume financial responsibility for managing all primary care services needed by patients who are enrolled in managed care plans, and to retain any payments in excess of costs for these patients. Some of these contracts also allow the department to earn payment bonuses for reducing the need for emergency room visits and other specialty medical services among managed care enrollees.

Other Contributors to the Public Health System

State Health Agency

The Tennessee Department of Health administers an array of state programs involving both public health and personal health care for vulnerable and underserved populations. The largest program administered by the department is TennCare, the statewide managed care program initiated in 1994 for Medicaid beneficiaries and other eligible individuals who lack private health insurance coverage. Statewide, ~800,000 Medicaid beneficiaries and 400,000 uninsured / uninsurable persons receive health care coverage through this program. In Shelby County, this program serves 180,000 Medicaid beneficiaries and another 56,000 uninsured / uninsurable persons.

The state health agency also administers grants to support the provision of public health services by local health departments. These grants support childhood and adult immunization services; family planning services; sexually transmitted disease treatment and control; tuberculosis screening, diagnosis, and treatment; TennCare eligibility screening and outreach services; services for children with special medical care needs; and general environmental health services. Many of these grants derive from federal pass-through funds administered by the state. Additional public health activities carried out by state health agency include the following: licensing health care facilities and professionals, administering funding for alcohol and drug abuse services, operating a central public health laboratory, and maintaining outreach programs for special populations.

Interaction between the state health agency and the Memphis-Shelby County health department involves funding, technical assistance, and shared program administration. The local health department depends heavily on state grants for funding many of its categorical public health programs. Moreover, the state health agency provides advice and technical assistance to the local health department and to other community health organizations regarding issues of program design, planning, and evaluation. Often, this assistance is provided through regional planning and policy development groups that are convened by the state health agency around issues such as minority health, environmental health, and health care accessibility. Some local public health activities are jointly administered by the state health agency and the local health department. For example, the agencies jointly operate and staff Shelby County's public health laboratory, allowing the facility to serve both as a local public health resource and as a branch of the state's laboratory system. Other programs such as restaurant inspection, environmental health monitoring, and vital records collection are carried out by the local health department under state authority.

State-local interaction also occurs through special intergovernmental entities known as community health agencies, which were created by special state legislation in the early 1990s. These agencies were created to plan and develop coordinated local systems for primary care delivery by bringing together the many community organizations involved in these activities. Each region of the state is served by one of these agencies, with Memphis and Shelby County constituting one such region. The Memphis and Shelby County Community Health Agency operates under state authority and with state funding that is administered by the Shelby County government. Representatives from the local health department, local hospitals, community health centers, local medical societies, and other community agencies serve on the governing board for the agency. The agency leads community health assessment and surveillance efforts within the county, conducts community-wide planning and priority-setting initiatives, and implements community health interventions within the county that target health issues not adequately addressed by individual community organizations.

Much of the agency's work to date has focused on documenting the needs of medically underserved populations within the county and developing interorganizational strategies to serve these populations. As part of this effort, the agency has fielded a survey of community health providers and clients within the county and developed an innovative transportation program that serves local beneficiaries of the TennCare program. Managed care plans contract on an individual basis with the community health agency to provide transportation services for their members.

Hospitals

The hospitals serving Memphis and Shelby County make important but varied contributions to the local public health system. The Regional Medical Center at Memphis, commonly referred to as The Med, has historically provided the bulk of health services for vulnerable and underserved populations in the community. As a county-affiliated facility, the Med provides access to health services regardless of insurance status or ability to pay. Historically operated by the city of Memphis, The Med is now organized as a nonprofit corporation with a governing board that is appointed by the Shelby County mayor. As the only hospital located in inner-city Memphis, The Med has historically faced a large demand for care from Medicaid beneficiaries and from the uninsured. Shelby County provides annual grants to the hospital to help finance its uncompensated care burden.

The Med consists of a 321-bed hospital, an array of 40 specialty outpatient clinics, and a network of community-based primary care clinics. The Med's hospital and clinics are staffed by ~500 faculty and residents at the University of Tennessee at Memphis medical school. The Med also jointly operates a managed care plan that serves TennCare beneficiaries in collaboration with the University of Tennessee faculty practice. During 1997, the hospital handled almost 22,000 admissions, 93,000 outpatient visits, and 79,000 emergency department visits. The jointly operated managed care plan served ~51,000 TennCare members during this same period.

The Med plays important roles in assuring access to primary care and preventive health services in addition to its roles in acute care and specialty services. In carrying out these roles, The Med works closely with the local health department. For example, The Med and the health department jointly operate a program to screen hospital patients for eligibility in the federal Supplemental Food Program for Women, Infants, and Children. Under this program, the hospital provides the nutritionists and clerical staff necessary to perform eligibility certification, while the health department administers the process of enrolling eligible patients in the program.

The Med also works closely with the health department in providing access to primary care services for vulnerable populations. For example, the two organizations joined with the local children's hospital and medical school to launch a new community health center in an area of Memphis that previously lacked geographic access to primary care services. All four organizations contributed financial resources and clinical staff to the center and assisted the center in securing external funding for ongoing operations. The Med has also worked collaboratively with the health department in siting its own community-based primary care clinics in areas of the county having the greatest need for services.

Additionally, the Med and the local health department have historically maintained a joint referral program for managing chronic diseases among vulnerable and underserved adults. Under this arrangement, health department physicians treating patients with chronic diseases could secure consultations and referrals from specialty physicians operating at The Med's outpatient clinics. Similarly, The Med physicians could refer patients to health department clinics for routine management and follow-up of chronic disease treatment. Historically, the physicians at the two organizations have worked closely to deliver seamless disease management services for patients who are unable to obtain needed care from private providers. This arrangement deteriorated somewhat with the 1994 implementation of the TennCare program for Medicaid beneficiaries and other medically indigent residents. TennCare imposed restrictions on the referral activity between The Med and the local health department, because patients covered under TennCare must follow the referral requirements established by their health plans. Patients treated at health department clinics can be referred to The Med only if their managed care plan maintains a contract with this hospital. Likewise, physicians at The Med can make health department referrals only for patients enrolled in plans that include health department clinics in their provider networks.

To help address this problem, the local health department participates on the provider network of The Med's jointly owned managed care plan, known as TLC Health Plan. Under this arrangement, TennCare members enrolled in TLC receive access to clinics operated by The Med and those operated by the health department. However, both The Med and the local health department contract with other managed care plans—some of which place restrictions on referrals to one or the other institution. The two organizations are now developing a joint contracting strategy that would encourage managed care plans to establish a single contract with both The Med and the health department. This integrated delivery approach would preserve the ability of the two organizations to coordinate their clinical service delivery activities.

Independent of its relationship with the local health department, The Med operates an array of health education and wellness programs that target broad segments of the community. First, the hospital conducts a series of ongoing wellness workshops and health screening programs at area community centers and senior centers within the county. Appropriate individuals are referred to these community programs by hospital discharge planners, outpatient clinic physicians, and emergency room staff. Additionally, the hospital operates a weekly radio show on health promotion that aims to raise awareness about basic health promotion and disease prevention practices, as well as available community services. Finally, the hospital operates several school-based health initiatives to address the health needs of children and adolescents in the community. In one initiative, the hospital sends a team of nurses to a local elementary school each month to conduct a health education program. As part of this program, the hospital also provides periodic dental screenings for children. In another initiative, the hospital operates a program for pregnant and parenting teens at an area high school. This program provides case management services to assure the delivery of prenatal care and well child services, as well as to encourage appropriate parenting skills among young parents. The program is designed to improve birth outcomes and child health, as well as to support the efforts of young parents to continue their education.

Administrators at The Med indicate that these types of community health activities have become increasingly difficult for the hospital to maintain over the last few years owing to a steadily declining revenue base. Some activities, such as a program for training and supporting church-based lay health advisors, have been discontinued or curtailed in recent years owing to revenue shortfalls. The Med has steadily lost its Medicaid patient base since the launch of TennCare in 1994, largely because the program offers these patients more choices for hospitals and physicians through participating managed care plans.[9] The state also eliminated the hospital's direct subsidy for graduate medical education, further constraining the organization's budget. As a result of these changes, the hospital has been forced to cut back on some of its independently financed community health initiatives and to rely more heavily on collaborative efforts such as those maintained with the local health department.

Other local hospitals make important contributions to community health in Memphis as well. The two largest private hospital systems, Methodist Healthcare and Baptist Memorial Healthcare System, are actively involved in community health planning and priority-setting activities through the state-sponsored Memphis and Shelby County Community Health Agency. Both organizations are represented on the governing board of this agency. Both hospitals are also important supporters of one of the area's community health centers, the Church Health Center, by contributing financial assistance, donated supplies and equipment, and volunteer clinical labor. These organizations work closely with the local health department and other area hospitals in supporting this center.

Methodist Healthcare has experienced a growing need for involvement in community health issues as a result of its increasing market share among TennCare recipients. Methodist's contracts with managed care plans and its proximity to several underserved areas within Memphis have allowed the hospital to assume a growing role in serving the often vulnerable and underserved beneficiaries of TennCare. Two of the 12 hospitals included in the Methodist system are located in central city areas of Memphis. To better serve this population, the hospital has initiated several community-based programs aimed at promoting health and preventing disease. One of these programs is a community-level outreach and education intervention designed to improve birth outcomes by expanding the uptake of prenatal care services in several underserved communities. Another program involves a community health educational intervention aimed at preventing and controlling sexually transmitted diseases—a growing source of emergency room visits for the hospital. As yet another community-level intervention, the hospital is currently working with the local health department to develop a jointly operated primary care clinic in one of Memphis' medically underserved areas. These community health interventions serve as strategies for reducing costs and improving health status among the populations served by Methodist.

Memphis' last remaining Catholic hospital system, Saint Joseph's Hospital, has developed a growing focus on the community health needs of the geriatric population over the past decade. Having discontinued its obstetrics and pediatrics programs in the early 1990s, the hospital serves a combined Medicare and Medicaid patient base that comprises 90% of its service population. Consequently, the hospital has become active in sustaining health promotion and disease prevention programs targeted at the aging inner-city residents of Memphis. In partnership with a local senior services agency, the hospital operates a health education program that addresses topics such as nutrition, physical activity, chronic disease management, and medications management with groups of seniors in the community. The hospital is also a primary partner in an effort to develop a new senior health and human services center offering information and referral services as well as health screening services for seniors. This effort is also being sustained in collaboration with local senior services organizations. In a third effort, Saint Joseph's is collaborating with another local hospital (Saint Francis) and the catholic diocese in Memphis to develop a church-based community nursing program. Through this project, part-time community health nurses based in several local churches will provide an array of health services to the larger community, including health education and outreach services, health assessments and screening services, and periodic home visitation services. Like The Med, St. Joseph's faces difficulties in sustaining some of its community health initiatives in the wake of TennCare, which has reduced revenues and patient demand somewhat since 1994.

Saint Francis Hospital is also involved in an array of community health initiatives, including the church-based nursing program operated jointly with Saint Joseph's. Although historically affiliated with the Catholic church and operated jointly with Saint Joseph's, Saint Francis is now owned and managed by the for-profit hospital chain Tenet Healthcare. Under its agreement with the local Catholic diocese, Tenet maintains many of the hospital's community service activities, including its long tradition of providing health screening and wellness services within the community. The hospital operates two mobile health clinics that travel to local community centers and work sites and offer screening and educational services to area residents. Administrators concede that this activity serves as much as a marketing devise for the hospital as it does a preventive health intervention for the community. Such dual-purpose activities are increasingly important for the hospital, as its market share (12%) lags far behind Baptist (32%), Methodist (27%), and The Med (20%). With the initiation of TennCare, the hospital is serving growing numbers of Medicaid beneficiaries and previously uninsured patients (a 50% increase since 1994), creating additional pressures for involvement in community health activities. The hospital now operates a transportation service to assist these patients in accessing hospital services, which are located in a suburban area of Memphis. The hospital is also actively working to increase its capacity to deliver primary care services to these patients, through the acquisition of primary care physician practices within the community.

Memphis is also served by a major not-for-profit children's hospital, LeBonheur Health Systems, which contributes substantially to the local public health system. As a major provider of care to Medicaid beneficiaries and other traditionally underserved populations, the hospital jointly operates a pediatric primary care evening clinic together with the local health department. This clinic helps to reduce emergency room volume at the hospital and to increase the delivery of preventive health services within the community—such as childhood immunizations, lead poisoning screenings, and childhood developmental examinations. Similarly, LeBonheur helped establish the Church Health Center in partnership with the local health department and several other organizations. This center provides comprehensive primary care services to both adults and children in one of Memphis' underserved communities. The hospital also operates a child abuse and violence prevention center that provides treatment, case management, and prevention activities in collaboration with local social services and law enforcement agencies. A poison control and drug information center maintained by the hospital provides treatment as well as preventive interventions, in collaboration with the University of Tennessee at Memphis medical school. The hospital also operates an array of public education and awareness campaigns around injury prevention, including a "Safe Kids" campaign that engages numerous community organizations in publicizing child safety strategies. As part of this program, the hospital administers a number of "mini-grants" each year to community organizations involved in developing and testing injury prevention programs. Finally, LeBonheur is an important contributor to the community health assessment and planning activities that take place through the state-sponsored Community Health Agency. Representatives from the hospital serve on the governing board for this agency.

Managed Care Plans

Memphis and Shelby County are served by both large commercial health plans and smaller plans that have developed primarily to serve the state's TennCare beneficiaries. Most of the commercial plans do not to participate in the TennCare program, with the notable exceptions of Prudential and the state's Blue Cross plans. Those plans that do not participate in TennCare maintain little if any direct contact with the local health department and the local public health system. These plans, such as the local United Healthcare affiliate known as Complete Health, suggest that their primary contributions to the local public health system derive from their influence on local clinical practice. Complete Health contracts with large numbers of the community physicians that serve Memphis and Shelby County, and it maintains systems for monitoring and encouraging the delivery of clinical preventive services by these physicians. These systems include routine provider feedback reports on topics such as immunization delivery and mammography; as well as physician education and guideline initiatives that inform providers about the most effective clinical practices.

Plans that participate in the TennCare program generally maintain a more direct involvement in the local public health system. To begin with, many of these plans contract with local public health providers—including the local health department and area community health centers—to provide and manage primary care and preventive services for their TennCare members. To date, the department holds contracts with five of the seven managed care plans that are licensed to enroll TennCare beneficiaries in Shelby County. Under the contracting arrangements, the health department provides both case management and primary care services to TennCare enrollees who choose the health department as their primary care provider (PCP). The health department receives a capitated per member per month payment for each enrollee who selects the health department as their PCP. In exchange for this fee, the health department agrees to provide all medically necessary primary care services. Physicians and advanced practice nurses at the department's six full-time primary care clinics deliver these services. Enrollees that have access to Memphis' school-based clinics may also receive services at these sites.

Health department physician do not follow their patients in the hospital when inpatient care is needed. Rather, the health department maintains subcontracting arrangements with private physicians that have admitting privileges at the hospitals affiliated with the enrollee's managed care plan. Subcontracting physicians serve as links between the health department physicians and the hospitals. Health department physicians decide whether inpatient care is needed for their patients, but they often consult with the subcontracting physicians for difficult and unclear cases.

The health department receives capitated per-member per-month payments for managing the delivery of primary care services to managed care enrollees. These payment arrangements create clear financial incentives for delivering care efficiently and effectively so that unnecessary care and avoidable health conditions are minimized. The health department assumes a measure of financial risk for health plan enrollees who choose the department as their PCP, because it must meet the costs of providing all necessary primary care services, even if these costs exceed the monthly capitation fees paid by the managed care plans. Health department staff reports that their organization's experience working within constrained governmental budgets and in providing preventive care allow the department to operate successfully under managed care. Staff suggests that their public health clinics have long faced a necessity for efficiency under the often limited governmental appropriations for public health services. These clinics have also amassed substantial expertise in providing and encouraging the utilization of disease prevention and health promotion services. This expertise ranges from encouraging pregnant women to utilize timely prenatal care to providing health education to clients and community members in areas such as nutrition, family planning, and sexually transmitted disease control. The department's extensive capacity for community outreach reinforces its ability to act as an efficient and effective primary care case manager under managed care systems.

The health department benefits financially from its ability to operate as an efficient and effective case manager for TennCare health plans. Several plans withhold a portion of their revenues as "bonus pools" to be distributed to health care providers that demonstrate effectiveness and efficiency in managing services needed by their patients. At the end of each quarter, funds remaining in the bonus pools are disbursed to providers based on their performance in care management. In this way, even though the health department is not capitated or "at-risk" for hospital services, the department still receives financial rewards for efficiently managing use of services in these settings. The health department has received substantial bonus payments from TennCare HMOs stemming from their success in managing services such as emergency room utilization and hospital inpatient stays.

To improve its ability to function as an effective primary care case manager, the local health department has made substantial improvements to its patient tracking and billing systems. Building the necessary information systems required substantial effort to secure the necessary funding, space, and operational expertise for these new systems. The department reports that its investment of time and resources has paid off in an enhanced ability to monitor the care received by patients and to interface easily with multiple managed care plans.

Some of the managed care plans serving Memphis make important public health contributions that extend beyond their formal relationships with the local health department. For example, several TennCare managed care plans have developed specialized interventions designed to improve health among the vulnerable populations that they serve. TLC Health Plan, which is operated jointly by The Med and the local medical school, operates a enrollee incentive program for encouraging pregnant women to utilize timely prenatal care visits. Under the program, enrollees that maintain timely prenatal visits receive special gifts such as grocery coupons and infant care products. The plan also maintains an active patient education program designed to inform enrollees about health promotion and disease prevention practices and about how to access services within the health plan. Finally, the plan is in the process of designing an in-home nurse visitation program for new parents, to be financed with the savings anticipated from shorter patient stays in the newborn nursery. The HMO is hopeful that such a strategy will improve perinatal health outcomes by providing better education and training to new parents.

The local affiliate of Prudential Health Plans has also implemented several innovative initiatives for assuring access to care for vulnerable populations within TennCare. First, the plan has initiated an extensive research initiative to identify barriers to prenatal care among its TennCare members, drawing on the expertise of Prudential's national Center for Health Care Research in Atlanta, Georgia. The plan has assembled an array of other community organizations to contribute to the study, including local churches, a parenting center, community health centers, and the local and state health department. This study promises to inform clinical practice not only at Prudential but at many other health plans that serve vulnerable and traditionally underserved populations.

Prudential also uses an array of patient interventions designed to enhance health care accessibility and effectiveness for vulnerable populations. For example, the plan employs social workers at each of its clinic sites to provide case management, information, and counseling to members regarding health and social support needs. The plan also operates an innovative health assessment program that sends self-administered health assessment kits to each new member, along with an incentive for returning the assessment. This program allows the plan to collect baseline health measures that are used to identify health risks and inform care management. This program also allows the plan to collect current member contact information that is not available from the state TennCare agency, so that telephone contact and follow-up programs can be initiated where needed. Prudential also uses automated physician and patient reminder systems for scheduled immunizations, well child examinations (the federal Early and Periodic Screening, Diagnosis, and Treatment program), mammograms, and pap smears.

Community Health Centers

In addition to the clinics operated by the local health department, Memphis and Shelby County are served by a network of nonprofit health centers that provide access to primary care, preventive health services, and social support services in medically underserved areas. Five centers operate seven different clinic sites within the area. Three of these centers receive federal funds through the Bureau of Primary Health Care for operating as comprehensive primary health care centers. One of the nonfunded centers, the Church Health Center, operates primarily with volunteer staffing and the support of the local health department, hospitals, and the medical school. The other nonfunded center maintains a primary affiliation with The Med.

All of the health centers maintain close working relationships with the local health department. Informal agreements allow the centers to make referrals and share supplies and staff. The health department formally contracts with some of these centers for providing categorical public health services such as sexually transmitted disease control and family planning. All of the health centers also maintain service contracts with managed care plans for serving TennCare beneficiaries. Unlike some other communities, there is little evidence that relationships among the health centers and the local health department are strained by competition for managed care contracts and patients. Close working relationships among the centers before TennCare implementation appear to have forestalled such problems.

Other Organizations

The University of Tennessee at Memphis' medical school and faculty practice is clearly a major contributor and catalyst for local public health activities. The local health department interacts frequently with the university regarding activities such as referral arrangements between health department clinics and faculty medical specialists, joint sponsorship of community health centers, and evaluations of local public health interventions. The university also maintains close affiliations with area hospitals such as The Med and LeBonheur children's hospital, contributing to the community health initiatives maintained by these organizations.

The local health department maintains cooperative relationships with the local medical community, primarily through the department's health officer. The local medical society is accommodative to local public health initiatives, but it does not appear to play active roles in initiating or sustaining such initiatives beyond contributing to local planning and policy development processes. The department's relationships with individual members of the local medical community have grown closer in recent years under the TennCare program. In serving the enrollees of private managed care plans, the health department has developed strong relationships with the private physicians that participate in these health plan networks.

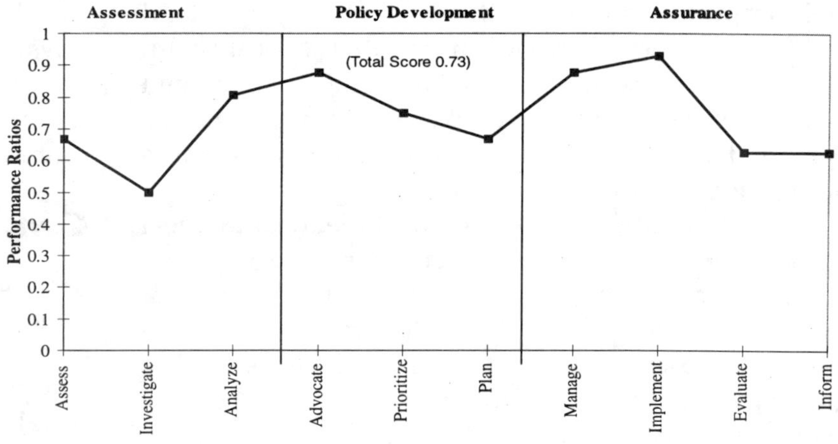

Figure 1. Public health performance scores for Memphis-Shelby County, 1993.

Local chapters of voluntary health associations such as the American Heart Association and the American Cancer Society sponsor an array of public awareness campaigns and health fairs on a periodic basis in collaboration with the health department, local hospitals, and other organizations. The local chapter of the United Way is active in funding community health and human service projects within Shelby County, and a local health department representative serves on the board of directors for this chapter. Local churches also maintain a tradition of involvement in community health issues ranging from chronic disease prevention to domestic and community violence prevention. An association of religious organizations known as the Metropolitan Interfaith Association uses funding from the United Way and member organizations to provide health and social support services for disadvantaged populations. The association funds a full-time nurse to address health issues among the homeless population, and it operates a transportation network to enhance access to community services. A local foundation known as the Community Foundation of Memphis also provides funding for grass-roots health and human services projects that benefit the population of Memphis. Numerous other community organizations are involved in education, counseling, and advocacy activities around community health issues.

Measures of Local Public Health System Performance

Results of the Local Public Health Performance Assessment Survey

Total public health performance within the Memphis-Shelby County jurisdiction appears higher than many other public health jurisdictions under study, based on reports from the local health department director during 1993. Results from the 81-indicator *Local Public Health Performance Assessment Survey* (see Appendix A) indicate the jurisdiction performs at 73% of the maximum possible level (**Figure 1**). This score is substantially higher than the median score of 51% found among a selection of 63 local public health jurisdictions during 1992-1993. Performance scores appear highest for the core public health function of *assurance* and lowest for the function of *assessment*. Among the set of ten public health practices, performance appears highest for the practices of *implementing policies and plans to address health needs, managing community health resources,* and *advocating for public health needs*. Performance appears lowest for the practices of *investigating health threats, evaluating public health programs and services,* and *informing and educating the public*.

When only the contributions of the local health department are considered, public health performance still appears above average for the health departments included in this study (**Figure 2**). The Memphis-Shelby County health department performance score of 58% substantially exceeds the median score of 39% found among the selection of departments studied during 1992-1993. When this score is expressed as a proportion of the total community score, it appears that the local health department contributes ~79% of the total public health effort expended within the jurisdiction. This share of total effort is substantially higher than those observed for other health departments under study. Health department performance appears highest for the public health practices of *implementing policies and plans to address health needs, advocating for public health needs,* and *analyzing data on health status and health risks*. Health department performance appears lowest

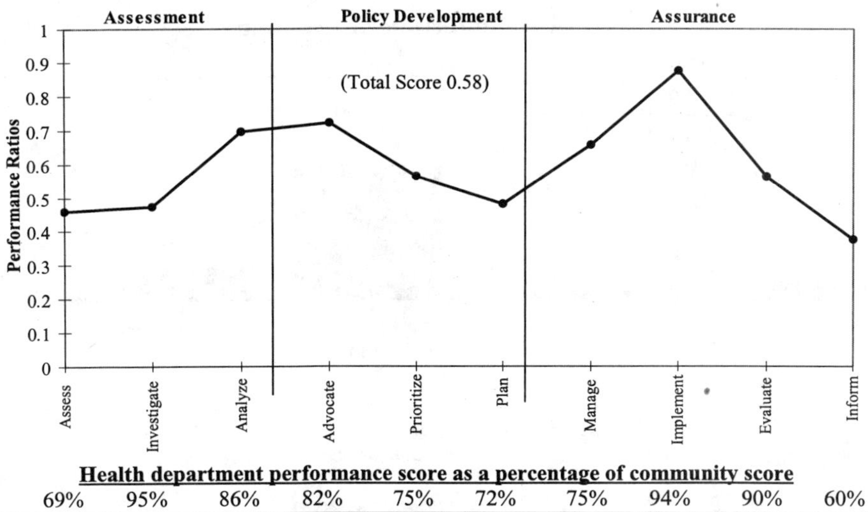

Figure 2. Health department performance scores for Memphis-Shelby County, 1993.

for the practice of *informing and educating the public.* Conversely, the public health contributions of organizations other than the local health department appear highest for the practice of *informing and educating the public*—as these organizations contribute 40% of the total community effort. Such extradepartmental contributions appear lowest for the practices of *investigate* and *implement*.

When we examine the proportion of public health activities in which specific types of community organizations participate, it appears that most organizations participate in *policy development* activities more than in *assessment* or *assurance* activities (**Figure 3**). State health agencies are the notable exception to this trend, as they are reported to participate more in *assessment* activities than in the other areas. State agencies also appear to participate in *assurance* activities more so than any other type of organization. Interestingly, nonprofit and voluntary agencies are reported to participate in the broadest array of policy development activities, followed closely by hospitals and local government agencies. Universities and federal agencies are reported to participate in a relatively narrow range of public health activities. Most types of organizations do not appear to be substantially involved in assurance activities.

Discussion of Performance Results

Community performance scores indicate that core public health functions are being effectively carried out within the jurisdiction. These results also reflect the dominant role that the local health department plays in local public health practice within Memphis and Shelby County—particularly for the *assurance* function. Nonetheless, performance in the *assessment* function appears to lag behind performance in other areas. Other than the state and local health departments, few community organizations appear to contribute substantially to these activities. In light of the substantial changes that TennCare is creating in the organization and financing of health services, strong assessment activities are needed in Memphis and Shelby County to ensure the early detection and correction of gaps within the evolving health system. Enhancing the performance of these assessment activities should be a priority for the community in the coming years. Recent activities being undertaken by the state-sponsored Memphis and Shelby County Community Health Agency suggest that such enhancements may already be underway.

Future Prospects and Projections

The local public health system serving Memphis and Shelby County, Tennessee has adapted rapidly to a changing health care environment that has heavily invested in the concept of managed care. The local health department has responded effectively to the short-term dynamics of this reform, but the long-term equilibrium of this system remains uncertain. For the foreseeable future, health department staff expect to continue their organization's involvement in providing primary care services to vulnerable and underserved populations. Many health care organizations in Memphis support this continued role for the local health department—particularly the managed care plans that participate in TennCare. The local health department has demonstrated its effectiveness in managing health services and health care needs within fixed budgets. Private health care providers do not appear ready to assume many of the health department's current roles in serving Medicaid recipients and the uninsured. Other traditional safety-net providers, such as The Med and Memphis' array of community health centers, face difficulties in meeting the health care needs of the community's uninsured population while simultaneously adapting to TennCare reforms. In this complex and evolving health care environment, the local health department plays a vital role in reinforcing Memphis' health care safety net and ensuring coordination and continuity within this system.

Perhaps the greatest challenge facing the local public health system in Memphis lies in the ability to sus-

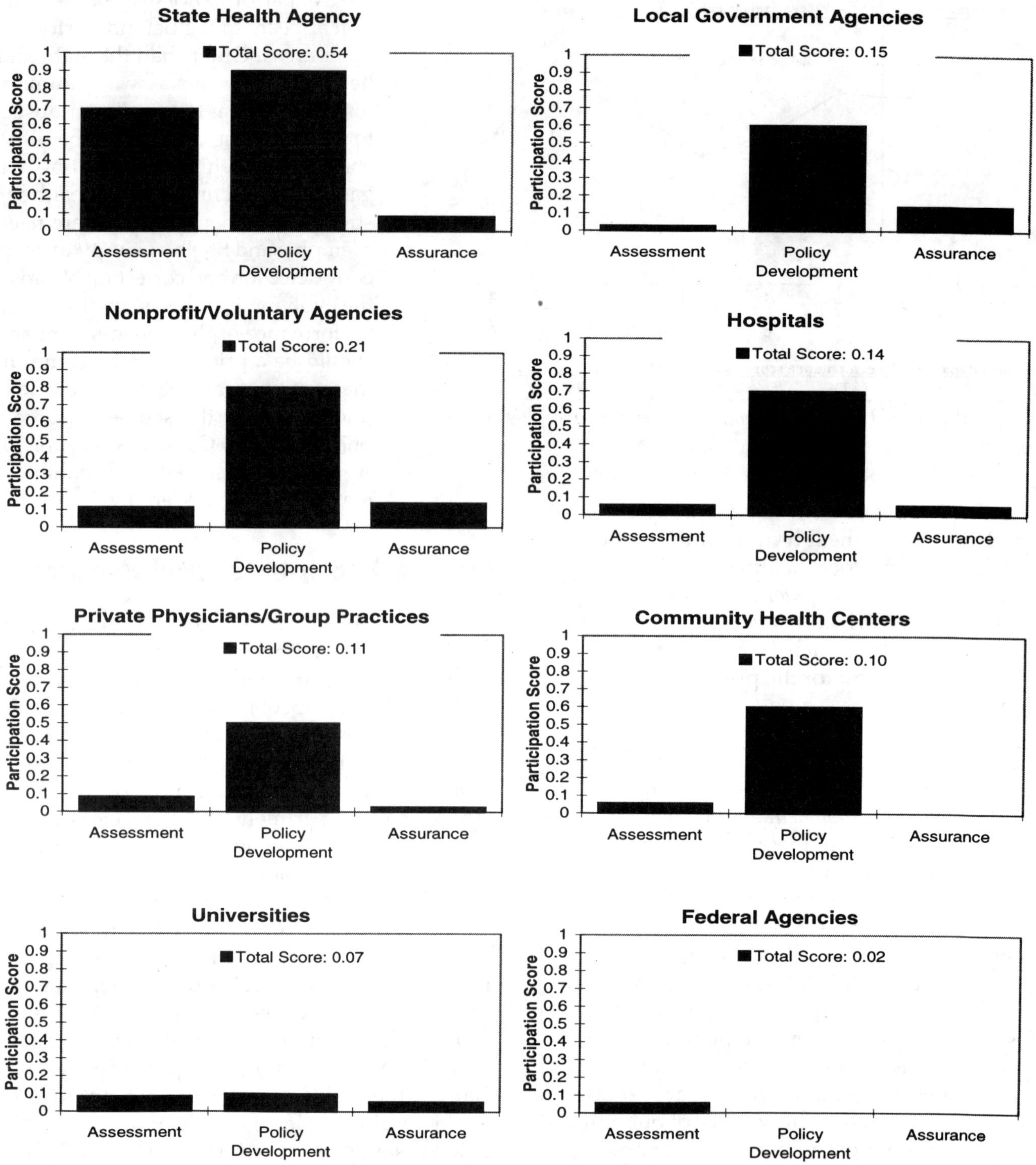

Figure 3. Participation in local public health activities by other organizations, 1993 (as reported by the local health department director).

tain and expand population-based public health functions while continuing to address the community's personal health care needs. Results from the public health performance survey suggest that an emphasis on population-based assessment activities are especially needed. Securing the necessary resources and expertise to mount new and expanded assessment activities is a daunting task for any public health agency. Accomplishing this task alongside substantial responsibilities in primary care delivery appears particularly difficult. A promising strategy for building assessment infrastructure may involve alliances with other organizations that could also benefit from this infrastructure Memphis' local health department maintains an impressive history of successful inter-organizational partnerships and a broad network of allies. The strong linkages between public and private health organizations in Memphis—together with the effective leadership of the local health department—promise to provide an effective structure for addressing the community's evolving health needs.

References

1. Memphis and Shelby County Health Department. *1995 Vital Statistics.* Memphis, TN: Memphis and Shelby County Health Department; 1995.
2. American Medical Association. *Physician Data by County*. Chicago, Ill: AMA; 1992.
3. American Hospital Association. *AHA 1997 Guide to the Health Care Field*. Chicago, Ill: AHA; 1997.
4. Group Health Association of America. *1995 Directory of HMOs*. Washington, DC: GHAA; 1995.
5. National Association of County and City Health Officials (NACCHO). *1992-93 National Profile of Local Health Departments*. Washington, DC: NACCHO; 1995.
6. US Department of Commerce. 1995 Consolidated Federal Funds Report. Washington, DC: Census Bureau; 1997.
7. Mays GP. Reconfiguring Memphis' public health system for managed care. In: Halverson PK, Kaluzny AD, McLaughlin CP, eds. *Managed Care and Public Health*. Gaithersburg, Md: Aspen Publishers; 1998:243-251.
8. Memphis and Shelby County Health Department. *Annual Report Fiscal Years 1992-93*. Memphis, Tenn: Memphis and Shelby County Health Department; 1995.
9. Roman LA. Tenncare recipients forsaking The Med. *Memphis Business J*. March 30, 1998.

Chapter 13

Case Study of Milwaukee, Wisconsin

Key Attributes

- Local health department transitioning of some personal health services to other community providers.
- Growing involvement of hospitals and managed care plans in community health initiatives.
- Strong network of community health centers that provide care for vulnerable and underserved populations.
- Collaborative approaches for community health assessment and policy development.

Community Characteristics

Demographic and Socioeconomic Characteristics

The city of Milwaukee lies at the heart of a four-county metropolitan area with more than 1.4 million residents, making it the nation's 32nd largest metropolitan area. Milwaukee is located in southeastern Wisconsin on the western shore of Lake Michigan. The city of Milwaukee contains 612,700 residents as of 1997, down from 628,088 in 1990 due largely to migration to suburban areas. Census data from 1997 indicate that 56% of Milwaukee residents are White, 35% are African American, 2% are Asian, and 1% are Native American (**Table 1**). Approximately 8% of Milwaukee residents report Hispanic ancestry. The area's unemployment rate stood at 4.2% in 1994 and has remained below the national average for more than a decade. Per capita income stood at $32,973 in 1997.

Community Health Status Indicators

Vital and health statistics data indicate that maternal and child health issues remain a concern for many city residents (**Table 2**). The 5-year infant mortality rate for the period from 1991 to 1995 stood at 11.8 per 1000 live births, substantially above state and national averages. This rate has improved to 11.2 deaths per 1000 live births in 1996, but it remains substantially above average. During the 1991-1995 period, 29% of women giving birth did not begin prenatal care in the first trimester, and more than 7% received no care or care only in the third trimester. Prenatal care delivery has improved in recent years such that by 1996 more than 21% of women received care within the first trimester. More than 10% of births during 1991 to 1995 registered as low birth weight (under 2500 g), compared with 8.7% of births in 1996. Contributing to these problems are relatively high rates of births to adolescents. Births to mothers age 10-17 comprised 7.8% of all births in 1996.

Table 1
Demographic Characteristics: Milwaukee, Wisconsin

Population (1997)	612,700
Median age in years (1990)	30.3
Percent 65 years and older (1990)	12.4
Percent non-White (1997)	43.6
Percent speaking a language other than English at home (1990)	10.9
Percent completing high school degree (1990)	71.5
Percent of individuals below federal poverty level (1989)	22.2
Median household income (1997)	$32,973
Average percent unemployed (1994)	4.2

Data from Department of Commerce, Bureau of the Census.

Table 2
Health Status Indicators: Milwaukee, Wisconsin, 1996

Infant mortality rate per 1000 live births	11.2
Percent of births to mothers age 10-17	7.8
Percent of infants with low birth weight	8.7
Percent of births with prenatal care later than first trimester	21.1
Deaths per 100,000 population, crude rates	959.4
Cancer, all types	229.2
Lung cancer	59.8
Female breast cancer	16.5
Heart disease	293.3
Cerebrovascular diseases	73.6
Chronic obstructive pulmonary diseases	41.2
Suicide	11.4
Pneumonia and influenza	35.0
HIV/AIDS	8.0
Diabetes mellitus	24.2
Homicide	14.1

Data from Wisconsin Department of Health and Family Services (unpublished data, 1997).

As in many communities, chronic diseases pose substantial threats to health and well-being among Milwaukee city residents. Cancers, heart diseases, and cerebrovascular diseases exist as the leading causes of death. Homicide, unintentional injuries, and HIV/AIDS infection also emerge as leading health threats when the years of potential life lost are considered. Almost 1700 "premature" deaths due to heart diseases were recorded between 1991 and 1995 (defined as deaths before age 65), compared with more than 700 deaths from homicide, 600 deaths from unintentional injuries, 500 deaths from lung cancer, 400 deaths from HIV/AIDS, and 200 deaths for breast cancer. Clearly, the predominant health threats confronting Milwaukee's population include a difficult mix of well-documented chronic diseases and varied acute conditions, many of which have their roots in social, behavioral, and environmental characteristics.

Local Health Resources and Manpower

Milwaukee's relatively large constellation of health care providers are rapidly organizing into three large integrated delivery systems (**Table 3**). This process has been accelerated by the 1995 privatization and merger of the county-owned Doyne Hospital, an action that removed 350 hospital beds from the community's total supply of over 6000 beds. All of the area's 11 remaining community hospitals are private, nonprofit corporations, and most of these are affiliated with one of the three emerging multihospital systems. Many of these hospitals are located outside the central city of Milwaukee, and several major facilities—including the local children's hospital and the area's premiere tertiary care and teaching hospital—lie outside the city of Milwaukee entirely. Only one hospital remains in the city's downtown area. The city is also served by a Veteran's Affairs medical center and several psychiatric and rehabilitation facilities.

A total of 3159 nonfederal physicians practice in Milwaukee County, which encompasses the city of Milwaukee as well as surrounding suburban municipalities. The physician-to-population ratio of 332 per 100,000 population suggests that the area confronts a slight work force shortage when compared with the US average. Of these physicians, ~31% provide patient care in the primary care disciplines of family practice, general practice, general internal medicine, pediatrics, and obstetrics/gynecology. A collection of four federally funded community health centers, one federal Health Care for the Homeless program, and one state-supported health center, provides access to personal health services for residents who are unable to access health services from private providers because of financial, geographic, or cultural barriers. These community health centers provide the bulk of primary care services to Milwaukee's uninsured and underinsured populations and also to many of the city's Medicaid beneficiaries. Although most Medicaid beneficiaries in Milwaukee are enrolled in health maintenance organizations (HMOs) as part of the area's mandatory man-

Table 3
Health Resources: Milwaukee County, Wisconsin

Number of nonfederal physicians (Number per 100,000 population) 1992[a]	3159 (332)
Family practice	239 (25)
General practice	65 (7)
Internal medicine	533 (56)
Obstetrics/gynecology	167 (18)
Pediatrics	200 (21)
Number of community hospital beds (FY1995)[b]	3884
Beds per 100,000 population	408
Number of community hospitals (FY1995)[b]	14
Number of HMOs (1994)[c]	9
Number of federally qualified health centers (1994)[d]	5
Total number of clinic sites	17
Local public health expenditures (1997)	$35,076,359
Percent from direct federal sources	9%
Percent from state sources (including federal pass-throughs)	<10%
Percent from local sources	47%
Percent from Medicaid	<1
Percent from Medicare	31%
Total federal funding for community health centers (1996)[e]	$1,930,290
Total federal funding for migrant health centers (1996)[e]	0
Total federal block grant funds for preventive health services (1996)[e]	0
Total federal block grant funds for maternal and child health services (1996)[e]	0
Total federal block grant funds for substance abuse services (1996)[e]	$5,245,097
Total federal funding for homeless health services (1996)[e]	$899,451
Total federal funding for National Health Service Corporation (1996)[e]	$292,932

[a]*Data from American Medical Association Physician Masterfile.*[1]
[b]*Data from American Hospital Association.*[2]
[c]*Data from Group Health Association of America.*[3]
[d]*Data from US Bureau of Primary Health Care (unpublished data, 1994).*
[e]*Data from US Department of Commerce.*[4]

aged care enrollment initiative, the community health centers maintain contracts with many of these HMOs for serving their Medicaid enrollees.

Milwaukee has a long history of managed care among both the commercial and Medicaid populations. Nearly half of the area's population is enrolled in HMOs. Milwaukee's Medicaid managed care initiatives began in 1984 under a demonstration waiver from the US Health Care Financing Administration. All of the city's women and children who received the cash assistance program Aid to Families with Dependent Children were enrolled in managed care plans over a 6-month period. By 1993, ~115,000 Medicaid beneficiaries received care through the six plans that participated in the program. Several of the large, for-profit corporations that dominate Milwaukee's commercial managed care market also participate in the Medicaid program, including the following:

- CompCare Health Plan, the state's oldest HMO with 160,000 total enrollees and a network-model structure that includes 805 primary care physicians;
- Prime Care Health Plan, the largest HMO in the state with almost 200,000 enrollees and 986 primary care physicians in its network; and
- Family Health Plan Cooperative, the area's only staff model HMO serving almost 110,000 enrollees with 88 staff physicians and an additional 200 contract physicians.

The area's long experience with Medicaid managed care has also fostered the development of several specialized managed care plans that tailor their service delivery and management approaches to the Medicaid population. For example, the Wisconsin Independent Physicians' Group (WIPG), a nonprofit managed medical provider network, has pioneered several health education and outreach initiatives for the Medicaid population, including programs in prenatal care coordination and child health screenings that have become models for the community and state. Similarly, Genesis Health Plan, an independent practice association (IPA) HMO, developed innovative social support services for its Medicaid enrollees such as free transportation and translation services, as well as reduced fee and free care to uninsured community members not eligible for Medicaid. Genesis was acquired by MHS, another HMO serving the local Medicaid population, in 1997.

The Local Health Department

Milwaukee's strong network of community health centers, Medicaid HMOs, and nonprofit hospitals has allowed the city's health department to move away from the direct provision of many types of personal health services. The Milwaukee Health Department currently provides only basic personal health services through its four health clinics in endeavors such as sexually transmitted disease control, immunization, and tuberculosis control. While transitioning responsibilities in personal health services to private providers, the local health department has engaged in deliberate efforts to strengthen its capacities in areas such as community health assessment, oversight, enforcement, and policy development.

Organizational Structure

The Milwaukee Health Department exists as one of nine departments within the City of Milwaukee municipal government. The department is headed by a commissioner of health who is appointed by the mayor and approved by the city council. The health department does not operate under a local board of health for advisory or governance purposes; rather, the mayor carries out these functions subject to the legislative powers of the city council. Paul Nannis served as Milwaukee's health commissioner for most of the past decade, until his recent move to a federal health post prompted the appointment of Seth Foldy, MD, as the city's top health official. Reporting directly to the commissioner of health, a physician-trained medical officer oversees all medical functions within the department. These areas of responsibility include patient care, laboratory, disease surveillance and reporting, and environmental hazards response.

The health department comprises four divisions that collectively carry out the agency's public health mission. A *bureau of public health services* administers all personal health services provided through the department's three health clinics and maternal and child health programs, as well as the city's population-based health education and nutrition programs. Included among the department's nutrition programs is the federally funded Special Supplemental Nutrition Program for Women, Infants, and Children (WIC). A *bureau of consumer protection and environmental health* administers activities related to environmental inspections, food and water safety, lead abatement, health code enforcement, and vector and nuisance control. A *bureau of laboratories* provides the scientific expertise and technical capacity for the department's initiatives in detecting, investigating, and tracking health threats within the city. Chemistry, virology, and microbiology subdivisions allow the department to respond to a wide range of environmental hazards and disease risks in the community. The remaining division within the health department provides administrative support for public health activities, including programs for public health planning, vital statistics, management information systems, and special projects such as a medical care program for low-income elderly residents and a lead poisoning prevention program.

Service Areas

Community Health Clinics

The local health department's involvement in personal health care delivery has declined over the past two decades, as the department has strengthened relationships with community health centers, hospitals, managed care plans, and other providers that have expanded care to underserved populations. Traditionally, the department operated health clinics in several underserved areas of the city to provide primary care services to residents without access to private providers. During the 1980s, the health department began to transfer the provision of many types of services to a network of four federally qualified community health centers and two university-sponsored primary care centers. A variety of mechanisms have sustained this transition, including contractual agreements, grants, and joint referral arrangements. These arrangements are discussed later in this chapter.

Currently, the health department continues to provide several types of personal health services that are not adequately available and accessible to all city residents. Services that continue to be provided through health department clinics include the followings: childhood immunizations; infant and child health screenings (EPSDT); adult screenings for cardiovascular disease and breast cancer; tuberculosis testing and treatment; sexually transmitted disease testing and treatment; and nutritional services under the WIC program. The department provides these services through four geographically dispersed clinics staffed by teams of public health nurses. One of these clinics focuses exclusively on the delivery of testing and treatment services for sexually transmitted diseases and HIV / AIDS. The other three clinics provide access to general health promotion, prevention, and detection services for children and adults.

The majority of patients who utilize personal health services from health department clinics are uninsured or underinsured residents. However, substantial numbers of individuals who receive health care coverage through Medicaid, Medicare, and private health insurance also access services through these clinics. Health department administrators suggest that these individuals may choose to access services from department clinics because of their geographic accessibility, their skills in treating individuals with diverse cultural and linguistic backgrounds, and their low fees in comparison to many private providers. The health department maintains contracts with several Medicaid HMOs for receiving reimbursement for specified types of health services—namely childhood immunizations and lead poisoning screening services—when their enrollees seek care from health department clinics. For uninsured clients, the department uses a sliding fee scale for personal health services delivered through the clinics, with free care being provided to patients without the ability to pay. In 1996, the department received almost $920,000 in insurance reimbursement and patient fees for personal health services (almost 6% of the health department budget). During this same year, the health department's clinics handled more than 174,000 patient visits and delivered more than 22,000 immunizations.

Home-based Services

The department maintains an extensive staff of public health nurses who provide health promotion and disease prevention services in the home, school, and community to vulnerable and high-risk populations. Approximately 48 full-time equivalent nurses provide over 30,000 home visits annually, most of which are for communicable disease control, outreach for low-income pregnant women, infant and child health assessments, and lead poisoning prevention and control. Other home-based services provided by the health department include the following: case management for substance-abusing women and their families; counseling and education for first-time parents; follow-up visits for infants with sickling disorders, galactosemia, and hypothyroidism; and HMO enrollment counseling for potential Medicaid eligibles. Additionally, more than 2500 of the home visits provided through the health department target the prevention and control of chronic diseases among adults, through screenings and disease management services. All of the department's home visitation efforts focus on clients who are isolated and difficult to reach, clients who are unable to access other established public or private services, and clients who require direct instruction and/or observation in their homes.

School-based Services

The health department's public health nurses also provide a range of public health and primary prevention services to school-age children enrolled in Milwaukee public schools. These services are provided through a "consultation and case management" arrangement with the public school department, wherein school personnel and public health nurses collaborate in designing and implementing school-based public health initiatives. Through one of these initiatives, the health department provides pregnancy prevention education, assessment, and second-time pregnancy prevention services to middle and high school students. Approximately 1600 students receive services through this program annually. Another program, designed to build on the successes of the pregnancy intervention, provides education, assessment, and counseling services to students in the areas of high-risk behaviors, violence prevention, communicable disease management, and chronic disease prevention. Other school-based services provided by public health nurses include childhood and adolescent vaccinations; and hearing, vision, and disease screenings. In total, the health department provides ~60,500 nonscreening services to public school students annually, and an additional 4000 screening services.

Community-based Services

The health department operates a range of programs that target broad segments of the community and operate through multiple sites within the city. The department's health education and public health nursing divisions play critical roles in developing and implementing these services in partnership with a broad array of community-based organizations. The health department's community-based services and programs include the following:

- A violence prevention program, which conducts community presentations and professional in-service workshops at area schools, colleges, health and social service agencies, and neighborhood and community groups;

- A community-wide infant mortality reduction program, which implements community-wide health education projects with funding from the local March of Dimes chapter;
- A breast cancer awareness project, which provides health education and mammography screening services at multiple community locations using a specially equipped van funded jointly by the local health department and Wisconsin's state health agency;
- A community-wide immunization tracking system, which is underway in collaboration with local hospitals, community health centers, and managed care organizations using initial funding from the Robert Wood Johnson Foundation and the Centers for Disease Control and Prevention; and
- A number of communitywide task forces that have developed to provide planning, policy development, and advocacy for specific health issues such as tuberculosis, lead poisoning, adolescent pregnancy, minority health, and avoidable hospitalizations.

Infrastructure and Resources

Overall, the local health department appears to be adequately funded and staffed for the public health activities it undertakes. A total departmental budget of almost $16.5 million was approved for 1997, which represents a 2% increase over the 1996 budget. This figure produces a per capita public health expenditure of $26, which is slightly higher than the median local health department expenditure of $20 identified through a national survey of departments in 1992.[5] Almost 80% of this budget ($15.5 million) is derived from federal, state, and private grant sources. This fact reveals the department's marked success in securing external grant support for many of the programs and services it operates. Another 16% of the health department's budget ($2.4 million) derives from city contributions to matching-fund grants. The remainder of departmental revenue flows from third-party reimbursement for health services, patient fees, and the sale of licenses and permits. For fiscal year 1997, the department was authorized for 426 full-time equivalent employees, a 4% decrease from the previous year. Health professionals on staff at the health department include 115 public health nurses, 8 health educators, 26 laboratory technicians, 1 epidemiologist, and 1 physician (the department's medical director).

The health department has heavily invested in its information resources in recent years. The department began construction of a computerized client tracking system in 1993 to enable common access to patient-level data on all clients using public health services provided by the department. The system enables automated scheduling of patient appointments and clinical staff time, client registration, tracking of clinical services and outcomes, client and third-party billing, utilization profiling, and case load management. The department is currently working to integrate this client tracking system with the community-wide immunization tracking system now under development. The immunization tracking system, which is also designed to be computer-based, endeavors to integrate immunization data from multiple providers, including the health department, managed care plans, hospitals, community health centers, and physician practices. The department's client tracking system is also designed to interface with the WIC registration and draft issuance system, which was computerized statewide in 1993.

Along with its computerized tracking system, the health department has implemented a standardized documentation system for all clinical services delivered by the department. This system provides a standardized methodology for documenting client knowledge, behavior, and health and functional status in the clinical records maintained within the tracking system. Health department administrators suggest that this standardized system will improve the organization's ability to monitor health outcomes in response to public health interventions.

The health department also maintains a comprehensive program evaluation system for all public health activities underway within the department. This system is part of the department's evolving total quality management initiative, which has been underway since 1991. In addition to using a standardized organizational assessment protocol, the National Association for County and City Health Officials' *Assessment Protocol for Excellence in Public Health*, health department administrators chose to devise their own evaluation system. Administrators suggest that this approach yields greater flexibility in tailoring the evaluation system to local needs and resources, as well as greater support from departmental staff who are part of the system's creation and evolution. The health department's evaluation system is structured around five core departmental objectives that were identified through a citywide planning process led by the mayor.[6] For each of these objectives, a series of outcome indicators are identified and used to track progress toward the objectives. These indicators include the community infant mortality rate, low birth weight rate, lead poisoning case rate, exposure rates to food-borne diseases, and rates of premature death attributable to chronic diseases. Because only a limited range of outcome indicators are readily measurable on an annual basis, the department uses a number of additional, process-level indicators to track health department performance toward its core objectives. These process indicators include measures of service volume in the health clinics, home visit programs, school-based programs, community-based programs, and environmental inspection and investigation programs. The department also computes efficiency measures for each service, which are based on the cost per service unit produced, and aggregates these measures to generate an efficiency measure for each of the department's core objectives.

As part of the evaluation system, the health department has developed an environmental quality index to serve as an outcome indicator for the core objective relating to environmental health. Included in the index are environmental health indicators such as the following: the incidence rates of exposure to various environmental hazards; incidence rates of acute and chronic diseases and injuries caused by environmental hazards; and the volume of resident complaints in the areas of water and sewer quality, pest control, animal nuisances and bites, solid waste and hazardous materials control, and noise. Increasingly, this index serves as a model for other local health agencies to monitor environmental health status at the community level.

Other Contributors to Local Public Health Practice

State Health Agency

Milwaukee's local health department maintains a close working relationship with the state agency that administers public health activities in Wisconsin. Wisconsin's state health agency exists as a division within the larger Department of Health and Family Services, which also houses state agencies for mental health, alcohol and other drug addiction services, child welfare services, disabilities services, health facilities licensing, and Medicaid financing. Milwaukee health department officials interact most frequently with the state Bureau of Public Health, a subdivision within the Division of Health that holds responsibilities in communicable disease prevention and control, maternal and child health, occupational health, chronic disease prevention, and emergency medical services. Administratively, local health departments in Wisconsin operate as decentralized units of local government, with the state health agency exercising only limited oversight and authority powers over these departments. The state agency assumes direct responsibility only for the local public health function of contact tracing for communicable diseases. Interaction between Milwaukee's local health department and the state Bureau of Public Health often occurs through grant-in-aid programs that support local public health services. For example, Milwaukee's breast cancer screening van is funded in part through a grant from the state's office for chronic disease prevention and health promotion.

The two agencies also interact frequently for planning, policy development, and technical assistance purposes through both formal and informal mechanisms. Policy issues regarding the Milwaukee's Medicaid managed care program have motivated much of this interaction. As the state's first local public health agency to operate under a Medicaid managed care initiative, the Milwaukee health department has provided the state with valuable feedback regarding intended and unintended program effects over the past decade. Milwaukee's health department has also worked closely with the state bureaus for Medicaid and public health to address identified gaps within the managed care initiative. For example, the local health department has played a critical role in obtaining modifications to the state Medicaid contract with HMOs. These modifications have included the following: reporting requirements for the delivery of core public health services like childhood immunizations, lead screenings, and tuberculosis control services; requirements for the provision of enabling services such as transportation and language translation services; and provisions for encouraging service agreements between HMOs and local health departments. Additionally, the state health agency has played an instrumental role in establishing a Medicaid managed care policy forum in Milwaukee that includes participation by the local health department and all of the major HMOs serving Medicaid beneficiaries in the area. Together, the local and state health agencies have effected substantial improvements to Milwaukee's Medicaid managed care initiative since its inception in 1984. These improvements have greatly facilitated the process of expanding this initiative to other areas within the state.

Other Local Health Departments in the Metropolitan Area

Milwaukee's county government does not operate a local health department separate from the municipal department. However, 13 other suburban cities and towns within the county operate their own local health departments. These departments vary widely in their resources and infrastructure, with some departments having less than 10 full-time equivalent staff positions and others employing more than 100 staff. As public health agencies serving the Milwaukee metropolitan area, these departments confront many similarities in their public health needs, threats, and opportunities. As a result, these departments have cultivated strong working relationships in areas of shared interest. For example, several of Milwaukee health department's public health initiatives, such as the immunization registry project and the lead poisoning prevention task force, have been implemented countywide through collaboration with other local health departments. Additionally, Milwaukee's local health department maintains service agreements with several other local health departments in the county for providing such services as hazardous material spill cleanup and laboratory testing. Milwaukee health department administrators admit that the current arrangement of local health departments in Milwaukee County results in some service duplication and inefficiency. Nonetheless, the concept of local health department consolidation meets with strong resistance from suburban municipalities that cherish their home rule authority and fear consolidation would siphon off their local health resources to the problems of inner-city populations.

Hospitals

Many hospitals serving the city of Milwaukee appear strongly committed to community health issues. For many of the private hospitals, this commitment flows from their affiliation with religious organizations and the missions of charity and public service that these organizations maintain. Nonetheless, recent turbulence in the local hospital market has caused many hospitals to restructure their involvement in community health issues and their roles within the local public health system. Milwaukee's county-owned general hospital, the John L. Doyne Hospital, was privatized in mid-1995 and then acquired by an existing private hospital, Froedtert Memorial Lutheran Hospital. These actions forced Milwaukee's private hospitals to reevaluate their responsibilities in indigent care and services for Medicaid beneficiaries. With acquisition of the former county facility, Froedtert Hospital assumed an expanded role in community health activities, including the provision of care to uninsured and underinsured residents. Historically, Froedtert has emphasized the provision of highly specialized inpatient and outpatient services, mainly to individuals with health insurance coverage. While this emphasis will be maintained, Froedtert administrators report that the acquisition of the county facility has motivated the hospital to expand capacity for providing primary care and preventive services to a broader scope of the community population. As part of this strategy, hospital administrators hope to develop referral arrangements, service agreements, and other interorganizational arrangements with community health centers, local health departments, and other providers with expertise in serving indigent patients and other vulnerable populations. As a member of Horizon Healthcare, one of Milwaukee's three multihospital systems, Froedtert also hopes to use its affiliations with other hospitals and clinics within this system to develop appropriate systems of care for these population groups. Because the hospital is located in a suburban and relatively affluent area of Milwaukee, administrators hope that these arrangements will enable vulnerable populations to receive much of their care in their own communities, rather than at the hospital's distant facility.

With the closure of the county hospital, other Milwaukee hospitals have also increased their involvement in community health issues. As the only hospital remaining in Milwaukee's downtown area, Sinai Samaritan Hospital has served as a major source of care for indigent populations and Medicaid beneficiaries for much of the past decade. Even before the closure of the county hospital, Medicaid beneficiaries comprised almost 50% of Sinai Samaritan's patients. The hospital's commitment to this population is evident even in its mission statement, which confirms that the organization is "committed to our location in the heart of the city, and dedicated to improving the health status of the diverse people we serve." Although inpatient specialty services remain an area of emphasis, the hospital has expanded its involvement in primary care and preventive services that have become increasingly unavailable in the central city communities served by the hospital. For example, the hospital provided more than 49,000 patient visits through its primary care, pediatric, and family care clinics during 1994. The hospital has also developed special capacities for providing women's health services, handling more than 34,000 visits through its women's health assessment clinic and its obstetrician/gynecology clinics during 1994. The hospital's nurse-staffed women's health information telephone line handled over 35,000 calls during this same period.

As part of its community health mission, Sinai Samaritan maintains strong linkages with other community-based organizations. The hospital provides funding and management services for one of Milwaukee's four federally funded community health centers, an activity that frequently leads the hospital to interact closely with the Milwaukee health department. Sinai Samaritan also funds members of its medical staff to serve as medical directors for family planning clinics operated by Planned Parenthood, an activity that has caused the hospital to lose affiliations with several local Catholic hospitals. The hospital maintains a team of community health nurses that participate in the community initiatives of local churches, synagogues, schools, and neighborhood associations. Through this team, the hospital identifies emerging community health needs and concerns and works to tailor hospital programs and services to address these issues.

Sinai Samaritan also maintains an extensive network of relationships with managed care organizations in the community, especially those that serve Medicaid beneficiaries. The hospital gained early experience in the managed care arena by operating its own HMO for several years, before eventually selling this plan to an established managed care corporation. The hospital now maintains contracts with more than 28 plans for providing hospital and/or ambulatory care services, including most of the Medicaid HMOs in Milwaukee. Almost 40% of the hospital's revenues derive from managed care contracts, many of which are now capitated contracts. This growth in managed care involvement has occurred in tandem with the hospital's integration within Aurora Health Care, one of Milwaukee's three major multihospital systems. Sinai Samaritan's administrator suggests that these arrangements create financial incentives for some of the hospital's health promotion and community health activities that previously were motivated only by the organization's charitable mission. Under capitated contracts with HMOs, these services can help the hospital retain revenues by reducing the need for intensive and costly health services among the HMO enrollees it serves. Additionally, the wide scope of primary care and preventive services offered by Sinai Samaritan helps the organization attract and maintain contracts with HMOs and other managed care organizations that desire an emphasis on prevention and health promotion.

Several other hospitals make substantial contributions to community health in Milwaukee. St. Mary's Hospital, Wisconsin's oldest private general hospital, maintains a long history of providing inpatient and ambulatory care services to Milwaukee residents, with a special focus on addressing indigent care needs. The hospital maintains national affiliation with the Daughters of Charity Catholic health system, and local affiliation with the Horizon Healthcare multihospital system. In addition to handling more than 11,000 hospital admissions annually, the hospital operates three geographically dispersed primary care clinics in partnership with the University of Wisconsin's medical school. These clinics are major sources of preventive and primary care services to Medicaid beneficiaries and indigent populations and maintain referral agreements with Milwaukee health department clinics and the area's community health centers. The hospital also provides both financial and management support to one of Milwaukee's four federally qualified community health centers. In addition to providing an annual $25,000 grant for operating expenses, the hospital equips the health center with its management and clinical information systems and provides the center's clinical staff with fringe benefits, malpractice insurance, and continuing education opportunities.

The hospital also contracts with Health Care for the Homeless of Milwaukee, a local homeless health center operator, to provide clinical assessment, diagnosis, and pharmacy services at two clinic locations within the city. The hospital provides 24-hour emergency coverage for the clinics as well as medical case management services. Nurse practitioners from St. Mary's provide these services with medical backup and consultation from volunteer physicians affiliated with the hospital.

St. Mary's hospital also plays a major role in providing critical enabling services to Milwaukee's vulnerable populations. Milwaukee's only hospital-based WIC program is maintained at St. Mary's main hospital facility. Additionally, the hospital operates an extensive transportation program that provides free transportation to St. Mary's inpatient and ambulatory care centers for community residents lacking convenient transportation. In partnership with Sinai Samaritan Hospital and several community health centers, St. Mary's operates a case management program for high-risk pregnancies. This program provides in-home counseling, education, and follow-up for women identified as at-risk for adverse birth outcomes. Finally, the hospital jointly operates a program for providing family-centered care and support services to medically indigent populations in Milwaukee, in collaboration with the family practice residency program of the Medical College of Wisconsin. Under this program, a range of interventions is maintained for improving care to vulnerable population groups through family-oriented support services. These interventions include the following: a clinic-based computer system that allows providers to link the medical records of family members, family counseling sessions that address a range of health issues, and special scheduling and staffing systems that allow all members of a family to receive needed health services during a single clinic visit.

St. Mary's Hospital maintains a large and growing involvement in managed health care for both commercial populations as well as Medicaid beneficiaries. The hospital cofounded Wisconsin's first HMO in 1972 and now contracts with many of the area's managed care plans for providing inpatient and ambulatory care services to their enrollees. These contracts currently represent approximately one quarter of the hospital's inpatient revenue. The hospital's main family practice center, which is staffed by residents from the Medical College of Wisconsin, contracts with multiple Medicaid HMOs on a capitated basis for providing primary care and case management services to their enrollees. Through these arrangements, the center acts as an independent practice association (IPA) by serving enrollees from multiple HMOs as well as providing fee-for-service and free care. The hospital also operates another family practice center that contracts exclusively with a local HMO for providing the full continuum of services needed by the plan's commercial and Medicaid enrollees—including pharmacy and mental health services. This arrangement is often referred to as a group-model HMO arrangement. St. Mary's Hospital is actively involved in evaluating the health outcomes, costs, and patient satisfaction levels of these two managed care arrangements in order to determine which model provides superior service to the Medicaid and commercially insured patients it serves. This strategy of experimentation and evaluation allows the hospital to remain cautious and flexible in its expanding involvement in managed care.

Another private hospital serving Milwaukee, Children's Hospital of Wisconsin, assumes a major role in sustaining local and statewide community health interventions for children. Despite its historical emphasis on inpatient care, Children's Hospital engages in a wide range of health promotion and disease prevention activities that support and extend the work of the local health department. The hospital funded during 1992-1993 a community health nurse to conduct educational sessions on lead poisoning testing and treatment practices in the private practices of local family physicians and pediatricians. The hospital also collaborates with the local health department in operating childhood immunization clinics and in assigning clinical staff from the hospital to provide immunizations at the local community health centers. Similarly, Children's Hospital serves as a primary contributor to the Robert Wood Johnson-funded initiative to develop a community-wide immunization tracking system. Like a growing number of health care organizations across the county, the hospital sponsors a bicycle safety program that includes the provision of subsidized and free bicycle helmets to children. The hospital also conducts a wide range of public health education and advocacy campaigns on issues such as water safety, accidental poisonings, firearm risks, and adolescent pregnancy. The hospital disseminates educational messages through local print, radio, and television media as well as special materials such as coloring books distributed to Milwaukee public school students. In almost all of these initiatives, hospital administrators report strong collaboration and coordination with Milwaukee's local health department.

Children's Hospital also supplements the work of the local health department and community health centers in providing personal health services to vulnerable populations. The hospital operates two homeless health care centers in Milwaukee that specialize in serving the unique health care needs of homeless children. The hospital also operates a lead poisoning clinic and a child abuse clinic at accessible, downtown locations. In addition, the hospital serves substantial numbers of Medicaid beneficiaries through its hospital-based pediatric clinics.

Like other Milwaukee hospitals, Children's Hospital maintains a strong and growing involvement in managed health care. Unlike these other organizations, however, Children's remains independent of the three multihospital systems that dominate Milwaukee's local health care market. Hospital administrators report that this independence allows the hospital to work with the full range of health care providers in the community, rather than operate under an exclusive relationship with a single system of care. Children's Hospital maintains contracts with many of the managed care plans serving the Milwaukee area, especially those plans that enroll Medicaid beneficiaries. Having operated its own Medicaid HMO during the 1980s, Children's Hospital maintains substantial expertise in the delivery of care under capitated reimbursement systems. Although most of the hospital's current managed care contracts are for inpatient and specialty services only, hospital administrators are now working to develop the capacity to provide a comprehensive set of child health services—including preventive services, primary care, and specialty care—under a managed care arrangement. Eventually, the hospital hopes to develop capitated subcontracting arrangements with HMOs that give the hospital responsibility for providing a full range of services to their pediatric enrollees. Administrators suggest that this level of community coverage would enable the hospital to implement health promotion and disease prevention interventions on a much broader scale within the community and to leverage more resources to address indigent care needs in the community.

Milwaukee's other community hospitals report modest but growing involvement in community health issues. The area's third major multihospital system, Covenant Healthcare, includes several of Milwaukee's Catholic hospitals in its membership (St. Joseph's, St. Michael, and St. Francis). Administrators at these hospitals stress their organizations' traditional commitments to serving vulnerable populations within the community. However, their organizations have only recently begun to consider the ways in which they may carry out this commitment beyond the walls of their facilities. All of these hospitals report a strong working relationship with the local health department and cite the outreach efforts of Milwaukee health commissioner Paul Nannis as a principal reason for their organizations' growing interest in addressing community health issues outside the domain of traditional hospital services. As a result of these efforts, hospitals represent important participants in the community-wide task forces formed around childhood immunization, lead poisoning, tuberculosis control, and adolescent pregnancy.

Milwaukee area hospitals also report a growing interest in community health assessment as a process for identifying and responding to local health issues. Much of this interest derives from a joint effort by the Wisconsin Hospital Association and the state Bureau of Public Health to assist hospitals and other health care organizations engage in coordinated efforts to assess health needs and develop plans for their communities. During late 1994, these two organizations developed a coordinated process for assessing health status, needs, and risks in local communities and for developing interorganizational initiatives to address these issues. This process was based in large part on the *Assessment Protocol for Excellence in Public Health* developed by the National Association of County and City Health Officials, as well as the Hospital Association of Pennsylvania's community assessment process. Beginning in 1995, the Wisconsin Hospital Association began conducting seminars and training sessions on community health assessment with its member hospitals. As a result of this effort, many of Milwaukee's hospitals now anticipate developing the capacity to conduct community health assessment activities as part of their strategic planning and community benefit efforts. The extent to which these activities may be conducted in a collaborative and coordinated manner remains to be seen. Competitiveness in the local hospital market—particularly among the three multihospital systems—continues to grow and may pose challenges for interorganizational collaboration. Despite this competitiveness, the local health department has experienced marked success in convening the full extent of local health care providers around community health issues. Hospitals seeking to undertake collaborative assessment activities may therefore wish to tap the local health department's expertise as convener and facilitator for these efforts.

Community Health Centers

Milwaukee's community health centers lie at the heart of the local community health system. These centers provide the bulk of primary care services for the city's uninsured populations and are also important providers of care to Medicaid and Medicare beneficiaries. Three of the city's four federally funded community health centers began operation in the late 1960s and early 1970s under the US Office of Economic Opportunity's neighborhood health centers program. After several federal program changes during the 1970s and 1980s, the centers now receive funding as community health centers under section 330 of the US Public Health Service Act. Two of the centers also receive financial and administrative support from local hospitals: the Sixteenth Street Community Health Center is supported by St. Mary's Hospital, and the Johnston/Sinai Health Center is supported by Sinai Samaritan Hospital. Rainbow Community Health Center also receives federal funding from the Indian Health Service. Milwaukee Health Services provides services at two clinic sites: Isac Coggs Community Health Center, and Martin Luther King Jr. Heritage Center. The city is also served by a homeless health center, which receives funding under Section 340 of the federal Public Health Service Act.

In addition to these federally funded centers, several other locally supported health clinics provide primary health care services to low-income and underserved populations within the city. The Medical College of Wisconsin's family practice residency program operates a health center that provides primary care predominantly to Medicaid beneficiaries and the uninsured. Milwaukee's local health department maintains service contracts and referral agreements with this clinic for serving patients who seek care within the health department's clinic system. As discussed earlier, St. Mary's Hospital also operates three neighborhood health clinics in cooperation with the Medical College's residency program. These clinics also serve large numbers of Medicaid beneficiaries and indigent patients. Finally, the local health department provided initial funding to the area's two nursing schools—at the University of Milwaukee and Marquette University—to operate two nurse-managed health clinics. Each clinic is staffed by a nurse practitioner and a team of registered nurses and nurse trainees and provides basic primary care and preventive services to residents of underserved areas within the central city of Milwaukee. The local health department operates several of its mobile public health programs at these clinics on a rotating basis, including services for childhood immunizations, breast cancer screenings, and lead poisoning testing.

Several of Milwaukee's community health centers play key roles as service providers and case managers in the local Medicaid managed care initiative. When this initiative first began in 1984, the three federally funded community health centers formed their own HMO in partnership with the local health department. Although this HMO became insolvent after several years of operation, the community health centers acquired valuable knowledge and skills through this experience that would later facilitate their interaction with surviving managed care plans. The health centers now operate much like traditional IPAs by establishing capitated contracts with Medicaid HMOs for providing primary care and case management services to their enrollees. Alongside these contracts, the centers continue to serve patients on a fee-for-service basis and to provide free care to the indigent.

Milwaukee's community health centers maintain strong relationships with the local health department. The department provides grant funding to the centers for delivering selected preventive services such as prenatal care for high-risk pregnancies, childhood immunizations, and breast and cervical cancer screenings for age-appropriate women. The department also maintains referral agreements with the health centers for services that the department's public health clinics are not be able to provide, such as sick care for children and adults, prenatal care, many types of diagnostic testing and evaluation, and family planning services. Finally, the community health centers are critical participants in the community-wide task forces that are convened by the health department around issues such as immunization, HIV, infant mortality, lead poisoning, and tuberculosis control.

Managed Care Plans

Milwaukee's managed care plans have long served as important contributors to the local public health system, although their relationships with state and local public health agencies have been tense at times. A detailed examination of Milwaukee's local managed care market has been conducted elsewhere.[7] Observations about the public health contributions made by local managed care plans are given below.

Relationships between the local health department and the local managed care market have improved and expanded substantially during the past decade. A measles epidemic in Milwaukee during 1989 and 1990 called attention to substantial gaps in the local health care system and created tension between the public health and managed care communities. During this epidemic, large numbers of measles cases emerged among children enrolled in Medicaid HMOs. The health department administered free vaccinations to more than 20,000 patients during the outbreak, including 11,000 HMO enrollees who failed to be immunized by their private providers. While responding to the public health crisis, the health department was vocal in its criticism of the managed care community over this issue. In addition to the bad publicity, Milwaukee HMOs incurred substantial financial costs due to the 232 hospital admissions and 3 fatalities that resulted from the epidemic.

The measles outbreak and its aftermath generated some animosity between the managed care and public health communities, but it also called attention to need for closer relationships between these two fields of practice. In the wake of the epidemic, the health department successfully negotiated contractual arrangements with Medicaid HMOs that allowed the department to receive payment for immunizing HMO enrollees who seek care at health department clinics. Soon after this, the local health department established a similar arrangement with several HMOs which allowed the department to receive payment for conducting blood lead screenings among age-appropriate HMO enrollees who present at health department clinics. The health department continues to negotiate with HMOs regarding the provision of sexually transmitted disease services and tuberculosis screening and treatment services to HMO enrollees. All of the HMOs prefer for their enrollees to receive care within their provider networks, where services can be coordinated and managed to improve quality and contain costs. The health department contracts demonstrate that many of Milwaukee's HMOs recognize the complexities of managing care among traditionally underserved populations and the need to explore creative, collaborative approaches for improving health care accessibility.

The local health department has now formed relationships with managed care plans that go beyond the delivery of personal health services to address population-based community health issues. For example, Milwaukee's health director has involved the local HMOs in a community-wide task force that oversees the implementation of community-wide immunization tracking system. The HMOs make important contributions to this effort given their expertise in clinical information systems and given their powerful roles in securing physician participation in the tracking system. The health department also involves HMOs in a community-wide environmental health task force that is seeking stronger relationships between private health care providers and the health department's environmental inspection and abatement programs. The goal of this effort is to ensure that when medical care providers detect environmental health issues such as childhood lead poisoning, the health department can be mobilized quickly for lead abatement activities. HMOs also collaborate with the local health department through community-wide task forces that address issues such as domestic and community violence, adolescent pregnancy, and infant mortality.

Several of Milwaukee's managed care plans have initiated community health activities independently of the local health department. One of Milwaukee's largest Medicaid managed care providers, the Wisconsin Independent Physicians' Group (WIPG), is particularly active in public health activities. WIPG is a nonprofit independent practice association (IPA) of more than 800 physicians serving primarily Medicaid enrollees in Milwaukee's managed care program. Early in the life of this program, WIPG developed an innovative prenatal health support program designed to improve birth outcomes within Milwaukee's low-income Medicaid population. The program consisted of in-home nursing visits to assess maternal and fetal health as well provide advice and counseling on health and lifestyle choices. The program also offered social support services such as child care and transportation to encourage the receipt of timely prenatal health care. After several years of operation, an external evaluation demonstrated the program's effectiveness in improving birth outcomes. The state Medicaid agency soon adopted the program as a standard benefit for all pregnant Medicaid recipients.

WIPG has produced other innovative public health interventions during its 15-year history. Collaborating with another Medicaid HMO, WIPG developed a system for encouraging and tracking the delivery of childhood developmental screening services by physicians. WIPG uses the system to remind physicians of the preventive services that need to be delivered, and to pay physicians for these services once all scheduled screenings have been completed. The system is also used to compare and profile physicians based on their success in delivering these preventive services, as an additional strategy for improving physician performance. Administrators at WIPG note that the system is now used widely among private physicians that participate in Milwaukee's Medicaid program.

Like WIPG, several other managed care plans have emerged specifically to serve Medicaid beneficiaries as part of Milwaukee's managed care program. These plans are notable for the specialized services and delivery mechanisms they have developed to serve the special health care needs of vulnerable populations. Managed Health Services Corporation (MHS) began operations in 1984 as a small HMO formed by a local nonprofit hospital to protect its traditional role in serving Medicaid beneficiaries. The HMO formed a subcontracting arrangement with an established commercial HMO so that it could operate under an existing HMO license and meet the federal requirement of having at least 25% of its enrollees from commercial (non-Medicaid) contracts. During the past decade, MHS's founding hospital closed and the organization converted to for-profit status in order to obtain additional access to capital. Despite these changes, the plan has retained its original focus on serving Medicaid beneficiaries.

MHS uses several service delivery strategies that are tailored to the needs of vulnerable population groups. The plan emphasizes the delivery of care through traditional safety-net providers, and therefore contracts with all of Milwaukee's federally qualified health centers to serve as primary care providers and case managers. The plan also contracts with the local health department for providing immunizations, lead screenings, and sexually transmitted disease control services to its enrollees. MHS provides free health education classes to its Medicaid beneficiaries in the areas of smoking cessation, weight control, childbirth, and parenting skills. Administrators note that while these benefits are commonly provided to commercial enrollees for additional fees, most plans do not provide these types of services as basic benefits to Medicaid enrollees. Finally, MHS provides a range of support services designed to encourage the appropriate utilization of health promotion and disease prevention services among its Medicaid enrollees. These services include the following: free transportation to and from all of MHS service providers; telephone and postcard reminder systems for scheduled preventive services such as infant and child health check exams and childhood immunizations; and a staff of patient advocates who assist individual beneficiaries in accomplishing tasks such as choosing and switching providers and scheduling appointments.

Another specialized Medicaid managed care plan, Genesis Health Plan, began operations in 1994 as a small, for-profit plan organized as a hybrid IPA and staff-model HMO. In tailoring its plan to the vulnerable populations it serves, Genesis placed emphasis on establishing primary care clinics in low-income ethnic neighborhoods and in staffing clinics with members of the ethnic communities that it serves. For example, several of its clinics are staffed by groups of foreign medical graduates and nurses, as well as support staff who reside in the neighborhoods where the clinics are located. This strategy is designed to improve access to services for traditionally underserved populations by reducing cultural and linguistic barriers to care. Genesis also directly provides support services such as transportation and language translation services to its enrollees. As a unique feature of this health plan, Genesis offers reduced-fee and free primary care services through its health clinics to low-income community members who are not eligible for Medicaid, in an effort establish these clinics as community health resources. This practice is rare for most staff-model HMOs, which typically serve only enrolled members. Genesis' founder and administrator reports that these community health activities are motivated in part by belief in the cost-effectiveness of these activities and in part by a desire to be a good corporate citizen and earn a reputation as a community resource. In 1997, Genesis was acquired by MHS, a competitor health plan. Although the two plans appear compatible in their missions, it remains to be seen how this arrangement will affect the operation of Genesis.

In addition to the specialized Medicaid managed care plans, many of Milwaukee's traditional commercial plans have begun to experiment with community-based initiatives in health promotion and disease prevention as a strategy for improving health outcomes and reducing long-term health risks among their enrolled populations. Milwaukee's largest HMO, PrimeCare Health Plan (owned by the for-profit United Health Care Corporation), operates a number of specialized case management and health education interventions for its 55,000 Medicaid enrollees and 200,000 commercial enrollees. The plan's in-home education and training program for pediatric asthma cases has reduced the proportion of pediatric asthma patients who utilize the emergency room annually from 30% to less than 5%. PrimeCare's administrator suggests that this program has been particularly effective among the plan's Medicaid beneficiaries, who are often at greater risk for experiencing acute asthma symptoms and who may have greater difficulty in complying with recommended asthma treatments.

The plan has also begun to emphasize programs to encourage the utilization of health promotion and disease prevention services, especially among its Medicaid enrollees who may experience more barriers to accessing and utilizing these services. To encourage the utilization of scheduled infant and child health check exams (also called EPSDT exams), the plan conducts a monthly random drawing among all members who are up-to-date on their exams, with the prize being a $100 gift certificate to a local department store. PrimeCare also participates in community-wide initiatives designed to improve health status at the population level. Along with the local health department and other community providers, the plan sponsors the Milwaukee Healthy Women and Infants Project which hosts neighborhood block parties across the city that provide education on prenatal care, pregnancy, and childbirth to community members. The HMO participates in a number of other community-wide task forces convened by the local health department, such as those on immunization, lead poisoning, adolescent pregnancy, and avoidable hospitalizations.

Another local plan, the Wisconsin Health Organization (WHO), now owned by the national for-profit company Humana, has only recently decided to place an emphasis on health education interventions for its 25,000 Medicaid enrollees and 75,000 commercial enrollees. The plan has begun work to develop the capacity for operating educational interventions in the areas of asthma management, diabetes management, childhood immunization, prenatal care, adolescent pregnancy prevention, and parenting skills. WHO's administrator reports that this new emphasis on health education has been motivated by several co-occurring factors: (1) the "critical mass" of Medicaid beneficiaries who have recently enrolled in the plan; (2) the plan's desire to expand its role in serving vulnerable population groups while remaining financially solvent; (3) the willingness of the local health department to work collaboratively with the plan in developing these interventions; and (4) the administrator's prior experience as a public health educator and his belief in the efficacy of health education interventions. The administrator notes that health plans may derive short-run marketing benefits from these types of interventions, in addition to the longer-run health benefits. Interestingly, WHO also operates a pilot HMO program for serving disabled individuals, in partnership with a local nonprofit agency. This experience may eventually assist the plan in serving other types of Medicaid beneficiaries that are currently excluded from Milwaukee's Medicaid managed care demonstration project, such as supplemental security income beneficiaries. WHO's administrator hopes to develop sufficient skills and capacities for providing health education and support services so that the complex needs of these new population groups can be effectively and efficiently addressed within the HMO system.

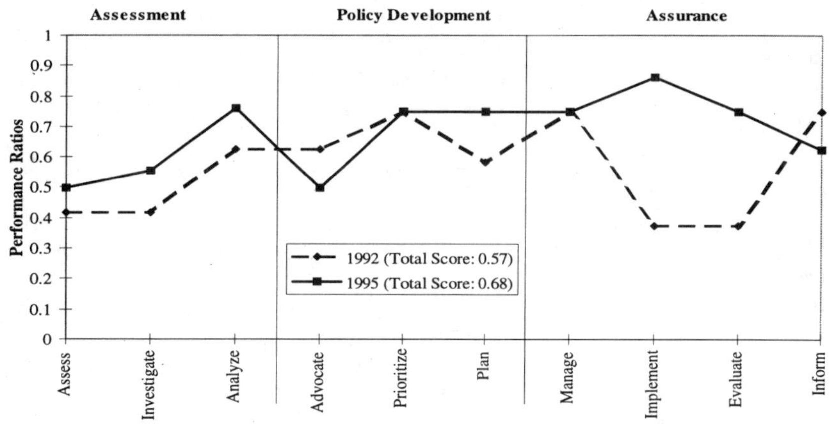

Figure 1. Community public health performance scores for Milwaukee, Wisconsin, 1992 and 1995.

Other Community Organizations

A number of other community-based organizations make substantial contributions to the local public health system in Milwaukee. Local chapters of the Rotary International and Junior League service organizations jointly operate a health education center which disseminates health information and conducts seminars, presentations, and workshops on a variety of community health issues. The Rotary club is also a key participant on the immunization task force that is developing the community-wide immunization tracking system for Milwaukee. The United Way also maintains a strong presence in Milwaukee's community health system by conducting periodic needs assessments of the local health care infrastructure and by contributing funding and administrative assistance to a wide range of community-based service projects. The local chapter of the American Lung Association provides leadership on a community-wide initiative to increase awareness of asthma and its appropriate treatment and control methods, in collaboration with the Medical College of Wisconsin and other local health care providers. The Milwaukee chapter of Planned Parenthood exists as a major source of family planning services within the community and collaborates with the health department and other organizations on a number of community health issues, including the task forces on adolescent pregnancy and infant mortality. Additionally, several community-based organizations that have formed around minority health issues, including the Black Health Coalition and the Latino Health Organization, play vital roles in advocacy and policy development at the local and state levels.

Measures of Public Health System Performance

On the basis of the local health director's responses to the public health performance assessment survey in 1992 and 1995, community-wide performance of public health activities in Milwaukee appears to have increased substantially over this 3-year period (**Figure 1**). In 1992, Milwaukee's health commissioner reported that public health activities were being performed in the jurisdiction at a level representing 57% of the maximum possible performance. In 1995, the reported performance level increased to 68%. Increases in performance were reported for the all of the public health practices accept *advocating* for public health issues and *informing and educating* the community about public health issues. The largest increases in performance between 1992 and 1995 appear to have occurred for the practices of *implementing* policies and programs to address health needs, and *evaluating* health services and resources for their impact on public health.

When we examine the public health practices directly performed by the local health department, performance appears to have increased for five practices, decreased for three practices, and remained relatively stable for two practices (**Figure 2**). Increases in health department performance are reported for the practices of *investigating* health threats, *developing plans and policies* to address health issues, *managing* health resources and services, *implementing* programs and services, and *evaluating* programs and services. The largest increases in health department performance appear to have occurred for these last two practices, suggesting that the health department has increased its role in public health assurance activities. When health department performance is expressed as a percentage of total community performance, it appears that the proportion of community effort that is carried out by the local health department has increased for six of the public health practices and decreased for four others. Increases in this proportion are reported for all of the *assurance* practices, suggesting that health de-

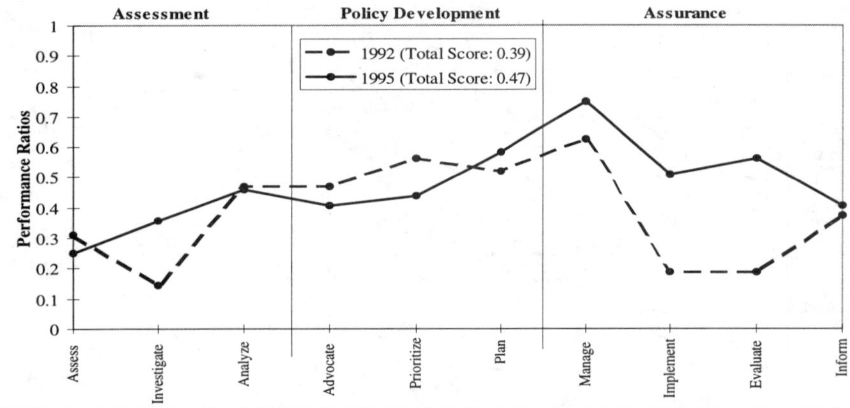

Health department performance score as a percentage of community score

	Assess	Investigate	Analyze	Advocate	Prioritize	Plan	Manage	Implement	Evaluate	Inform
1992:	75%	35%	75%	75%	75%	89%	83%	50%	50%	50%
1995:	50%	64%	61%	81%	58%	78%	100%	59%	75%	65%
Chng:	-33%	+84%	-19%	+08%	-22%	-13%	+20%	+18%	+50%	+30%

Figure 2. Local health department performance scores for Milwaukee, Wisconsin, 1992 and 1995.

partment efforts are largely responsible for the reported growth in community performance of assurance activities. Decreases in the proportion of total effort carried out by the local health department are reported for the practices of *assessing* health needs, *analyzing* health risks, *prioritizing* health needs, and *developing* plans and policies. This finding suggests that organizations other than the local health department are responsible for the increases in total community performance that are reported for these practices.

Participation in public health activities by organizations other than the local health department appears to have increased between 1992 and 1995, according to the local health director's reports (**Figure 3**). Overall, these organizations appear to participate in a greater proportion of the *policy development* activities than in the *assessment* or *assurance* activities. Interestingly, participation by the state health agency appears to have declined between 1992 and 1995 for all three public health functions. This decline appears to have been offset by increases in participation by local government agencies, hospitals, private physicians, community health centers, universities, and federal agencies. The only other area of declining participation appears to be among nonprofit and voluntary agencies for *assurance* activities. Interestingly, managed care plans appear to have become important participants in many types of public health activities by 1995 (not shown in Figure 3). The health director reports that these organizations were involved in 24% of the *assessment* activities listed on our survey, 50% of the *policy development* activities, and 17% of the *assurance* activities. These organizations were not listed as participants in any of the public health activities during the 1992 survey.

Results from the 1992 and 1995 public health performance assessment surveys appear to reflect many of the trends noted in our case study analysis of Milwaukee's public health system. Improving relations between the local health department and the managed care community are reflected in the high levels of managed care participation in public health functions. Moreover, the local health department's general strategy to perform more public health activities through collaborative arrangements with other organizations appears clear. Two observations regarding this strategy are notable.

First, the results of the 1992 and 1995 performance assessments indicate that the health department's policy of encouraging other organizations to share greater responsibilities in local public health practice has coincided with an overall increase in community performance. These results are consistent with an earlier, cross-sectional analysis of public health performance in 63 jurisdictions during 1992 and 1993,[8] and suggest that successful methods can be found to transfer responsibility for certain public health functions outside the domain of governmental public health agencies. It should be noted, however, that Milwaukee's approach to collaboration does not entail an across the board reduction in health department responsibilities. Rather, it appears that reductions in the *policy development* and *assessment* responsibilities of the local health department between 1992 and 1995 are offset by substantial increases in its *assurance* responsibilities — especially in the areas of *evaluating* programs and services and *implementing* policies and programs.

Second, our results indicate that the increase in community public health performance in Milwaukee has occurred alongside the decreasing involvement of the state health agency in local public health activities. This result stands in contrast to several cross-sectional studies that have found higher levels of public health performance in centralized local health departments compared with decentralized departments.[9,10] Milwaukee demonstrates that strategies do exist for successfully responding to the growing trend in devolution of governmental authority from state to local levels. A key component of Milwaukee's strategy appears to be the participation of other community organizations in local public health functions.

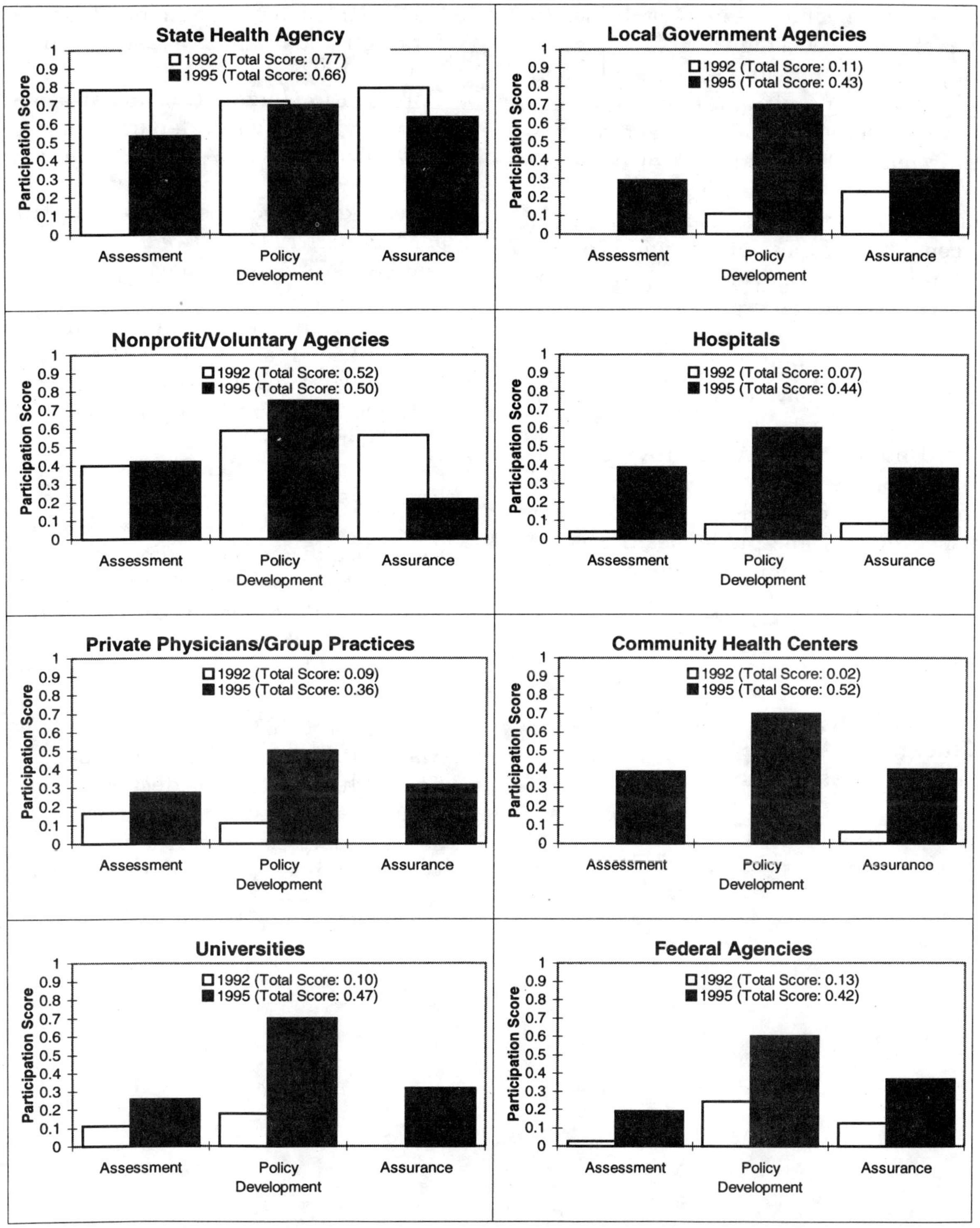

Figure 3. Participation in public health activities by other organizations (as reported by the local health director).

Conclusions and Future Prospects

Having achieved enviable levels of infrastructure and expertise, Milwaukee's public health system has begun to pursue the more intangible objectives of improved effectiveness, efficiency, and relevance within an evolving health care system. In pursuing these goals, the local health department benefits from its strong leadership, local political support, and carefully cultivated respect from the private health care community. The local health department has clearly adopted a strategy of interorganizational collaboration in carrying out its public health responsibilities. Despite the turmoil of competition and consolidation in Milwaukee's private health care market, the health department has experienced a high degree of success in encouraging collaboration among the public and private organizations that contribute to public health activities in Milwaukee. Much of this collaboration is occurring in the relatively early stages of planning and policy development—especially for those that involve Milwaukee's managed care organizations. It remains to be seen whether these efforts will produce meaningful community interventions to address Milwaukee's existing and emerging public health issues. Nevertheless, the changes in the health department's approach to public health practice over the past decade appear to have elevated the level of public health performance in Milwaukee by involving an increased number of private providers. Although the nature of the health department's work has changed over time, its overall level of performance is not diminished. Rather, the public health system has achieved a high level of community involvement.

References

1. American Medical Association. *Physician Data by County*. Chicago, Ill: AMA; 1992.
2. American Hospital Association. *AHA 1997 Guide to the Health Care Field*. Chicago, Ill: AHA; 1997.
3. Group Health Association of America. *1995 Directory of HMOs*. Washington, DC: GHAA; 1995.
4. US Department of Commerce. 1995 Consolidated Federal Funds Report. Washington, DC: Census Bureau; 1997.
5. Gordon RL, Gerzoff RB, Richards TB. Determinants of local health department expenditures, 1992 through 1993. *Am J Public Health*. 1997; 87(1):91-95.
6. Milwaukee Department of Administration. *City of Milwaukee 1997 Plan and Budget Summary*. Milwaukee, Wis: Milwaukee Department of Administration; 1997.
7. Mays GP. The local health department's role in Milwaukee's managed care market. In: Halverson PK, Kaluzny AD, McLaughlin CP, eds. *Managed Care and Public Health*. Gaithersburg, Md: Aspen Publishers; 1998:252-260.
8. Halverson PK, Miller CA, Kaluzny AD, Fried BJ, Richards TB, Schenck SE. Performing public health functions: the perceived contributions of public health and other community organizations. *J Health Human Serv Admin*. 1996;6:288-303.
9. Richards TB, Rogers JJ, Christenson GM, Miller CA, Taylor MS, and Cooper AD. Evaluating local public health performance at a community level on a statewide basis. *J Public Health Manage Pract*. 1995;1(4):710-783.
10. Mays GP. Availability and adequacy of local public health services: the effect of state-local administrative relationships. In: *Association for Health Services Research Annual Meeting Abstracts*. Vol 13. Washington, DC: Association for Health Services Research; 1996:148.

Chapter 14

Case Study of Multnomah County, Oregon

Key Attributes

- Medicaid health maintenance organization operated jointly by local health department and hospital.
- Primary care capacity maintained by the local health department.
- Competitive and collaborative relationships among local health department, hospitals, and managed care plans.
- Growing involvement in community health activities among hospitals and managed care plans.

Community Characteristics

Demographic and Socioeconomic Characteristics

Portland, Multnomah County, and the surrounding metropolitan area contain a population of more than 1.6 million people, making the it Oregon's largest urban area. Approximately 625,000 people reside in Multnomah County, the urban core of the metropolitan area (**Table 1**). Steady gains in employment and household income during the 1990s have bolstered the socioeconomic status of many Portland residents. Census data from 1990 indicate that 13% of the county population lived below the federal poverty level in 1990. The population has become increasingly diverse, with Census data indicating that 6% of the population are African American, 4.7% are Asian, and 3.1% are of Hispanic origin. Almost 83% of the county population have attained 12 or more years of formal education.

Community Health Status Indicators

Portland and Multnomah County face many of the same health problems and risks that plague other large metropolitan areas (Oregon Department of Human Resources, Center for Disease Prevention and Epidemiology, unpublished health statistics, 1996). Approximately 6.1% of births in 1996 were low birth weight (less than 2500 g), and this rate has remained relatively stable and consistently higher than the statewide rate during the past 10 years. Infant mortality stood at 6.0 deaths per 1000 live births in 1996 (**Table 2**), down from 9.6 deaths per 1000 live births in 1993. Births to teenage women (age 10 to 19) comprised 12.5% of the total births in 1996. The teenage pregnancy rate in Multnomah County has declined during the last 3 years but remains at 23%. Nearly 22% of pregnant women in Multnomah County did not receive prenatal care during their first trimester.

Communicable diseases remain a concern for some population groups within Multnomah County (Multnomah County Health Department, unpublished data, 1996). Almost 2000 HIV and AIDS cases have been diagnosed among county residence through February

Table 1
Demographic Characteristics: Multnomah County, Oregon

Population (1996)	625,000
Median age in years	34.5
Percent 65 years and older (1990)	13.6
Percent non-White (1990)	13.0
Percent speaking a language other than English at home (1990)	9.2
Percent completing high school degree (1990)	82.9
Percent of individuals below federal poverty level (1989)	13.1
Median household income (1989)	$26,928
Average percent unemployed (1992)	7.0

Data from US Department of Commerce, Bureau of the Census.

Table 2
Health Status Indicators: Multnomah County, Oregon, 1996

Infant mortality rate per 1000 live births	6.0
Percent of births to mothers age 10-19	12.5
Percent of infants with low birth weight	6.0
Percent of births with prenatal care later than first trimester	21.9
Deaths per 100,000 population, age-adjusted	880.9
Cancer, all types	205.3
Lung cancer	60.4
Female breast cancer	29.2
Heart disease	226.4
Cerebrovascular diseases	78.6
Chronic obstructive pulmonary diseases	45.9
Suicide	15.4
Pneumonia and Influenza	30.8
HIV/AIDS	23.7
Diabetes mellitus	21.5
Homicide	7.2

Unpublished data from Oregon State Health Department, 1997.

1995, and a 58% death rate has been observed among these cases. The incidence of primary and secondary syphilis has substantially declined in recent years, with only 17 cases reported in 1994 compared with 146 cases in 1990. Gonorrhea continues to affect substantial numbers of county residents, with 681 cases reported during 1994. Incidence for both measles and pertussis have remained low in recent years (0 and 8 cases reported in 1994, respectively), and the tuberculosis case rate has dramatically declined in recent years (from 88.9 per 100,000 in 1993 to 38.9 per 100,000 in 1994).

Heart disease remains the leading cause of death among Multnomah County residents, although death rates from heart disease have declined from 290.7 per 100,000 residents in 1989 to 226.4 per 100,000 in 1996 (Table 2).[1] Other leading causes of death include cancer (205.3 per 100,000), cerebrovascular diseases (78.6), chronic obstructive lung disease (45.9), and unintended injuries (34.4). Mortality rates from female breast cancer have increased from 15.8 in 1989 to 29.2 in 1996. Motor vehicle fatality rates have declined from 16.2 in 1989 to 10.9 in 1992.

When deaths are expressed in terms of years of potential life lost, the five leading causes of lost years of life include (in order): cancer, unintentional injuries, heart disease, AIDS, and suicide.[1] Among African Americans, Hispanics, and Native Americans, the two leading causes of lost years of life are unintentional injuries and homicide.

Local Health Resources and Manpower

Three private hospital-based health care systems and a public university hospital system provide most inpatient care and a substantial amount of ambulatory care for the Portland area. The Sisters of Providence Health System, a nonprofit corporation affiliated with the Catholic Church, operates two medical centers in Multnomah County with a combined inpatient capacity of over 700 beds.[2] The two facilities managed over 34,000 inpatient admissions and 900,000 outpatient visits during 1994. Another nonprofit system, Legacy Health System, operates two hospitals in the county with a combined capacity of 739 beds and a volume of almost 25,000 admissions and 354,000 outpatient visits in 1994. Kaiser Permanente Northwest, a regional arm of the nation's largest health maintenance organization (HMO), has historically been a major provider of inpatient care in Portland as well. Since the 1995 closure of its 216-bed facility in central Portland, the nonprofit organization operates only one hospital in a suburban area outside Multnomah County. Increasingly, Kaiser contracts with Legacy and Providence for hospital services needed by its more than 300,000 enrollees in the Portland area. The Oregon Health Sciences University operates a 350-bed hospital facility in Portland, which includes a children's hospital and a number of tertiary and quaternary care departments. This facility serves as the major teaching hospital for the University's medical and nursing schools and served

Table 3
Health Resources: Multnomah County, Oregon

Number of nonfederal physicians (Number per 100,000 population) 1992[a]	3015 (501)
Family practice	137 (23)
General practice	43 (7)
Internal medicine	596 (99)
Obstetrics/gynecology	154 (26)
Pediatrics	178 (30)
Number of community hospital beds (FY1995)[b]	3125
Beds per 100,000 population	519
Number of community hospitals (FY1995)[b]	10
Number of HMOs (1994)[c]	5
Number of federally qualified health centers (1994)[d]	4
Total number of clinic sites	21
Local public health expenditures (FY1996)	$108,000,000
Percent from direct federal sources	<1%
Percent from state sources (including federal pass-throughs)	<5%
Percent from local sources	32%
Percent from Medicaid	58%
Percent from Medicare	<1%
Total federal funding for community health centers (1996)[e]	$2,861,284
Total federal funding for migrant health centers (1996)[e]	$9500
Total federal block grant funds for preventive health services (1996)[e]	$1,393,150
Total federal block grant funds for maternal and child health services (1996)[e]	$6,243,055
Total federal block grant funds for substance abuse services (1996)[e]	$3,866,653
Total federal funding for homeless health services (1996)[e]	$958,319
Total federal funding for National Health Service Corps (1996)[e]	$179,228

[a]*Data from American Medical Association Physician Masterfile, 1992.*
[b]*Data from American Hospital Association, 1997.*
[c]*Data from Group Health Association of America, 1995.*
[d]*Data from US Bureau of Primary Health Care, 1994.*
[e]*Data from US Department of Commerce, 1997.*

more than 17,000 inpatients and 275,000 outpatient visits in 1994. In addition to these facilities, Portland is served by a 270-bed nonprofit hospital affiliated with the Adventist church, a Shriner's hospital for children's orthopedics, and a Veteran's Affairs medical center.

Data from the American Medical Association indicate that 3015 active nonfederal physicians practice in Multnomah County, leading to a ratio of 501 physicians per 100,000 population (**Table 3**).[2] Approximately 37% of these physicians practice in the primary care disciplines of family practice, general practice, internal medicine, obstetrics/gynecology, and pediatrics. As in many urbanized areas, a maldistribution of physicians leaves some areas of the county underserved by private health professionals. The county health department operates a network of nine primary care health centers that provide access to ambulatory health services in many of the county's underserved areas. In addition, a coalition of seven nonprofit health centers provides primary care services to low-income residents of the Portland metropolitan area. This coalition provides over 25,000 patient visits annually to homeless individuals and families and other low-income residents of the Portland metropolitan area.[3]

Including Kaiser's group-model HMO and the managed care systems operated by Legacy and Providence, more than 15 HMOs operate in Multnomah County.[4] In total, ~40% of the population in the Portland metropolitan area are enrolled in HMOs. Almost 90% of Medicare beneficiaries and 60% of Medicaid beneficiaries are served by these plans. An estimated 113,775 residents of Multnomah County (or 18.5% of the population) did not have any health insurance coverage in 1993.

The Local Health Department

Health Officer and Staff

The Multnomah County Health Department operates as one of seven county departments under the authority of a four-member elected board of commissioners. The board of county commissioners serves as the local board of health for the department, as a separate board does not exist. The department is headed by an administrative director who is responsible for the overall management of the agency and by a health officer who is trained as a physician and oversees the department's regulatory health functions. The long-time administrative director, Billi Odegaard, maintained a 30-year history with the department before retiring at the end of 1998. Trained in public health nursing, Ms. Odegaard began her tenure as a nursing supervisor and later a director of nursing within the health department. When the health department was combined organizationally with the human services department in 1973, Ms. Odegaard became administrator of the health division within the larger umbrella agency. In 1991, the health department was again established as a separate county department, and Ms. Odegaard was appointed its administrator. Ms. Odegaard managed a total departmental budget of $108 million (fiscal year 1997) and a total staff of 815 full-time equivalent positions.

State law requires each county to appoint a physician to perform the statutory-defined functions of a local health officer. Multnomah County's health officer also serves as head of the regulatory health services division within the health department. The health officer holds statutory authority under state law for issuing quarantine orders and other regulatory mandates regarding health risks within the county. The health officer also supervises the medical examiner's office and the emergency medical services program for the county.

Service Areas

Organizationally, the health department consists of nine divisions, seven of which administer public health services or activities and two of which provide administrative and support services for the department as a whole. Service divisions include offices for primary care services, HIV/sexually transmitted disease services, community health services (referred to as specialty health and field services), dental services, regulatory health services (including environmental health services, violence prevention, and emergency medical services), corrections health, and the county's Medicaid managed care program. A business office division and a support services division perform administrative and technical functions that are needed by multiple service divisions within the department.

Primary Care Services

The primary care services division administers the department's programs for providing preventive and curative primary care services to both children and adults who do not have adequate access to health services from private providers. This division operates nine community-based primary care clinics located in underserved areas of Portland and Multnomah County. These clinics are staffed by teams of physicians and nurse practitioners, as well as ancillary personnel such as community health nurses, social workers, nutritionists, dietitians, pharmacists, and technicians. The department currently has 27 physicians on staff and contracts with an additional 6 physicians. The department employs 46 nurse practitioners, 3 physician assistants, and 239 nurses who work in the clinics as well as in other divisions. Several medical specialties are offered through the clinics, including optometry, dermatology, podiatry, endocrinology, pediatric pulmonology, colposcopy, ENT, rheumatology, and obstetrics/gynecology.

Each of the community clinics offer a comprehensive range of preventive and primary care services that include medical care for acute and chronic illnesses, immunizations, family planning, prenatal care, nutrition services, and well child exams. Clinics also administer the Women, Infants, and Children program (the federal Special Supplemental Food Program for Women, Infants, and Children). Several of the clinics operate special programs in addition to their full range of primary care services. The Westside Health Clinic operates an urgent care center and an after-hours primary care clinic. The Northeast Health Center administers a diabetes program that consists of intensive health education sessions on topics such as nutrition, exercise, medical complications, and goal setting. The division is currently working to expand this program to all of the primary care clinics. Another clinic, La Clinica de Buena Salud, specializes in the health needs of Latino children and their families. The Southeast Health Center administers a prenatal substance abuse intervention program designed to help women who are at risk of abusing alcohol and other drugs to deliver healthy babies. Finally, the Northeast Health Center participates in a federally funded project that links individuals with chemical dependency problems to appropriate treatment services and programs in the community.

In total, the primary care clinics operated by the health department provided ~138,000 patient care visits to 109,000 patients during the 12-month period from November 1993 to October 1994.[2] The majority of patients served by the clinics are individuals who do not have health insurance coverage. Medicaid beneficiaries comprise the second-largest group of clients served by the clinics and include individuals who are members of the department's own Medicaid managed care plan, individuals who are members of other Medicaid managed care plans, and individuals who are covered under the state's Medicaid fee-for-service program. The clinics also serve substantial numbers of patients who have health insurance coverage through Medicare, private HMOs and other third-party insurers, worker's compensation plans, and the federal refugee assistance program.

HIV/STD Services

Through the HIV/STD services division, the health department administers a range of services for the prevention, detection, and control of HIV/AIDS and other sexually transmitted diseases. The department operates a community testing site that offers both confidential and anonymous HIV testing. For Multnomah County residents testing positive for HIV, the department operates an HIV clinic where staff conduct health assessments and develop care plans for patients, provide a full range of primary care services, and provide case management services. The clinic participates in several special projects aimed at improving services to HIV patients, including a case management initiative that links the clinic with 12 other HIV service organizations in a six-county area; a project to improve the delivery of mental health and substance abuse services to HIV patients; and a program designed to promote wellness among HIV patients and their noninfected partners. In addition to the HIV clinic, the department also operates a STD clinic that provides testing and treatment for STDs and also conducts activities related to health education, active partner notification, disease surveillance, and training for health care providers.

Specialty and Field Services

The health department administers a range of additional disease control programs through its specialty and field services division. The department's tuberculosis (TB) clinic conducts regular TB screenings and educational programs in high-risk neighborhoods, provides directly observed therapy to noncompliant cases, and conducts contact tracing for identified cases. During fiscal year 1995, the TB clinic provided more than 16,500 patient encounters and identified 73 active TB cases. Also within this division, the department operates an international health center that provides communicable disease screenings and health assessments for newly arriving refugees. The clinic also provides primary care services and specialty care referrals for refugee clients residing in Multnomah County and neighboring Washington County. Originally funded through the federal refugee resettlement program, this clinic is now supported largely through state funds from the Oregon Health Plan, the statewide program for Medicaid beneficiaries and medically indigent populations.

The department also operates a network of 12 school-based health centers located in public middle schools, junior high schools, and senior high schools within the county. These clinics offer primary care for acute and chronic illness, well child exams, immunizations, family planning, health promotion, and mental health services. Clinics are staffed with a nurse practitioner, a community health nurse, a mental health consultant, and a secretary. One additional school-based clinic is located in an elementary school and is designed specifically to target children who are homeless or are at risk for homelessness.

An occupational health office within the department administers programs and services to improve health and safety in the workplaces of both public and private employers. Services include annual flu vaccination clinics, hepatitis B vaccination clinics, bloodborne pathogen education sessions, and tuberculosis screening clinics. In one recent year, over 45 flu vaccination clinics were held at public and private work sites, serving over 1800 employees.

The health department provides an extensive array of community health services through a network of six geographically dispersed field teams within the county. Teams consist community health nurses, outreach workers, mental health consultants, and office assistants. Team members conduct health education and information sessions in the community, teach health-related classes, serve on community boards and committees, and provide a variety of health services through visits to individuals, families, and groups. Services are delivered wherever the client is located, including homes, field team offices, county clinics, hospitals, schools, shelters, and other neighborhood locations. Services include assessment and case management for teenage pregnancies, postpartum care and education for teen parents, counseling for students with behavioral and attendance problems in school, care for children with chronic health care needs, and services for homeless individuals and families.

A final component of the specialty and field services division, the communicable disease office assumes responsibility for surveillance, case tracing and investigation, and health education regarding a wide range of communicable diseases. In carrying out these responsibilities, staff from the communicable disease office work closely with staff from other offices, including school health nurses, sanitarians, and primary care clinic staff. Communicable diseases most commonly targeted by the office include hepatitis A, shigella, meningococcal disease, hepatitis B, tuberculosis, and HIV / AIDS.

Dental Health Services

The health department operates a network of community-based dental clinics and a school-based dental program to provide access to urgent and routine dental care for county residents who are unable to access needed services from private providers. The department operates five community-based dental clinics staffed by teams of dentists, dental hygienists, and dental assistants. Four of these dental clinics are colocated with primary care clinics also operated by the health department. The health department also operates a dental managed care organization that served over 12,728 enrollees as of June 1995. This organization, referred to as MultiCare Dental, serves low-income beneficiaries of the Oregon Health Plan who are eligible for dental services. The state provides the organization with a capitated, per-member per-month reimbursement amount in exchange for addressing all the dental health needs of beneficiaries choosing to enroll in the organization.

The department's school-based dental health program provides primary preventive dental services to students in county elementary and middle schools. Services include oral screening, oral wellness education, and the provision of fluoride supplements and dental sealants. During 1995, a total of 32,045 students participated in the fluoride supplementation program, and 3270 students participated in the dental sealant program. A total of 49 volunteer dentists participated in providing the necessary screening services prior to the application of dental sealants.

Medicaid Managed Care

The Multnomah County Health Department has maintained a relatively long history of involvement in managed health care. In the early 1970s under the leadership of health officer Hugh Tilson, MD, the county implemented a managed care program for serving low-income individuals and families who could not receive health insurance coverage through public programs or employers. This program, known as Project Health, allowed qualified individuals and families within 115% of the poverty level to enroll in one of six prepaid managed care plans which contracted with the county to provide a specified range of benefits.[5] Contracting plans included those operated by the Kaiser Foundation, the Sisters of Providence System, Oregon Health Sciences University, and the local Blue Shield association. The county health division also operated its own prepaid health plan under this program.

In the late 1980s, the Oregon legislature adopted amendments to the state Medicaid program which allowed primary care organizations (PCOs) to contract with the state on a partially capitated basis for providing a basic set of primary care services and case management to Medicaid beneficiaries. The Multnomah County Health Department developed its own PCO, called MultiCare, to operate under this demonstration program and compete with the other PCOs formed by private physician practices, community health centers, and other primary care providers in the area.

Multnomah County began its most recent managed care initiative during the early 1990s as the state of Oregon developed its plans for reforming the Medicaid program. While the state government worked during 1991 to finalize the much publicized list of priority health conditions to be covered under Medicaid, the local health department began formal discussions with the Oregon Health Sciences University hospital (OHSU) regarding a collaborative effort in managed care. In January 1993, the neighboring Clackamas County Public Health Division joined the Multnomah County health department and OHSU in their planning for a Medicaid managed care strategy. The Oregon Primary Care Association, a statewide network of community health centers, soon joined the planning effort as well. The group developed plans for a jointly operated, fully capitated HMO that could serve Medicaid beneficiaries under Oregon's pending application with the US Health Care Financing Administration for an 1115 waiver to institute statewide Medicaid managed care. This waiver was approved in August 1993 as a 5-year demonstration program, and 1 month later the planning group's application to become a fully capitated Medicaid health plan was approved by the state Office of Medical Assistance Programs.

A detailed discussion of the County's managed care strategy is provided elsewhere.[7] Below we summarize key elements of the local health department's current involvement in the Medicaid managed care plan. The jointly-operated HMO was designed to provide inpatient and specialized outpatient services from OHSU's medical center, while offering primary care and case management services through a network of providers that comprise health department clinics, affiliated community health centers, and OHSU clinics staffed by residents and faculty. In total, the service network consisted of 17 organizations with 43 primary care clinics serving 11 Oregon counties.

The collaborating organizations chose to establish the HMO as a unit of county government under the administrative authority of the local health department. This strategy allowed the HMO to use the administrative machinery already in place within the health department for managing the delivery of primary care services, including its systems for scheduling, billing, and quality assurance. This strategy also required Multnomah County to administer a health plan that operated beyond county boundaries, because the network included community health centers located across the state. The legality of this arrangement was reviewed with the state attorney general's office and ultimately upheld. In mid-1997, the HMO was established as a separate nonprofit corporation but maintained its administrative ties to the founding organizations.

The plan began with 9500 enrollees who "rolled over" from their membership in PCOs that the health department and the community health centers operated under Oregon's existing managed care program. By the end of 1994, enrollment in CareOregon had doubled. Since its first year of operation, the CareOregon health plan has continued to expand its enrollment. Initially only beneficiaries of the Aid to Families with Dependent Children were enrolled in the plan, but in January 1995 the state extended eligibility to include the aged, blind, disabled and foster children who are eligible for Medicaid. Currently, almost half of the plan's enrolled population resides within Multnomah County, and a full 85% reside in the three-county Portland area.

Other Service Areas

Other service areas administered within the health department include a corrections health division that provides medical, dental, and psychiatric health services to adult and juvenile offenders who are in the custody of county correctional facilities. The regulatory health division within the department houses the following programs: (1) the medical examiner's office that determines the cause of death for county residents under certain circumstances; (2) an emergency medical services program that responds to over 42,000 requests for emergency medical services and transportation; (3) an environmental health division that inspects restaurants, swimming pools, lodging facilities, and adult nursing homes for compliance with health and safety codes, and monitors community water systems and other potential environmental hazards; (4) a childhood lead poisoning prevention program that operates as part of a multicounty intervention and provides blood lead screening at all county primary care facilities, environmental testing prompted by cases with elevated blood lead levels, and health education sessions regarding environmental exposure to lead; (5) a violence prevention program that provides funding to community agencies for implementing peace promotion programs; and (6) a vital statistics office that manages birth and death records.

The health department's support services division administers a central public health laboratory and oversees the laboratory and x-ray testing services that are performed at the department's primary care clinics. This division also oversees six pharmacies that are operated in the primary care centers. Other support services provided through this division include: an information and referral program that operates several telephone referral lines and researches information regarding available health services in the community; a health education unit that develops and disseminates a wide range of informational materials on health and safety issues; and a language services office hat provides interpreter services for limited-English speaking individuals who seek assistance from health department programs.

Infrastructure and Resources

Multnomah County Health Department maintains a large and geographically dispersed infrastructure for delivering personal and population-based health services in the community. In total, the department administers its programs and services through 9 community-based primary care clinics, 13 school-based clinics, 5 specialty clinics, 6 dental clinics, 6 clinic-based pharmacies, 6 field offices for providing community health services; a centralized laboratory; and a centralized administrative office. A total of 815 full-time equivalent personnel positions are assigned to the department. Clinical personnel for the department include 27 salaried physicians, 6 contracted physicians, 239 nurses (both RNs and LPNs), 46 nurse practitioners, 3 physician assistants, and 61 clinical assistants, technicians, and aides.

The health department's budget for fiscal year 1997 totals $108 million, substantially larger than the department's budget of $52 million in fiscal year 1994, before the start-up of CareOregon. The dramatic increase in department revenue after CareOregon's launch can be ascribed largely to the fully capitated reimbursement system under which CareOregon operates. Under this system, the health department receives the full stream of capitated reimbursement payments from Medicaid that cover all services for all CareOregon enrollees. The health department then distributes these funds appropriately among the participating providers in CareOregon, including OHSU Hospital and clinics, the community health centers, and Clackamas County Health Department. As a result of this system, Medicaid reimbursement stands as the single largest funding source for the department, comprising ~58% of the department's budget when revenue from the Oregon Health Plan and from the fee-for-service Medicaid program are combined. Local government appropriations provide ~32% of the department's revenue, while direct federal sources (not including Medicare or Medicaid) comprise 9% of the revenue. Funding from client fees, Medicare, third-party insurers, other state sources, and private foundations account for less than 1% each of the department's total budget. Fee revenue for the department is generated through the provision of facility inspections (including restaurants, swimming pools, lodging facilities, food services, and adult nursing homes) and through the provision of personal health services to clients who are not fully insured through the Oregon Health Plan, Medicare, or private health insurance plans. For these clients, the department uses a sliding fee schedule that is based on ability to pay.

Approximately 53% of the department's total budget supports expenditures related to the direct provision of personal health services to clients. Health department administrators suggest that expenditures for direct service provision have grown slightly since the initiation of CareOregon, because enrollment growth in CareOregon has allowed the department to provide medical services to greater number of Medicaid beneficiaries. Another 45% of this budget is used to purchase personal health services from contracted providers. These contracting providers include acute care hospitals, federally qualified health centers, and private physician practices. This proportion has substantially grown with the initiation of CareOregon, since the department's fiscal year 1994 budget called for only 17.5% of the budget to be devoted to contracts, medical referrals, and other service reimbursements. The remaining 2% of the department's budget supports environmental health and other nonpersonal public health activities. Although the relative proportion of the budget devoted to nonpersonal services has declined with the initiation of CareOregon (due to the large increase in the total budget), health department administrators suggest that overall levels of funding for nonpersonal services have remained generally stable.

Other Contributors to Local Public Health Practice

State Health Agency

The state health agency for Oregon is organized as a division within a larger umbrella agency, the Department of Human Resources, which administers all state programs related to health, mental health, substance abuse, public assistance, and social services. The state health division maintains responsibility for administering all state public health programs, operating the state public health laboratory, monitoring emergency medical systems within the state, and licensing hospitals located within the state. A separate division within the department, the Office of Medical Assistance Programs, administers the state Medicaid program, which is referred to as the Oregon Health Plan.

Administrators at the Multnomah County Health Department view their agency's relationship with the state health division as interactive and mutually supportive. As the state's most populated local public health jurisdiction, Multnomah County often serves as a testing ground for new state public health initiatives. The local health department also exists as a valuable source of information for the state agency regarding emerging public health needs and viable strategies for addressing public health concerns. The county and state agencies collaborate on number of public health initiatives, such as the childhood lead poisoning prevention project funded by the US Centers for Disease Control and Prevention. In general, state and local health agency administrative relationships are decentralized in Oregon, meaning that the state health division's primary mode of interaction with local health departments is through consultation, technical assistance, and periodic performance review.

One of the state's major initiatives for performance review, the Oregon Benchmarks program, involves the biennial collection and analysis of outcome-based information regarding a variety of state and county programs and services.[6] More than 50 of the outcome-based indicators adopted by the state legislature involve public health, health care services, or the accreditation of child care facilities. Under the Benchmarks program, county health departments are required to prepare a health plan that includes the use of at least two of the state-identified indicators for tracking progress toward county health objectives. The state health division then uses these indicators to assess county health department performance. Although these indicators are not currently used by the state health division for making funding and reimbursement decisions, a local community foundation now uses information from the Benchmarks program in making grant award decisions.

As one of the largest participating managed care plans in the Oregon Health Plan, the Multnomah County Health Department also maintains frequent interaction with the Office of Medical Assistance Programs (OMAP), which administers this program. County health department administrators suggest that their interaction with OMAP, although frequent, is not as productive as they would desire. These administrators suggest that the speed with which Oregon's Medicaid managed care program was adopted and implemented has created challenges for OMAP in keeping up with the program's needs regarding information, oversight, and evaluation. From the health department's perspective, the information systems and quality assurance processes currently operating within the Oregon Health Plan are often inadequate for providing policymakers and contracting health plans with the information needed to assure that the health needs of beneficiaries are being met and that contractors are fulfilling all program requirements. Health department administrators also suggest that, as with many governmental regulatory agencies, OMAP confronts difficulties in retaining adequate numbers of qualified staff who are often offered lucrative employment opportunities by the managed care plans that contract with OMAP. As a result, department staff do not always feel that OMAP is able to respond adequately to their requests for information or their recommendations regarding contract enforcement under the Oregon Health Plan. As an example, the health department is unable to obtain information from OMAP regarding the enrollment trends of limited English speaking beneficiaries of the Oregon Health Plan, to determine if other managed care organizations are failing to enroll these beneficiaries in their plans. Likewise, health department staff suggests that OMAP is largely unable to verify that health plans choosing not to contract with county health departments for the provision of public health services have adequate processes in place for directly providing these services to their enrollees. The state's capacity to monitor these and other aspects of the Oregon Health Plan are clearly improving, but challenges remain in addressing outstanding information, evaluation, and enforcement needs of the program. Nonetheless, Multnomah County Health Department maintains a close working relationship with OMAP and plays a critical role in identifying outstanding needs and advocating for their remedy.

Hospitals and Managed Care Plans

OHSU Hospital

Several Portland area hospitals make substantial contributions to the local public health system and maintain strong relationships with the county health department. As a participant in the CareOregon health plan, the OHSU Hospital works closely with the health department in administering this jointly operated plan. However, OHSU Hospital and the health department maintain a long history of interorganizational collaboration that predates the CareOregon project by many years. The hospital itself had been owned and operated by Multnomah County until 1973, when county officials sold it to OHSU in order to free local resources for use in purchasing medical care for the working poor (under the Project Health initiative). Many of OHSU's medical school faculty have practiced in the county's primary care clinics for years, either on a voluntary basis or under contracts with the health department. Several of the health department's primary care clinics were originally staffed by pediatricians and nurse practitioners from OHSU, until sufficient numbers of clinical staff could be recruited by the department. Currently, a state prenatal project funds OHSU perinatologists to rotate through county health department clinics and provide support and consulting to clinic staff regarding infant mortality reduction strategies, prenatal care practices, and related clinical issues. This program operates not only in Multnomah County but also in other counties across the state. Interestingly, faculty from OHSU's family medicine department serve as medical directors for several county health departments, although this is not the case for Multnomah County.

OHSU also plays an instrumental role in designing and implementing a number of the community health interventions currently underway in Multnomah County and statewide. The hospital operates a public campaign to promote accident prevention through bicycle safety, which includes a bicycle helmet give-away program. The hospital also sponsors a head injury prevention program targeted at high school students, in cooperation with the Oregon Blue Cross and Blue Shield Association. Through this program, neurology faculty from OHSU joins with leaders from community groups and conduct educational sessions in area high schools on topics including seat belt use, driving while intoxicated, and the incidence of unintentional head injuries.

OHSU's hospital administrator suggests that the hospital's involvement in public health issues and its relationship with the county health department have been strengthened as a result of the jointly operated CareOregon health plan. In collaboration with the county health department, OHSU hospital has worked to establish its own network of primary care clinics to supplement those of the county and thereby improve access to services for Medicaid beneficiaries. These efforts have allowed the hospital to assume a growing role in providing access to primary care and preventive health services, in contrast to the provision of specialized medical services that typically dominate the agendas of academic medical centers. Moreover, the collaborative CareOregon project has created expanded opportunities for clinical staff from OHSU Hospital to learn basic public health principles and practices from the county health department. OHSU's hospital administrator suggests that, as a result of these learning opportunities, OHSU staff have adopted more effective and efficient clinical practices through an increased awareness of basic health promotion and disease prevention practices, and through a reduced dependence on the expensive and often excessive medical technologies available though the medical center.

OHSU's educational mission has also been affected by the hospital's close relationship with the local health department. As part of the medical school curriculum at OHSU, medical students are rotated into community practice settings and asked to design and implement public health improvement projects during their rotation. The county health department's clinics serve as settings in which students gain experience not only in clinical practice but also in the principles of community health improvement and public health practice.

Administrators from both organizations recognize that the relationships between OHSU and the county health department may require adaptation in response to larger changes in the local health care environment. To ensure the sustained competitiveness of the jointly operated CareOregon health plan, a new organizational structure for the plan may be required. OHSU administrators are currently working with the state legislature to change the organizational status of its hospital to that of a public authority, which would give the organization enhanced flexibility in such practices as purchasing, contracting, hiring, and employee compensation. If successful, this change might create a rationale for reorganizing the CareOregon health plan under OHSU ownership rather than under an independent organizational entity. Regardless of changes in the form of relationship between OHSU and the health department, it appears certain that the strength and durability of this relationship will remain intact.

Sisters of Providence Health System

The private health care systems operating in the Portland area also make important contributions to the local public health system, although their ties to the local health department may not be as strong or as formalized. The Sisters of Providence Health Care System lists community health improvement as an explicit component of its organizational mission. Pursuant to this mission, the system conducts an annual community health needs assessment of the Portland metropolitan area to determine the predominant health needs and risks in the community. The system uses data obtained from the county health department, the United Way, and other sources to compile a report on health service needs that is then used to shape program and service priorities for the system. Providence is also a major provider of uncompensated care to uninsured and underinsured residents of Multnomah County through its two hospitals and primary care clinic. The primary care clinic is staffed by physicians being trained in the hospital's internal medicine residency program and provides ~12,000 patient encounters per year to uninsured and underinsured patients. During the first quarter of 1995, Providence's two hospitals provided over $1500 in charity care and an estimated $800 in nonbilled services such as cash and in-kind donations, free health screenings and assessments, and other volunteer clinical work. Providence's hospitals and primary care clinic also serve as major sources of primary and specialty care for Medicaid and Medicare beneficiaries in the Portland area. Providence funds a state Medicaid eligibility technician to work onsite at its facilities to help patients determine their eligibility for public programs. In total, unsponsored services such as charity care, education and research, nonbilled activities, and the unpaid costs of Medicaid and Medicare participation amounted to 36% of the system's total operating expenses for the first quarter of 1995.

Providence also contributes to the accessibility of primary care services in medically underserved areas through the operation of a neighborhood health clinic in partnership with the county health department. Along with other contributors, Providence provides funding to support the operating expenses of this clinic and also donates the time of physicians and other clinical personnel to help in staffing the clinic. In 1992,

Providence dedicated $10,700 for clinic operating expenses and $289,777 in reimbursing contracted physicians for their charity care and community service. Through similar arrangements, Providence also contributes to the operation of a migrant health center and several dental clinics that serve low-income residents of a neighboring county.

Providence collaborates with the local health department on several other community health initiatives. The hospital and health department jointly sponsor two projects in underserved areas of Portland which are designed to encourage the utilization of prenatal care services among low-income pregnant women. In both of these projects, clinical staff from Providence works with community health teams from the health department to deliver targeted prenatal care services to high-risk women. Providence also collaborates with the health department on a communitywide breast and cervical cancer screening program, an initiative to deliver health care to homeless populations, and a childhood immunization initiative.

The Oregon Health Plan exists as another arena in which Providence interacts with the local health department. The Providence system operates its own managed care plan for serving Medicaid beneficiaries under the Oregon Health Plan. Therefore, Providence is a competitor with the health department's CareOregon plan in the market for these beneficiaries. Providence's plan served almost 12,000 Oregon Health Plan enrollees as of April 1995, making it the fourth largest Medicaid HMO in the three-county metropolitan area. Providence's history of serving vulnerable population groups and its experience in operating a commercial managed care product have allowed the system to operate successfully in the Medicaid HMO market, according to its administrators. Providence maintains an extensive health assessment and care management system for its Medicaid enrollees, which includes components such as administration of a health risk assessment to new members; targeted health-risk education for individuals with specific risk factors; patient tracking and reminder systems to improve the delivery of preventive services such as immunizations, mammograms, and pap smears; multidisciplinary health management programs for high-risk patients and those with chronic diseases; a 20-hour medical advice telephone system staffed by registered nurses; and a regular series of free health education classes on topics such as childbirth, smoking cessation, nutrition, weight control, stress management, and exercise counseling.

Despite being competitors in the Medicaid HMO market, Providence maintains several collaborative partnerships with the county health department for serving Medicaid HMO enrollees. Through one of these partnerships, Providence serves as a designated provider of hospital services to Medicaid enrollees in the health department's CareOregon health plan. CareOregon administrators report that their decision to contract with Providence for specified hospital services despite the existing partnership with OHSU Hospital accomplishes two objectives: (1) to expand access to hospital services for CareOregon enrollees who may be geographically isolated from the distant OHSU campus and (2) to remain competitive in enrolling Medicaid beneficiaries who may desire to seek care from a private provider such as Providence. Health department administrators also express confidence in the capacity and expertise developed by Providence for serving vulnerable population groups.

In another partnership between the two organizations, Providence subcontracts with the local health department for providing maternity case management services to Medicaid beneficiaries enrolled in its HMO. Under the Oregon Health Plan administrative rules, Medicaid HMOs may choose whether to provide maternity case management services directly to their enrollees or to subcontract with county health departments for these services (**Table 4**). Providence administrators indicate that their decision to subcontract with the health department for these services emerged from a desire to employ the most effective mechanisms available in the community for encouraging prenatal care utilization and improving birth outcomes among their enrolled Medicaid beneficiaries. Under the subcontract, community health nurses from the health department conduct home visits with expectant mothers enrolled in Providence's HMO. During these visits, nurses conduct prenatal health assessments and counseling and insure that the enrollees receive scheduled prenatal clinical exams from their primary care providers. These partnerships between Providence and the local health department illustrate the organizations' unique abilities to manage both competition and collaboration within the Medicaid managed care market so that both organizations meet their missions of community health improvement as well as their financial imperatives.

Legacy Health System

Another large hospital-based health care system in Portland, Legacy Health System, is expanding its involvement in the local public health system as it becomes more involved in managed health care generally and in the Medicaid market specifically. The system's two Portland hospitals have historically dominated its operations and its mission. As a result, the

Table 4
Excerpt from the Oregon Health Plan Administrative Rules Regarding Relationships Between HMOs and County Health Departments

Rule 410-141-120 (1) (h):
In order to make advantageous use of the system of public health services available through county health departments and other publicly supported programs and to ensure access to public health services through contract under ORS Chapter 414:

(A) Unless cause can be demonstrated to OMAP's satisfaction why such an agreement is not feasible, Contractors shall execute agreements with publicly funded providers for authorization of and payment for point-of-contact services in the following categories:
- immunizations;
- sexually transmitted diseases; and
- other communicable diseases.

(B) OMAP Members may receive the following services from appropriate non-Contractor providers:
- family planning services; and
- human immunodeficiency virus (HIV) and acquired immune deficiency syndrome (AIDS) prevention services.

(C) Contractors are encouraged to execute agreements with publicly funded providers for authorization of and payment for services in the following categories:
- maternity case management;
- well-child care;
- prenatal care;
- school-based clinic services;
- health services for children provided through schools and Head Start programs; and
- screening services to provide early detection of health care problems among low income women and children, migrant workers, and other special population groups.

(D) Recognizing the social value of partnerships between county health departments and other publicly supported programs and other health providers, Contractors shall take appropriate measures to involve publicly supported health care and service programs in the development and implementation of managed health care programs."

OMAP = Oregon Office of Medical Assistance Programs
Contractor = Managed care plan
Source: Oregon Department of Human Resources, Office of Medical Assistance Programs. Oregon Health Plan Administrative Rules. *Salem, Oregon: OMAP, 1995.*

system's contributions to public health have traditionally been limited to the provision of charity care to low-income residents in the Portland area. One of Legacy's hospitals, located in central Portland, has maintained a long history of serving the health care needs of low-income residents, making the hospital a disproportionate share hospital under Medicaid regulations and the second-largest provider of uncompensated care in Portland (behind OHSU Hospital). Over the past decade, Legacy's administrators launched several managed care products in order to remain competitive in a local health care market that has rapidly moved away from fee-for-service health care delivery systems. In partnership with the Oregon Blue Cross and Blue Shield Association, Legacy launched a commercial HMO and later a plan for serving Medicaid beneficiaries under the Oregon Health Plan. As revenues from hospital operations have continued to shrink under the expanding managed care market, Legacy's health plans have become increasingly important to the viability of the organization. These plans have also created imperatives for the system to begin emphasizing the delivery of health promotion and disease prevention activities within its enrollee populations.

A growing recognition of the importance of communitywide participation in health promotion and disease prevention activities led Legacy's administrator to found a group called Oregon Health Systems in Collaboration, comprising administrators from the major medical care providers operating in the Portland area. This group was convened to serve as a forum for conducting communitywide planning regarding health care delivery and for initiating collaborative interventions aimed at community health improvement. Although the group originally included only the major medical care systems in the community, Legacy's administrator soon recognized the need for involvement by public health agencies and therefore recruited the participation of the Multnomah County Health Department as well as the state health division. With leadership and support from Legacy, this group has attended conferences and seminars together on the topic of community health improvement and has sustained ongoing dialogue about systems of care for Medicaid beneficiaries and other vulnerable populations in the community. As most of the participating organizations operate Medicaid managed care plans, this group has also provided a forum for negotiating interorganizational service agreements and reimbursement schedules under the Oregon Health Plan. Although the group has not yet shown much success in launching broad-based public health interventions, it has appeared successful in improving awareness about community health issues and concerns and about organizational resources and capacities within the community. Legacy's administrator indicates that participants are now moving to commit a percentage of their earnings each year to the group, which will then be used to support communitywide health improvement interventions such as efforts to assess health status and health needs in the community at large.

Legacy and the local health department have maintained a mixed but improving relationship in the Medicaid managed care arena. The Legacy-Blue Cross joint venture HMO, called HMO Oregon, quickly achieved the status of the largest Medicaid HMO in the Portland area with almost 25,000 enrollees or 24% of the market as of May 1995. Much of this venture's enrollment success could be attributed to the large network of private physicians that joined the independent practice association model HMO in response to Blue Cross' active recruitment efforts statewide and its generous fee-for-service reimbursement schedules. Local health department administrators became concerned not only about the competitive threat that this HMO represented but also about the ability of the private physicians within HMO Oregon to address adequately the complex medical and social needs of the Medicaid population. Elevating these concerns was the fact that, during the first year of the Oregon Health Plan implementation (1994), HMO Oregon chose at first not to subcontract with the local health department for public health services such as maternity case management. After a year's experience with this population, administrators at HMO Oregon decided against providing the maternity case management services internally and established a contract with the local health department for these services. This development clearly improved relations between the two organizations and alleviated some of the local health department's concerns.

Some competitive tension remains between Legacy and the local health department, primarily regarding contracts for hospital services. Health department administrators would like to establish contractual arrangements that would enable CareOregon enrollees to access hospital services at Legacy's centrally located hospital. Their attempts at negotiating a discounted fee schedule with Legacy have so far proven unsuccessful, in part because CareOregon also maintains contracts for hospital services with Legacy's primary competitors, OHSU and Providence. Legacy administrators maintain that exclusive contracting arrangements are an important component of their organization's competitive strategy in the hospital and managed care markets. The system's ability to insure both quality and efficiency in health care delivery hinges upon being clinically and financially responsible for a defined population, according to these administrators. Consequently, Legacy has so far declined to establish discounted fee arrangements with CareOregon, which would not give the system exclusive responsibility for providing hospital services to CareOregon enrollees.

Kaiser Foundation Health Plan

Kaiser exists as the oldest managed care organization in the area as well as the nation, having its origins in serving workers of the Kaiser shipyards in Portland and Vancouver, Washington during World War II. Today, Kaiser stands as the largest HMO in the Portland area with more than 400,000 enrollees and the third-largest Medicaid HMO in the area with more than 13,000 enrollees. Although historically Kaiser has been a major provider of both hospital and ambulatory care services in the community, the closure of its centrally located hospital and the development of contracts with other hospital providers in the area suggest that the organization is diminishing its involvement in direct hospital care provision.

Kaiser's relationship with the local health department extends at least as far back as the early 1970s, when Kaiser served as a participating plan in the Project Health initiative by the health department that brokered prepaid health care for low-income uninsured individuals and families. Under the current managed care initiative of the Oregon Health Plan, Kaiser contracts for the local health department to provide maternity case management services to Kaiser's Medicaid enrollees. Kaiser is also an active participant on the Oregon Health Systems in Collaboration project and interacts frequently with health department administrators in this forum.

Kaiser administers a number of other initiatives that target community health issues. Kaiser contributes both clinical staff time and medical supplies to a coalition of seven nonprofit community health centers operating in the Portland area for serving uninsured and underinsured community members. A small grants program administered by Kaiser has contributed over $170,000 to community coalitions and nonprofit groups for community interventions involving child health and safety, teen parent education, teen pregnancy prevention, homelessness, and domestic violence. Many of these interventions include leadership and involvement from the local health department. Kaiser also operates a program that distributes free bicycle helmets to low-income children, along with a series of bicycle safety fairs which has reached over 30,000 residents during the past 2 years.

Portland Adventist Health System

Portland Adventist Medical Center stands as the other major hospital provider in the Portland area. Owned by a nonprofit hospital system affiliated with the Seventh Day Adventist Church, Portland Adventist also operates under an explicit mission of community service and community health improvement. Many of the organization's community initiatives focus on health education and health promotion. For example, the hospital operates a health van that travels to churches and other community organizations to perform free health assessments, including such services as cholesterol screening and blood pressure monitoring. Corporate donations are solicited from area businesses to help offset the costs of operating and maintaining this service. The hospital also collaborates with a local nonprofit organization in operating a telephone hotline for "latch-key" children who must stay home alone after school.

Interaction with the local health department had been minimal until the hospital decided in 1993 to establish a community health planning group for the central Portland area that is served by the hospital. As part of this effort, Portland Adventist began working with the local health department as well as with local schools, businesses, churches, physicians, and community groups to identify health needs in the central Portland area. The local health department proved instrumental in providing area health statistics that could be used by the group to identify the most pressing health needs and to develop collaborative interventions to address these needs. After almost a year of regular meetings, the group decided to develop an intervention for reducing child school absenteeism. Portland Adventist provided a one-time start-up grant of $250,000 to fund a case management team that comprised a family support worker, social worker, and school nurse to conduct child and family counseling in both the home and school for at-risk children. Additionally, the program contracts with a pediatric nurse practitioner for addressing specific clinical health issues. Now that this intervention is successfully underway, the community group continues to meet on a regular basis to explore other health issues and develop new projects within the community.

Administrators at Portland Adventist suggest that the hospital and its community health initiatives have not been dramatically affected by developments in the Medicaid managed care market. The hospital maintains contracts for providing hospital services to several Medicaid HMOs, and their Medicaid enrollees comprise ~10% of the patients served by Adventist. Administrators indicate that the hospital's involvement in community health issues stem primarily from an organizational mission of community service, rather than from financial or competitive motivations under managed care. Currently, most of the hospital's relationships with managed care plans do not entail financial risk-sharing arrangements or capitated reimbursement schedules. Hospital administrators speculate that these arrangements, if they were to develop, might create additional incentives for engaging in the types of community health activities that the hospital already has underway. Administrators at Portland Adventist do suggest that the Oregon Health Plan holds potential for reducing the uncompensated care burdens of its hospital, thereby freeing additional resources to commit to its community health mission. The state Medicaid office indicates that the Oregon Health Plan has already reduced hospital uncompensated care costs by 30% on average, suggesting that the plan may truly enable local hospitals such as Portland Adventist to increase their community health involvement.

Other Managed Care Plans

In the Multnomah County area, the local health department's CareOregon plan competes with 5 other HMOs that serve Medicaid beneficiaries. HMO Oregon, a plan operated by Oregon Blue Cross and

Blue Shield and Legacy Health System, maintains the largest Medicaid beneficiary enrollment in the area with almost 25,000 enrollees as of midyear 1995. CareOregon ranks second in enrollment with ~20,000 enrollees, with Kaiser Permanente's plan (13,625) and Providence's plan (13,294) also serving substantial numbers of beneficiaries. Local health department administrators attribute much of CareOregon's solid market position to its unique abilities to serve vulnerable populations. The health department is known in the community for its long history of providing access to quality health services for Medicaid and medically indigent populations. Administrators suggest that the health department's unique skills and reputation also create challenges for CareOregon to remain competitive in the Medicaid marketplace, because of the potential for adverse risk selection. As an example, the health department's extensive capacity for providing language translation services appears to encourage larger proportions of recent immigrants and other non-English speaking beneficiaries to enroll in CareOregon. More than 35% of CareOregon enrollees speak a language other than English at home. These enrollees may require more provider time for successful care management, and they may be at greater risk for certain health conditions than the average Medicaid beneficiary.

Several of the competing Medicaid HMOs maintain contracts with the local health department for the provision of core public health services to their enrollees. The state Medicaid agency encourages HMOs to subcontract with local health departments for these types of services. Figure 1 provides an excerpt from the state contract regarding this language. Some, but not all, of the Medicaid HMOs operating in Multnomah County choose to contract with Multnomah County Health Department for tuberculosis control services, sexually transmitted disease control services, and maternity case management. HMOs that choose not to contract with the health department for these services pose special problems, because the health department must turned away enrollees from these plans when they seek care from health department clinics. Health department administrators report that this policy is very difficult to enforce because of the organization's basic philosophy of open access to services, and because of the difficulties in verifying enrollment status for some patients.

Several of the managed care plans operating in Portland interact through a multi-organizational planning and policy development association known as Oregon Health Systems in Collaboration. Participants include the Providence and Legacy health systems, Blue Cross and Blue Shield of Oregon, Kaiser Permanente Northwest, the Oregon Health Sciences University, Adventist Medical Center, and the local health department. This association serves as a forum for identifying community health problems that affect all of the participating health systems, and for initiating jointly-sponsored initiatives to address these problems. Important initiatives sponsored by the association include a community-wide health assessment and priority-setting process known as the Healthy Communities Initiative, and a state-wide childhood immunization registry.

Community Health Centers

A network of seven nonprofit community health clinics operates within the Portland metropolitan area, providing health services to low-income residents of the Portland metropolitan area. These clinics participate in a collaborative venture called the Coalition of Community Health Clinics that serves as mechanism for pooling resources, coordinating services, and joint planning. The local health department also participates in the Coalition and contributes resources and manpower to the clinics, along with other organizations in the community. As a federally designated community health center (under Section 330), the health department maintains a long history of involvement in community health clinic activities statewide. The Sisters of Providence Health System and the Kaiser Foundation Health Plan are also major contributors to the Coalition. Member clinics provided over 25,000 patient visits during 1995 to Portland area residents. More than 800 professional and lay volunteers participated in providing health services through Coalition clinics during this same year.

The Coalition administers several special programs that support the provision of health services to vulnerable population groups. Through the Specialty Referral Project, the clinics maintain a pool of ~150 medical specialists who volunteer their services to clients of the seven clinics. The project allows the clinics to coordinate their referrals in order to assure that all clients receive timely access to specialists. The Coalition also administers a donations clearinghouse through which donated medical supplies, equipment, and medications are distributed to participating clinics. Many of the area's health care providers are important contributors to this program. Additionally, the Coalition operates a prescription assistance telephone hotline that assists low-income individuals in obtaining prescription medications.

Other Organizations

A range of other public and private organizations makes important contributions to the public health system in Multnomah County. Local health department administrators report that the local chapters of the Urban League and the United Way are particularly involved in activities such as assessing health needs in the community and supporting the implementation of community health interventions. A number of grassroots community and neighborhood groups are also active in the Portland metropolitan area, and the local health department works with many of these organizations through its six field teams. Likewise, many area churches participate in public health activities such as the community health assessment and intervention partnership supported by Portland Adventist Hospital. Public sector organizations also make substantial contributions to local public health activities such as the violence prevention program, which is sustained through the involvement of local public school systems, county family assistance centers, and city and county law enforcement agencies.

Measures of Public Health System Performance

Structured interviews with the local health department director during 1992 and 1995 suggest that performance of core public health functions within the jurisdiction remains consistently above average. These interviews, which used the *Local Public Health Performance Assessment Survey* (see Chapter 1), indicate that overall performance has declined from 64% of the maximum possible score in 1992 to 57% of the maximum in 1995 (**Figure 1**). Both of these results exceed the median score of 51%, which was found among the selection of 63 local public health jurisdictions surveyed in 1992 and 1993. Substantial declines in community performance appear to have occurred for the core public health practices of *informing and educating the community regarding health issues, managing resources and developing organizational structure,* and *evaluating programs and providing quality assurance*—all of which fall within the core public health function of assurance. A notable performance decline is also reported for the practice of *setting priorities among health needs.* Substantial increases in community performance are reported for the practices of *implementing programs and services,* and *developing plans and policies to address health needs.* On the whole, community performance in the core public health functions of assessment and policy development appears to have remained relatively stable during the 3-year period. Performance of assessment activities has remained lower than performance of other functions.

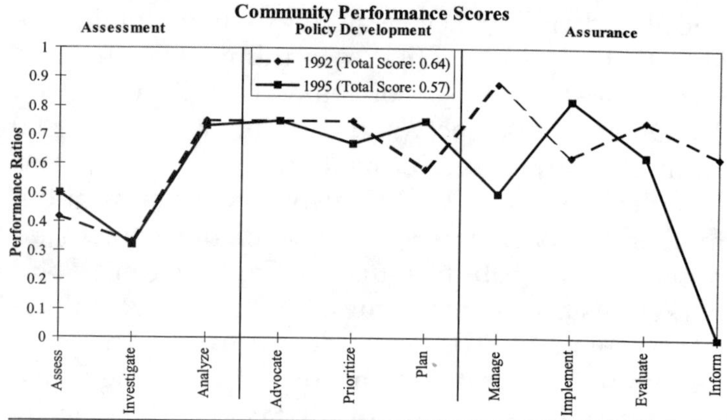

Figure 1. Community public health performance scores for Multnomah County, Oregon.

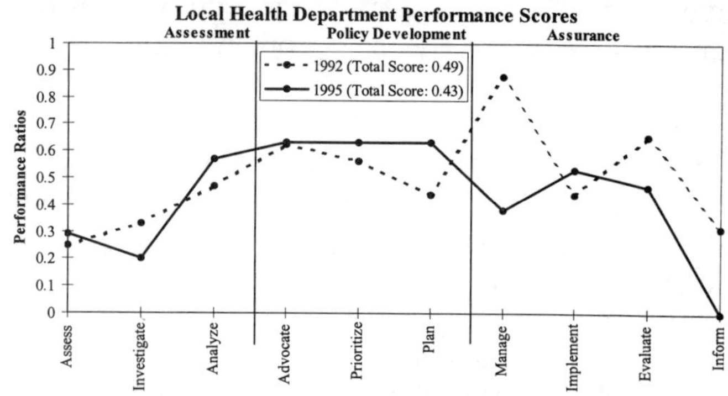

Health department performance score as a percentage of community score

	Assess	Investigate	Analyze	Advocate	Prioritize	Plan	Manage	Implement	Evaluate	Inform
1992:	60%	99%	62%	83%	75%	75%	100%	70%	87%	50%
1995:	58%	63%	78%	84%	94%	84%	76%	65%	75%	0%
%Chng:	-3%	-37%	25%	1%	25%	12%	-24%	-8%	-15%	-100%

Figure 2. Health department performance scores for Multnomah County, Oregon.

When we examine the public health activities contributed specifically by the local health department (**Figure 2**), performance appears to have declined somewhat during the 3-year period. The overall health department performance ratio drops from 49% of the maximum possible score in 1993 to 43% of the maximum in 1995. As with the community performance score, the most precipitous declines are reported within the core function of assurance. The only substantial increase in performance appears to occur for the practice of *developing plans and policies to address health needs.*

When we examine the extent to which other organizations participate in public health activities within the community, state and local government agencies appear to be involved in the largest proportion of these activities (**Figure 3**). State agencies appear to have maintained their overall level of participation in these activities between 1992 and 1995, but their involvement appears to have shifted somewhat from assessment and assurance activities to policy development activities.

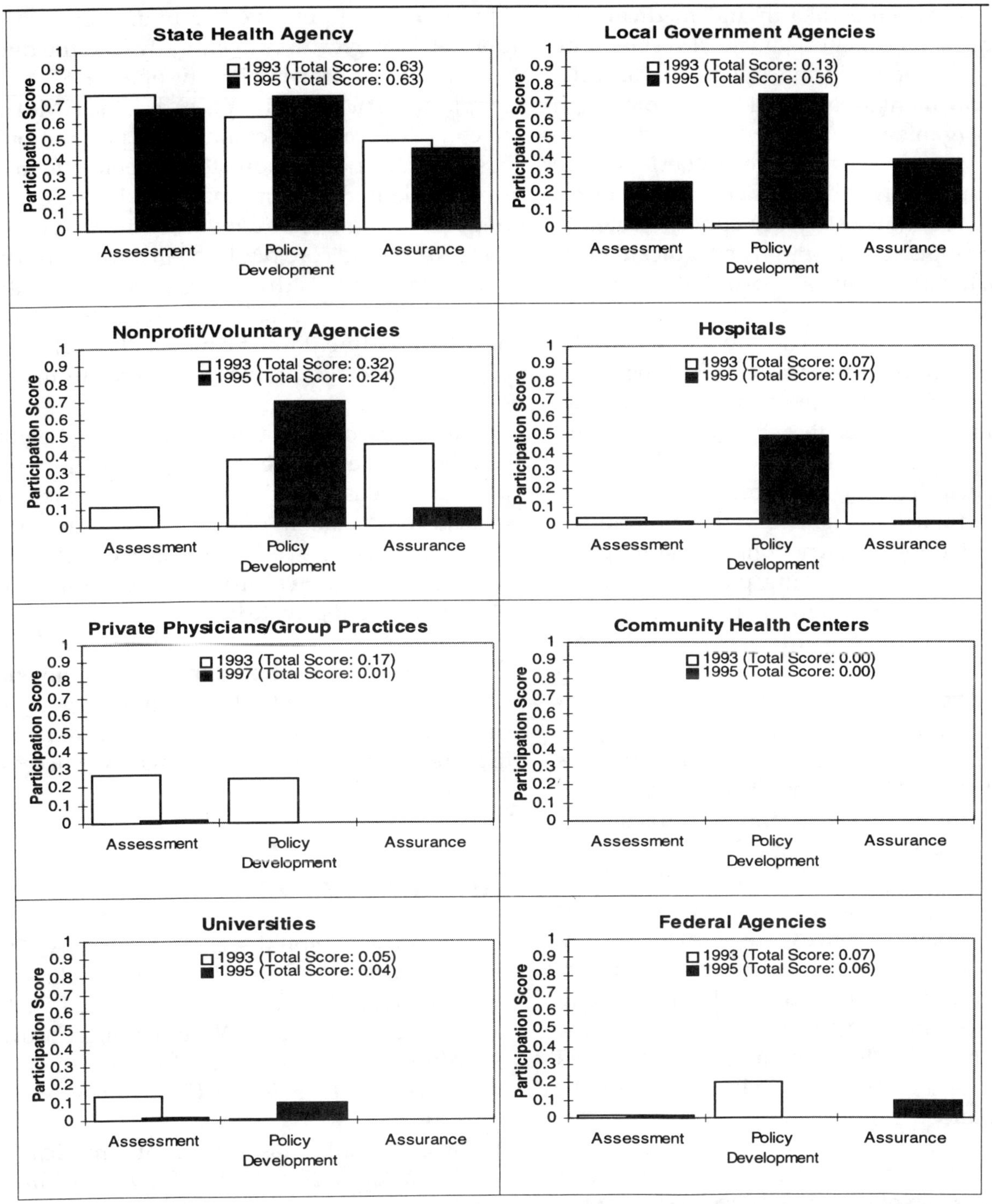

Figure 3. Participation in public health activities by selected organizations, 1992 and 1993 (as reported by the local health director).

Local government agencies appear to have increased their participation notably during this 3-year period, especially for policy development activities. Hospitals and nonprofit agencies are reported to have diminished their overall levels of participation in public health activities but to have increased their involvement specifically in policy development activities. Other organizations—such as physician groups, community health centers, universities, and federal agencies—appear to have participated in a relatively small proportion of public health activities throughout this time period.

The reported trends in public health performance occur during a time period that has seen dramatic changes in the local public health and medical care systems serving Multnomah County. The statewide implementation of Medicaid managed care, and the local health department's expanded involvement as a managed care organization, are two of the most notable changes. The observed declines in performance for some assurance activities and increases in performance for other assurance activities appear related to these larger developments. Through its Medicaid managed care plan, the local health department reports expanded roles in service delivery activities. At the same time, however, the department continues to show relatively low performance in assessment activities. Some of these assessment activities may have become more difficult to maintain under the statewide Medicaid managed care program, which has allowed a collection of private health plans to assume responsibilities in serving vulnerable and underserved populations.

With the health department no longer assuming primary responsibility for delivering public health services to these populations, new monitoring systems may be needed to assess health needs and threats among populations that are served through the collection of managed care plans. The state Medicaid agency holds primary authority for establishing reporting requirements for managed care plans and monitoring the care delivered through these plans. State agencies, however, are also reported to have diminished roles in assessment activities. The emerging collaborative effort among local health plans—the Oregon Health Systems in Collaboration—may offer an effective vehicle for expanding assessment activities within the community. As described earlier, this group is working to identify existing gaps in assessment and to establish a dedicated pool of resources to support communitywide assessment efforts. Clearly, assessment activities need to be addressed as a priority area in improving public health performance within the jurisdiction.

Future Prospects and Projections

Portland's local public health system thrives on a constellation of overlapping public and private efforts in health improvement—an arrangement which has developed over time through decades of effective leadership and informed management in the public and private sectors. The local health department is notable for its direct involvement in the operation of a managed health care enterprise for Medicaid beneficiaries. Through this involvement the local health department has achieved notable success in shaping the local Medicaid managed care market, rather than simply reacting to it. The imperative to remain competitive in this market, however, may eventually lead the department to rethink its role in the jointly-operated HMO. For example, administrators suggest that the HMO may need to consider enrolling commercial populations as well as Medicaid populations to compete effectively with private plans. Such a strategy may lead the local health department to become involved in activities that extend far beyond core public health issues and concerns, and that potentially draw resources and attention away from these core issues. In view of these risks, the local health department must continually evaluate the benefits and opportunity costs that accrue from its involvement in Medicaid managed care.

This study of Portland's local public health system suggests that a key area for future development lies in population-based health activities, and especially public health assessment efforts. Already the local health department is engaged in efforts to develop collaborative community health assessment initiatives with other public and private health care organizations serving Portland. Success in these efforts will be critical if the local public health system is to remain effective in addressing the community's evolving health needs and risks. Portland appears to have the leadership, expertise, and resources necessary to achieve success in these endeavors.

References

1. American Hospital Association (AHA). *1995 AHA Guide to the Healthcare Field*. Chicago, Ill: AHA; 1996.
2. American Medical Association (AMA). *Physician Data by County, 1994*. Washington, DC: AMA; 1996.
3. Multnomah County Health Department. *Annual Report 1994-1995*. Portland, Ore: Multnomah County, 1996.
4. Group Health Association of America (GHAA). *1995 National Directory of HMOs*. Washington, DC: GHAA; 1995.
5. Miller CA, Moos M-K. *Local Health Departments: Fifteen Case Studies*. Chapel Hill, NC: American Public Health Association; 1981.
6. Nelson DE, Fleming DW, Grant-Worley J, Houchen T. Outcome-based management and public health: the Oregon Benchmarks experience. *J Public Health Manage Pract*. 1995;1(2):8-17.
7. Mays GP. A public-sector HMO in Portland, Oregon. In: PK Halverson, AD Kaluzny, and CP McLaughlin. *Managed Care and Public Health*. Gaithersburg, MD: Aspen Publishers; 1998:233-242.

Chapter 15

Case Study of Southwest Washington Health District

Key Attributes

- Transfer of responsibility from the local health department to community providers for delivery of many personal health services.
- Local health department capacity building in population-based public health services.
- Formal community health assessment and improvement initiative with broad community participation.
- Strong collaborative relationships between the local health department, the community hospital, and the local division of a national managed care corporation.

Community Characteristics

Demographic and Socioeconomic Characteristics

The Southwest Washington Health District is located in the southwestern corner of Washington State, just north of the Oregon border and the Columbia river. Until January 1998, the district comprised three counties—Clark, Skamania, and Klickitat—which contained a combined population of ~335,000 residents. In January, the rural Klickitat County formed its own local health department, leaving the district as a two-county jurisdiction. Clark County accounts for the majority of this population with 310,000 residents. The district's largest city of Vancouver lies just across the river from Portland, Oregon, and contains ~130,000 residents. The remainder of the district's population is distributed in small towns and rural areas. The district's population continues to grow rapidly, with a total population increase of more than 20% between 1980 and 1990. During the 1990s, Clark County has been the fastest-growing county in Washington State, averaging annual population increases of ~4%.

The district's population contains relatively small racial and ethnic minority groups. White residents account for ~94.5% of the district population, followed by persons of Hispanic origin (2.7%), Asians and Pacific Islanders (2.3%), African Americans (1.2%), and Native Americans (1.2%). A small but growing immigrant population resides within the district, including many Eastern Europeans who have arrived during the 1990s. Approximately 3.6% of the population is estimated to be foreign-born.

On the whole, socioeconomic characteristics of the district's population mirror state and national norms, although specific geographic and demographic populations within the district experience substantial socioeconomic challenges. Per capita personal income for the district stood at $18,602 in 1992, which is marginally below state and national norms (**Table 1**). Per

Table 1
Demographic Characteristics: Southwest Washington Health District, Washington

Population (1990)	262,958
Percent 65 years and older (1990)	10.8
Percent non-White (1990)	5.5
Percent speaking a language other than English at home (1990)	5.6
Percent completing high school degree (1990)	82.8
Percent of individuals below federal poverty level (1989)	9.8
Per capita income (1992)	$18,602
Average percent unemployed (1993)	7.0

Data from US Department of Commerce, Bureau of the Census.

Table 2
Health Status Indicators: Southwest Washington Health District, Washington, 1996

Infant mortality rate per 1000 live births	6.3
Percent of adolescent females age 10-17 giving birth	3.9
Percent of infants with low birth weight	4.8
Percent of births with prenatal care later than first trimester	18.7
Deaths per 100,000 population, age-adjusted	793.5
Cancer, all types	196.9
Lung cancer	58.8
Female breast cancer	19.7
Heart disease	226.3
Cerebrovascular diseases	59.3
Chronic obstructive pulmonary diseases	47.1
Suicide	17.4
Pneumonia and influenza	35.7
HIV / AIDS	4.7
Diabetes mellitus	34.3
Homicide	1.7

Data from Washington State Department of Health (unpublished data, 1997).

capita income in the district's two predominately rural counties appears much lower, at $15,974 in Klickitat County and $17,133 in Skamania County. Census data for 1990 indicate that the proportion of the population below the federal poverty level was 9.8% for the district as a whole, which is somewhat lower than state and national averages. However, the poverty rate in Klickitat County far exceeds these norms, with 17.0% of the population living below the poverty threshold. Unemployment stands at 7.1% of the district's total civilian labor force, but it exceeds 13% in the district's two rural counties. Many residents of Vancouver and Clark County maintain employment in the diversified service and manufacturing industries of the Portland metropolitan area. In contrast, agricultural and timber operations are the dominant industries within Klickitat and Skamania Counties.

Approximately 83% of adult district residents have achieved 12 or more years of education, similar to state and national trends. However, only 16% of the population have 4 or more years of college education, which is substantially below state and national norms. Educational attainment in the district's two rural counties is substantially lower than in the more urbanized Clark County.

Community Health Status Indicators

The counties comprising the Southwest Washington Health District show substantial diversity in community health status. Disease-specific mortality rates for Clark County, the largest and most urban county within the district, generally fall below state and national norms. By contrast, Klickitat County confronts markedly higher mortality rates for pneumonia and influenza, chronic obstructive pulmonary diseases, lung cancer, suicide, and motor vehicle crashes. Skamania County faces substantially higher mortality rates from heart disease. Mortality rates from cerebrovascular disease, breast cancer, and HIV / AIDS are below the statewide averages in all three counties. The infant mortality rate for Clark county stands at 5 deaths per 1000 live births in 1995, which is slightly below state and national averages. Aggregate health status indicators for the district as a whole are shown in **Table 2**.

The low birth weight rate exceeds state norms in all three counties, with the highest rate of 8.3% occurring in the Klickitat County. Approximately 80% of Clark County mothers received prenatal care in the first trimester, compared with 73% in Klickitat County and 87% in Skamania County. Clark County confronts the highest adolescent birth rate of the three counties, with 31% of births occurring to females age 12 to 17 years. This rate exceeds the statewide average of 29%, as well as the rates in Klickitat and Skamania Counties of 22 and 24%, respectively. Clark and Klickitat Counties face similar rates of maternal smoking (18%) that exceed the statewide rate of 16% as well as the Skamania County rate of 13%.

Table 3
Health Resources in Southwest Washington Health District, Washington[a]

Number of nonfederal physicians (Number per 100,000 population) 1992	347 (121)
Family practice	50 (17)
General practice	11 (4)
Internal medicine	38 (13)
Obstetrics / gynecology	22 (8)
Pediatrics	21 (7)
Number of community hospital beds (FY1995)[b]	350
Beds per 100,000 population	122
Number of community hospitals (FY1995)[c]	3
Number of HMOs (1994)[d]	6
Number of federally qualified health centers (1994)[e]	0
Local public health expenditures (1997)	$10,673,197
Percent from direct federal sources	0%
Percent from state sources (including federal pass-throughs)	30%
Percent from local sources	28%
Percent from Medicaid	19%
Percent from Medicare	<1%
Total federal funding for community health centers (1996)[f]	0
Total federal funding for migrant health centers (1996)[f]	0
Total federal block grant funds for preventive health services (1996)[f]	0
Total federal block grant funds for maternal and child health services (1996)[f]	0
Total federal block grant funds for substance abuse services (1996)[f]	$996,561
Total federal funding for homeless health services (1996)[f]	0
Total federal funding for National Health Service Corp (1996)[f]	0

[a]*Statistics reflect the three-county jurisdiction of Clark, Klickitat, and Skamania Counties.*
[b]*Data from American Medical Association Physician Masterfile.*[1]
[c]*Data from American Hospital Association.*[2]
[d]*Data from Group Health Association of America.*[3]
[e]*Data from US Bureau of Primary Health Care (unpublished data, 1994).*
[f]*Data from US Department of Commerce.*[4]

Local Health Resources and Manpower

A diverse collection of health facilities and professionals operate within the three-county area of Southwest Washington Health District (**Table 3**). Because of the close proximity to Portland, some residents of the health district also obtain health services from providers located there. This is especially true for Vancouver residents who work for Portland area employers and obtain health insurance through these firms. Most residents, however, depend on the collection of providers located within the health district.

The nonprofit Southwest Washington Medical Center provides the majority of hospital-based services to area residents. The 297-bed facility provides acute medical and surgical care through its inpatient facility, outpatient clinics, emergency room, and urgent care center. The hospital also operates a home health agency and a community cancer treatment center. During calendar year 1995 the hospital handled 15,664 admissions and 161,292 outpatient visits. Also operating within the district are two small, nonprofit hospitals located in predominantly rural areas of Klickitat County. Klickitat Valley Hospital maintains 22-bed facility that handled 649 admissions and 9626 outpatient visits during 1995. Skyline Valley Hospital operates a 32-bed facility that served 731 inpatients and 11,541 outpatient visits during this period. All three hospitals offer obstetrical services.

A total of 347 active, nonfederal physicians practice within the health district, producing a physician-to-population ratio of 121 physicians per 100,000 population. Of these physicians, 41% practice in the primary care disciplines of general practice, family medicine, pediatrics, obstetrics / gynecology, and general internal medicine. In addition to private practice physicians, several other primary care resources exist within the community. Many local physicians practice in multispecialty groups, with Kaiser Permanente Medical Group being the largest and accounting for more than one quarter of all physician care in Clark County. The Southwest Washington Medical Center also serves as a major source of primary care services within the community, especially for traditionally underserved populations such as Medicaid beneficiaries and the uninsured. The medical center operates a family practice clinic staffed by 12 physicians participating in its family practice residency program. The hospital also operates a prenatal care clinic in collaboration with local physician groups and the local health department. Additionally, the hospital operates a pediatric clinic that serves primarily low-income Medicaid beneficiaries. Adding to the community's primary care resources, the local health department operates public health clinics in each of the district's three counties. These clinics provide adult and childhood immunizations, sexually transmitted disease services, and HIV counseling and testing services. A community clinic also operates in Vancouver two evenings per week, providing free and reduced-fee primary care services to uninsured residents on an episodic basis. Staff from the medical center, the health department, and a local health maintenance organization operate this clinic, which typically serves 35 to 40 patients per night. Finally, a local church operates a free primary care clinic in Vancouver with volunteer labor from local private physicians and nurses. This clinic operates by appointment only and serves approximately five patients per week.

Health insurance coverage for residents within the Southwest Washington Health District varies widely. A local division of Kaiser Permanente, the nation's largest nonprofit health maintenance organization, maintains the largest market share of residents with employer-provided health insurance. Kaiser's Vancouver division serves ~27% of Clark County residents through a network of four multispecialty medical clinics located across the county. In addition to Kaiser, several other managed care plans operate within the health district, most of which are based in Portland. Many residents of Southwest Washington receive their health insurance through Portland area employers and therefore maintain membership in Portland-based health plans. (See Chapter 14.)

Substantial numbers of Medicaid beneficiaries are also served through managed care plans, under a statewide mandatory Medicaid managed care program initiated in 1993. Under this Section 1915(b) Medicaid waiver program, beneficiaries eligible for Medicaid through the federal Temporary Assistance for Needy Families program (formerly the Aid to Families with Dependent Children program) or the Supplemental Security Income program are required to enroll in approved health maintenance organizations or provider-sponsored managed care plans. Kaiser Permanente is the largest Medicaid managed care provider within the jurisdiction, serving ~25% of the total Medicaid population. Several other plans based in Vancouver, Portland, Olympia, and Seattle also serve Medicaid beneficiaries residing within the health district. Under the state's Basic Health Plan, a number of low-income, formerly uninsured residents within the health district also receive care through managed care plans. This program provides low-income, uninsured residents not eligible for Medicaid with the ability to enroll in private managed care plans for a reduced premium payment which is based upon income. (See Chapter 16.)

The Local Health Department

The Southwest Washington Health District has undergone substantial reorganization over the past decade in an effort to adapt to larger policy and marketplace trends. Historically, the district provided a comprehensive range of personal health services along with its population-based public health activities. Beginning in 1990, the department initiated a process to transfer many of its personal health care responsibilities to other community providers. Over the past 7 years, this process has dramatically changed the organization and operation of the local health department. To date, the department appears to be functioning effectively in carrying out core public health functions through its new organizational structure.

Organizational Structure

Under its new two-county structure, the Southwest Washington Health District operates as a special intergovernmental agency under the authority of a 10-member board of health. The board consists of elected officials from both counties now participating in the district, as well as from the cities and towns that fall within the district. The board holds responsibility for establishing health district policy, approving the annual budget, reviewing the operational activities of the health district, and appointing the district's executive director. The executive director serves as the district's administrative head. A physician-trained medical director serves as the district's clinical chief and reports directly to the executive director. Washington state law requires every local health department to be staffed by a physician-trained health officer.

Thomas Milne maintained a 15-year history as executive director of the health district. Before his tenure at the health district, Mr. Milne spent 9 years as a senior manager within the local health department serving nearby Portland and Multnomah County, Oregon. Experience within this large, urban health department allowed Mr. Milne to anticipate some of the health policy and marketplace changes that would eventually diffuse to smaller jurisdictions such as Southwest Washington. Upon joining the health district in 1983, Mr. Milne led the agency's dramatic organizational and operational changes. Many of these changes were implemented in anticipation of trends such as managed care growth and the expanding involvement of private health care providers in community health services. In November 1997, Mr. Milne was tapped to head the nation's largest professional association for local health directors, the National Association of County and City Health Officials.

During Mr. Milne's tenure, the health district underwent substantial structural and operational change. This change reflected the district's move away from an emphasis on personal health care delivery and toward a focus on population-based health services. District administrators indicated that the rationale for this change was threefold. First, the district desired to increase its focus on population level issues in an effort to achieve larger improvements in community health status. Second, the health district desired to improve the continuity of care received by populations traditionally served through public health clinics. The district sought to accomplish this objective by finding ways to integrate underserved populations within the community's mainstream health care delivery systems. This strategy represented, at least in part, an attempt to anticipate the policies being discussed at the state level regarding health care reform and universal health care coverage. District staff felt that these policies would eventually eliminate the need for delivering personal health services outside of mainstream health care delivery systems. Third, the district faced a declining revenue base for local public health services during the 1980s. Medicaid revenues declined during much of this period in response to eligibility restrictions imposed by federal legislation. The district anticipated further reductions in Medicaid revenues as these beneficiaries enrolled in managed care plans and received services from private providers.

The health district began planning for its reorganization and privatization activities during the mid-1980s, but implementation did not begin until 1991. Before 1991, the local health department maintained four operational divisions. The *clinical services division* administered personal health care programs through the department's three public health clinics. Services delivered through these clinics included the following: prenatal care; preventive and primary care services for infants and children; preventive health services for adults; sexually transmitted disease services and HIV/AIDS testing and counseling; family planning services; and nutritional services supported through the federal Special Supplemental Food Program for Women, Infants, and Children (WIC). A home health nursing program also operated within this division, as did a prenatal care program providing prenatal services and postnatal follow-up to at-risk women and infants. The *community health division* housed health promotion and health education programs, the WIC program, and a community health nursing program. Programs involving food safety inspection, water quality monitoring, and solid and hazardous waste disposal were administered through the *environmental health division*. Finally, a *regional HIV/AIDS division* coordinated planning and resource allocation for programs involving HIV testing, counseling, and referral. An *administrative division* supported the work of these four operational divisions by housing activities such as billing, grants management, vital records, and information and computing systems. The managers of each division comprised a management team, which addressed strategic planning and policy development activities.

In 1991, the health district initiated a gradual process of transferring responsibilities in personal health service provision to other community providers. In this year, the district discontinued its prenatal care program and transferred its patients to a newly developed, community-based prenatal care clinic administered by the Southwest Washington Medical Center. Over the following 3 years, the district transferred responsibility to the medical center for operating a variety of health promotion and disease prevention services, including a diabetes screening and education program, and a cardiac screening and risk reduction program. In 1994, the department discontinued its primary care and preventive services programs for infants and children. A new child health clinic, also operated by the medical center, assumed responsibility for providing these services. Finally, the department transferred its responsibilities in operating a school-based dental health program to a private contractor in 1995.

The district now operates under a new organizational structure that reflects its diminished role in personal health services and its newly emerging emphasis on population-based services. This new structure consists of five administrative divisions and a regional office. A *community and family health* division houses the department's remaining clinical programs in family planning, communicable disease control, sexually transmitted disease control, and HIV / AIDS testing and counseling. The division also provides WIC services, community health nursing, and vaccine distribution and quality control. A new office of access assurance was also opened, which provides outreach and assistance to Medicaid beneficiaries and other vulnerable populations to ensure that they receive access to health care from community providers and health plans. The *assessment and epidemiology* division administers programs for assessing health needs within the community, evaluating public health services and programs delivered within the district, and investigating and controlling disease outbreaks—including communicable disease contact tracing and epidemiological surveillance. The district's medical officer provides oversight for this division's activities. The *health promotion* division operates programs involving health information dissemination and community health education initiatives. Finally, the divisions for *environmental health* and *administrative services* remain largely unchanged.

Overview of Programs and Services

Personal Health Services

The service transfers executed during the 1990s eliminated an estimated 50% of the health district's patient visits for personal health services. Nonetheless, the district remains responsible for delivering a number of important clinical services that are not adequately available from other community providers. These services continue to be provided through the district's public health clinics, which are located in each of the three counties comprising the jurisdiction. Services delivered through these clinics are described below.

- Childhood and adult immunization services. Walk-in childhood immunization services are provided through the district's main clinic in Vancouver 3 days per week. Walk-in clinics for childhood immunization are also held on a weekly or monthly basis at the district's five satellite clinic sites. Adult vaccinations for influenza and pneumonia are periodically delivered during the fall and early winter at these same clinic sites. Travel vaccinations, which historically had been offered at the district's main clinic, were discontinued in January 1997. Teams of public health nurses staff all immunization clinics. Although the district continues to offer immunization services, over 90% of childhood immunizations are now provided through other community providers. Much of the district's immunization activity now centers around distributing vaccine to physicians' offices, providing quality assurance services to these community providers (including the monitoring of vaccine storage and administration procedures), and assisting providers with strategies to improve immunization rates. The health district's involvement in directly providing immunization services has declined from 50% of childhood immunizations in 1991 to 6% by 1997, while immunization rates have steadily increased during this time period.
- Family planning services. The district operates a family planning clinic through its main clinic site on a daily basis. Clients may obtain pregnancy testing and counseling, sex education, complete physical examinations regarding reproductive health, confidential birth control services, and referrals for abortion services. A team of nurses and health educators staff this clinic. Health department administrators are currently working with community providers to explore the feasibility of transferring responsibility for these services to other providers.
- Sexually transmitted disease services. A sexually transmitted disease clinic operates 3 days per week through the district's main clinic site. This clinic provides confidential screening, testing, and treatment for sexually transmitted diseases. Health educators also provide counseling and education regarding disease prevention and control. A separate HIV / AIDS clinic operates weekly through the main clinic site, providing confidential testing, counseling, education, and case management for this disease. The clinic provides referrals to community providers for HIV / AIDS treatment services.
- Other communicable disease services. The department operates a tuberculosis screening and control program that provides testing at all district clinic sites. Diagnosed cases are referred to community providers for treatment, with program staff providing case management and follow-up to insure patient compliance with the full course of treatment. Staff from the division of health protection and disease control conduct contact tracing activities and directly observed therapy.
- Nutritional services. The district provides nutritional counseling, breast-feeding information and support, and food vouchers for low-income women eligible for the federal Special Supplemental Food Program for Women, Infants, and Children (WIC). These services are administered through the district's main clinic site.

Health Promotion Services

The district maintains a team of health educators as part of its division of health promotion. This team implements an array of community education campaigns—including activities in family planning, sexually transmitted disease control, HIV / AIDS awareness, and food safety—to supplement the district's clinical services programs. Most of these campaigns are carried out through community presentations and seminars held throughout the district. The district's health education team also works closely with staff at Southwest Washington Regional Medical Center and other community providers in implementing a broad range of health promotion and education initiatives in areas such as: cardiovascular health; physical fitness; cancer prevention and control; smoking cessation; diabetes education; violence prevention; and adolescent health and safety. Most of these initiatives are carried out through community presentations and seminars, and many are held at the medical center's health education center.

The district also operates a health information and referral telephone line staffed by public health nurses during weekdays. This program, operated through the division of community and family health, fields questions from residents on a variety of health-related topics, and offers referrals to appropriate community providers for health services. The program is designed to promote and improve health within the community by the following: encouraging appropriate utilization of health services; increasing community knowledge of self-care and beneficial health behaviors; and ensuring continued access to public health services—especially those that have been recently shifted from public to private providers.

Community Health Assessment

The local health department maintains involvement in an active community health assessment process designed to identify emerging health issues. This process was initiated in 1993 in Clark County, with funding from the Centers for Disease Control and Prevention, the health district, Clark County, the City of Vancouver, Southwest Washington Medical Center, and Kaiser health plan.[5] The local health department provided leadership for the assessment process and worked in close partnership with Southwest Washington Medical Center and Kaiser to convene a community process. The health department collected available data on community health status and conducted a series of focus groups with community members. From this information, the department produced a series of reports on demographic, social, and health trends within the jurisdiction. A wide range of local organizations and individuals were then recruited to participate in community planning and priority-setting sessions. Participants included county and city elected officials, health care providers, voluntary associations, businesses, educational institutions, neighborhood groups, law enforcement agencies, social service agencies, and religious organizations. Through this process, the group developed a strategic plan for addressing high-priority health issues during the next two decades. The plan, entitled *Community Choices 2010*, is reviewed and updated regularly by the three sponsoring organizations.

A private, not-for-profit corporation was established as a subsidiary of the Greater Vancouver Chamber of Commerce to formalize the process of implementing plan objectives and continually reassessing community needs. This organization, also named Community Choices 2010, continues to receive funding and staff support from the health department and the other participating organizations. The organization oversees over 400 volunteers working on a variety of community projects that are pursuant to the community strategic plan. The health department provides biannual updates to the community assessment process and leads the effort to develop performance benchmarks based on the strategic plan. The department initiated similar community assessment processes in Klickitat and Skamania Counties beginning in 1995.

The local health department's division of assessment and epidemiology also maintains an initiative to assess the effects of transitioning service delivery responsibilities from the health department to other community providers. This ongoing effort includes a telephone survey of previous health department clients to assess their ability to access services from other providers. Service utilization measures are also examined as part of this study.

As a final activity in community health assessment, the local health department continues to be an active participant in the state health agency's initiative in public health performance assessment (see Chapter 6 on state performance assessment efforts). As part of this initiative, the state agency conducted a survey of local health departments during 1996 to examine and compare their involvement in core public health activities. This information was then provided to participating local health departments. The Southwest Washington Health District has used this information to evaluate its performance in comparison to other health departments and to identify areas in need of improvement.

Environmental Health Services

The local health department's environmental health division maintains an array of programs for preventing exposure to hazardous substances and environmentally based diseases. The division's solid waste disposal program conducts assessments of waste disposal facilities and investigates illegal dumping incidents. The hazardous waste disposal program conducts monitoring and planning activities regarding the transport and disposal of hazardous wastes within the jurisdiction. On-site sewage systems and septic tanks are inspected through the department's sewage disposal program. The department tests the water quality of wells and public and private water systems through its safe drinking water program. The food handling program conducts mandatory training for food service workers and implements periodic inspections of all food service establishments. Through its land use program, the department reviews construction plans and provides consultation for subdivision developments within the jurisdiction to insure that these developments meet all health and safety codes. Health and safety inspections of schools, school cafeterias, recreational areas, swimming pools, and spas are conducted through the department's public facility inspection program. The department is also responsible for conducting investigations of noise and nuisance complaints. Finally, the department operates mosquito control activities in Clark County under a contract with the Clark County Mosquito Control District. The environmental health division maintains a full service laboratory to support these programs.

Infrastructure and Resources

The local health department's programs and services are carried out through a main administrative office and clinic located in the city of Vancouver, together with five satellite clinics located in outlying areas of the jurisdiction. A separate environmental health office and laboratory are also located in Vancouver. The department's main clinic operates 5 days per week, while the satellite clinics operate on schedules ranging from daily to weekly frequencies, allowing health department staff to rotate through the clinics.

The department employs a total of 180 staff who fill 158 full-time equivalent positions. Approximately 70% of the department's work force hold full-time positions, while 30% hold part-time positions. The department's clinical staff includes one physician (the medical director), 24 nurses, 3 nurse practitioners, and 7 nutritionists. Nonclinical professional staff include the following: 20 environmental health specialists, 6 health educators, 1 epidemiologist, and 2 social workers. Despite the discontinuation of several clinical services, the health department has largely avoided reductions in its work force. During the past decade, many of the department's clinical staff have been retrained to take on new responsibilities in community health practice. With reduced clinical responsibilities, these staff have assumed roles such as leading community health education and outreach campaigns; conducting public health assessment and evaluation activities; maintaining liaison relationships with other community providers; and providing health information and referrals to individuals via the telephone information line. Through these arrangements, the local health department maintains its clinical human resources in the event that they may be needed to supplement the capacities of community providers.

The local health department's expenditures totaled approximately $11 million in fiscal year 1997 and $10 million in fiscal year 1998 when the department changed to a two-county district. This amount produces a per capita local public health expenditure of approximately $32, which is higher than the average per capita expenditure of $20 found in a national survey of local health departments during 1992-1993.[6] The health director reports that departmental revenues from Medicaid have declined somewhat over the past 3 years as greater numbers of beneficiaries have enrolled in managed care plans, and as many of the department's clinical programs have been discontinued. As a result, revenues from federal, state, and private grants have become increasingly important for financing local public health services. However, the department has been successful in securing funds from a special Medicaid administrative match program, which supports nonclinical activities such as outreach, enrollment, and education for Medicaid-eligible residents. The health district receives approximately $800,000 per year in revenue from this source.

Other Contributors to Local Public Health Activities

State Health Agencies

The Southwest Washington Health District maintains cooperative relationships with Washington's state health agencies. Three different agencies have jurisdiction over health issues in Washington State (see Thurston County case study). The local health department interacts most frequently with the Washington Department of Health, which oversees traditional public health activities such as infectious disease control, maternal and child health, environmental health, epidemiology, health statistics, and health facilities and services licensing. The state's 33 local health departments are all organized as self-governed, decentralized administrative units of local governments. Consequently, they interact with the state Department of Health principally for funding and technical assistance needs. The Department of Health conducts much of its public health activities through contracts, grants, and cooperative agreements with local health departments such as Southwest Washington Health District.

Since 1994, much of the health district's interaction with the state Department of Health has occurred in conjunction with a statewide initiative to improve public health practice—the Public Health Improvement Plan. Begun in 1993 under newly adopted state legislation, this initiative has focused on identifying core public health functions, measuring their performance within the state, and developing interventions to improve this performance. The health district's executive director has served as a critical participant on the steering committee for this initiative by representing the perspectives of local health departments within the state. Through this committee, the district has played an important role in helping to define the core public health functions that local health departments are expected to carry out. The district has also been involved in developing an assessment tool used by the state for measuring local health department performance.

Southwest Washington Health District also maintains frequent contact with the Washington State Health Care Authority, the agency that oversees the state's health insurance plan for low-income uninsured residents. The district's executive director serves on the advisory committee for this program, giving the organization a voice in decisions regarding program eligibility, coverage policies, and quality assurance processes. This involvement has allowed the district to play an active role in encouraging local residents and local health care providers to participate in this program. According to district administrators, this involvement has also helped the district shape its policies for transferring clinical services programs to private providers.

The district maintains relatively limited interaction with the Department of Social and Health Services, which administers the state's Medicaid program. Most of this interaction involves reimbursement for clinical service delivery, an activity that has declined substantially in recent years as the district has discontinued many of its clinical services programs. In collaboration with county social services agencies, the district also works with this state department in securing the enrollment of eligible residents in the state's Medicaid program.

Hospitals

Hospitals appear to be expanding their roles in local public health activities within the Southwest Washington health district. The organizations providing hospital-based services to residents of Southwest Washington include three facilities located within the district and at least four facilities located across the state line in Portland, Oregon. The three locally operated facilities—Southwest Washington Medical Center, Klickitat Valley Hospital, and Skyline Hospital—generate the bulk of hospital contributions to local public health activities. Two of these facilities, however, are located in Klickitat County, which recently withdrew from the health district. The effects of this withdrawal on hospital contributions to local public health activities remain to be seen.

Southwest Washington Medical Center maintains a close working relationship with the local health department, evidenced by numerous jointly sponsored programs and services. Beginning in 1995, the local health department's executive director has served on the medical center's board of trustees—an arrangement designed to create a closer administrative link between the two organizations. The executive director chairs the board's quality assurance committee and serves on committees for physician recruitment, ethics, and executive affairs. The local health department is currently investigating the possibility of creating a trustee position for the medical center's chief executive officer.

In collaboration with the local health department, Southwest Washington Medical Center has assumed responsibility for providing many of the clinical public health services formerly provided the department. Prime among these services is a prenatal care clinic for serving low-income women. This clinic, staffed by nurse practitioners and nurse midwives, was collaboratively developed with the health district and three local obstetrician/gynecology practices. The medical center assumes primary responsibility for operating the clinic, while physicians from the health district, the medical center, and the private practices rotate responsibility for serving as the clinic's medical director. The health department participates on the community advisory board that oversees the clinic. The medical center also operates a pediatric clinic that has assumed responsibility from the health district for providing child health services to low-income and underserved families. Additionally, a family practice residency program developed by the medical center in 1995 provides a continuum of primary care services to low-income adults and children within the community.

The medical center's growing involvement in primary care delivery to vulnerable populations appears to be motivated both by financial concerns and community health concerns. Under the state's two managed care programs for underserved populations—the Medicaid program and the Basic Health Plan program for the uninsured—community providers face opportunities for earning substantial revenues by serving these program beneficiaries. Through its recently developed primary care programs, the medical center is able to compete for serving these beneficiaries by offering a full continuum of care. At the same time, these primary care programs appear to help the hospital reduce utilization of more costly hospital-based services such as emergency department services and specialized inpatient and outpatient care. Hospital administrators report that emergency room utilization has substantially declined since the implementation of Medicaid managed care in 1994.

The hospital's growing involvement in primary care delivery also appears to stem from a firm commitment to improving health within the community. As evidence of this commitment, the hospital plays a key role in operating the free community clinic for uninsured residents, in collaboration with the health district, Kaiser, and other health and social service agencies. Moreover, the hospital continues to serve as a major contributor to the community-wide health assessment and improvement effort known as Community Choices 2010. As one of the five main organizations responsible for founding and funding this effort, the hospital maintains a 5-year history of support for the community health initiatives launched through this effort.

The medical center's contributions to community health also include an expanding role in providing health promotion and disease prevention activities within the community. A diabetes management program operated by the medical center provides services for diagnosing the disease and educating patients about optimal disease management strategies. A nutrition clinic offers counseling and support for community residents needing weight management services and nutritional guidance for infants, children, and adults. The hospital's cancer center operates a cancer awareness and risk assessment program that provides community residents with information and counseling regarding prevention practices, diagnostic and therapeutic alternatives, disease management strategies, and risk factor assessments. The cancer center also organizes several peer-based support groups for cancer patients and their families. The medical center's health education center offers a wide array of community programs designed to improve health-related behaviors and decision-making among community residents. Programs include topics such as drug interactions, exercise and physical activity, community and domestic violence prevention, and injury prevention among children and adolescents. Other health education programs are sponsored through the medical center's prenatal care clinic on topics including infant care, childbirth preparation, and breastfeeding.

Klickitat Valley Hospital has also made substantial contributions to local public health activities within the Southwest Washington Health District. As one of the few sources of health care in the predominantly rural Klickitat County, this small hospital maintains a broad array of community health programs to address local health needs.[7] These programs include the following:

- an annual health fair sponsored in collaboration with local businesses, churches, physicians, and the district health department. The hospital provides free health screening services and assessments as well as health education seminars to community residents during this activity.
- a breast and cervical cancer screening program for low-income women, conducted through a partnership with the district health department and a grant from the US Centers for Disease Control and Prevention. This program includes an outreach and educational component that is maintained through the participation of area businesses, churches, physician groups, and Native American tribal councils.
- a community-wide HIV/AIDS awareness program that conducts community education seminars in schools and other community locations throughout the area. Other contributors to this program include businesses, churches, civic groups, and the district health department.
- a newborn immunization program that provides outreach and follow-up services to insure that children born at the hospital receive timely childhood vaccinations. The hospital collaborates with area day care centers, schools, physicians, and the district health department in tracking immunization status and administering vaccinations.

The array of community health programs maintained by the hospital is notable given its small size and limited resources. Presumably, these programs will continue in collaboration with Klickitat County's newly developed local health department.

Portland-based hospitals maintain relatively little involvement in public health activities within the Southwest Washington area. In many cases, these hospitals serve only as regional referral centers for residents of this area and therefore depend on the area's local community hospitals to serve as routine sources of health care. Many of Portland's hospitals are actively involved in public health activities underway in Oregon. (See Chapter 14).

Managed Care Plans

Several managed care plans operate within the Southwest Washington region, but Kaiser Permanente maintains a large majority of the market share. This nonprofit, group-model HMO is the nation's oldest and largest managed care plan, established during World War II to serve workers at Henry Kaiser's Vancouver shipyards. Kaiser Permanente currently serves ~25% of Clark County residents through a network of four multispecialty medical clinics located within the city of Vancouver. These clinics offer family practice, pediatrics, obstetrics/gynecology, internal medicine, pharmacy, radiology, vision care, and mental health/substance abuse services. Kaiser Permanente does not operate any hospitals or subspecialty clinics in Southwest Washington. Enrollees requiring these services are referred either to Southwest Washington Medical Center or to Kaiser-affiliated providers located in Portland.

Kaiser maintains a long history of involvement in community health issues and a strong relationship with the local health department. The HMO is a primary sponsor of the free community health clinic, in partnership with the health department and Southwest Washington Medical Center. Kaiser contributes both staff time and medical supplies to this venture. Additionally, Kaiser serves as a founding partner of the community health assessment and planning effort known as Community Choices 2010. Kaiser provides an annual grant of $50,000 to support the implementation and evaluation of community health interventions that are designed to address issues identified through the assessment and planning process. Kaiser staff assume active roles on the steering committee of this effort and is involved in shaping the public health policies developed by the committee. Kaiser staff report using the Community Choices effort to improve the targeting of HMO programs and services to community health needs. For example, the HMO uses information on immunization rates collected through this effort to develop strategies for reducing missed immunization opportunities among Kaiser providers. As another example, the health plan chose to adopt a smoking cessation counseling intervention for its members in response to the Community Choices objective to reduce smoking within the community. The HMO also relies on information and feedback from the Community Choices effort in making decisions about clinic locations and expansions.

Kaiser maintains an array of programs designed to increase the delivery and utilization of health promotion and disease prevention services. Although these programs are targeted specifically at the HMO's enrolled members, Kaiser's large market share within Southwest Washington insures that these programs have a substantial effect on community health. Many of these programs focus on health education interventions designed to improve the lifestyle decisions and care-seeking behaviors of Kaiser members. For example, Kaiser maintains a major educational effort in encouraging appropriate self-care practices among its members. As part of this program, new members attend an orientation session with Kaiser clinicians who provide an overview of basic prevention and self-care strategies and teach members to use an extensive self-care manual provided to all Kaiser members. A major component of this education session addresses appropriate care-seeking behaviors such as the utilization of routine primary care and preventive health office visits, as well as emergency room and urgent care services.

As a strategy for increasing access to routine primary care and preventive health services, Kaiser operates a walk-in nurse treatment room at its main medical office. This facility provides routine diagnostic and preventive services that do not require direct physician time, such as streptococcal tests, urinary tract infection tests, pregnancy tests, clinical breast examinations, well child examinations, and health education and counseling services. Kaiser staff suggests that this program increases access to care by reducing the waiting time and expense that would be incurred for a full primary care office visit.

Kaiser also operates several programs for providing targeted health education and counseling for members with special health conditions. A pregnancy counseling program provides home and office nurse visits to expectant mothers soon after a pregnancy is identified. Through these visits, trained nurses provide nutritional counseling, health assessments, and case management services to pregnant women while ensuring that they receive routine prenatal care. Kaiser also operates a health education and case management program for members diagnosed with diabetes, which provides routine group counseling and support sessions as well as periodic telephone follow-up sessions to encourage appropriate disease management practices among patients.

Kaiser also serves as an important source of care for Medicaid beneficiaries and other low-income individuals through Washington's managed care programs. Approximately 7500 Medicaid beneficiaries in the Southwest Washington region are enrolled in Kaiser's health plan, making Kaiser the region's largest Medicaid managed care provider. Kaiser also enrolls beneficiaries of the state's Basic Health Plan, a managed care program designed to serve low-income, uninsured individuals. Rather than develop separate systems of care for serving vulnerable population groups, Kaiser works to ensure that these groups receive needed health and support services through the same systems of care that serve beneficiaries of its commercial health plan products. Interventions such as Kaiser's walk-in nurse treatment clinic and its health education and case management programs serve all Kaiser members, although they are particularly important for vulnerable populations that face educational, economic, and cultural barriers to care. Similarly, Kaiser maintains a staff of bilingual clinicians to reduce linguistic barriers to care among its commercial enrollees as well as its public program beneficiaries.

Kaiser maintains strong relationships with the local health department and other community organizations that contribute to public health in Southwest Washington. In addition to the collaborative activities involving the Community Choices initiative and the community health clinic, the HMO works closely with the local health department and hospital in reviewing state health legislation. The three organizations cochair a health legislation committee within the local chamber of commerce. This committee formulates policy positions regarding pending and existing state legislation and advocates these positions before the state health agency and legislature once these positions are adopted by the Chamber board. This arrangement has allowed the organizations to achieve a strong voice in shaping state health policy. Additionally, the three organizations participate in a broad range of jointly sponsored public health initiatives as needs emerge within the community. For example, the three organizations rapidly came together in 1996 to jointly implement a school-based vaccination program during a measles outbreak. While the health department led the effort, each organization contributed the staff, supplies, and financial resources that enabled the effort to be implemented efficiently and effectively.

Collaboration between Kaiser and Southwest Washington Medical Center reached new levels in 1997 with an agreement that enables Kaiser beneficiaries to receive hospital services in Vancouver rather than from Kaiser-affiliated hospitals in Portland. The two organizations are jointly financing expansions of Southwest's emergency department and its family birthing center to accommodate the additional demand generated by Kaiser members. This agreement diminishes an historically competitive relationship between the two institutions, and allows greater interaction between the clinical staffs of Kaiser and Southwest. By reducing the number of Kaiser patients that receive hospital services outside the county and state, this agreement also improves the ability of the local health department to monitor disease trends and hospital utilization statistics among residents of the Southwest Washington jurisdiction.

Several other managed care plans operate within the Southwest Washington region, but none of these plans maintain strong relationships with the local health department. Most of these plans are based in Portland and serve individuals and families who receive health insurance through Portland-based employers.

Other Organizations

A broad array of other community organizations contributes to the public health system serving Southwest Washington. A number of voluntary health associations are based in Vancouver, including local chapters of the American Diabetes Association, American Red Cross, American Heart Association, and the American Cancer Society. These organizations sponsor public awareness campaigns and advocacy initiatives both independently and in coordination with the local health department and other organizations. Several health professions associations are active in the community, including a medical society, dental society, and nurses association. Washington State University's Vancouver campus maintains a presence within the local health district and provides technical assistance on projects such as the Community Choices initiative (through the business school and the president's office). The Seattle-based University of Washington School of Medicine works closely with the local medical center in operating its family practice residency program, while the University's comprehensive cancer center provides support and assistance to the medical center's cancer education, prevention, and control programs. An active local chapter of the United Way provides funding and assistance for a variety of health and social service projects, including an on-line and telephone referral program for community health and human services. Finally, several neighborhood and church-based organizations sponsor health promotion programs within the community, and engage in fund-raising activities to support the local community health clinic. Currently, no federally supported community or migrant health centers operate within the jurisdiction. An effort to establish such a center is now underway through a partnership between the local health department, the medical center, and the community health clinic. Should this effort be successful, the local health department may consider transferring the remainder of its clinical services to this health center.

Measures of Public Health System Performance

A survey conducted with the local health director in 1997 suggests that core public health functions are performed within the jurisdiction at slightly better than 50% of the maximum possible performance level (**Figure 1**). The overall performance level of 56% exceeds the average score of 51% found among a national selection of local health departments during 1992-1993. When community performance levels are examined within each of the three core public health functions identified by the Institute of Medicine, performance is reported to be highest for the *assurance* function, and lowest for the *policy development* function. When these functions are subdivided into ten individual public health practices, the practice of *informing and educating the public* is reported to be most adequately performed within the community, followed by the practices of *analyzing the determinants of health, advocating for community health needs*, and *managing health programs and resources*. The practice of *prioritizing health needs* is reported to be the least adequately performed within the jurisdiction.

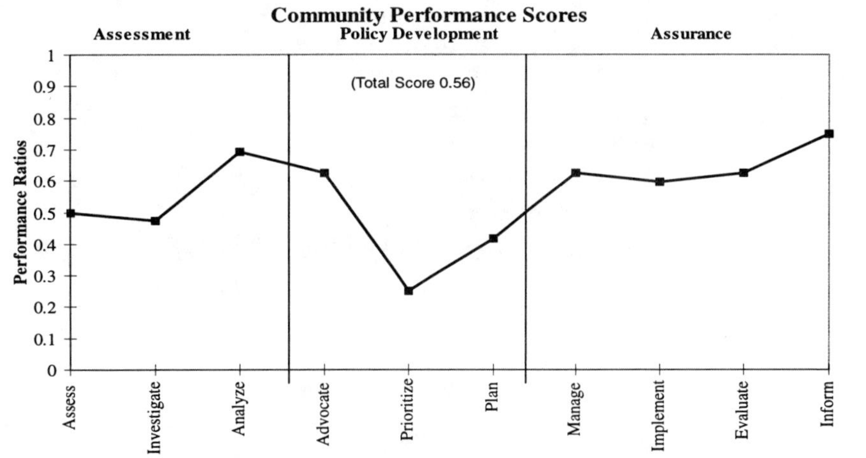

Figure 1. Community performance scores for Southwest Washington health district.

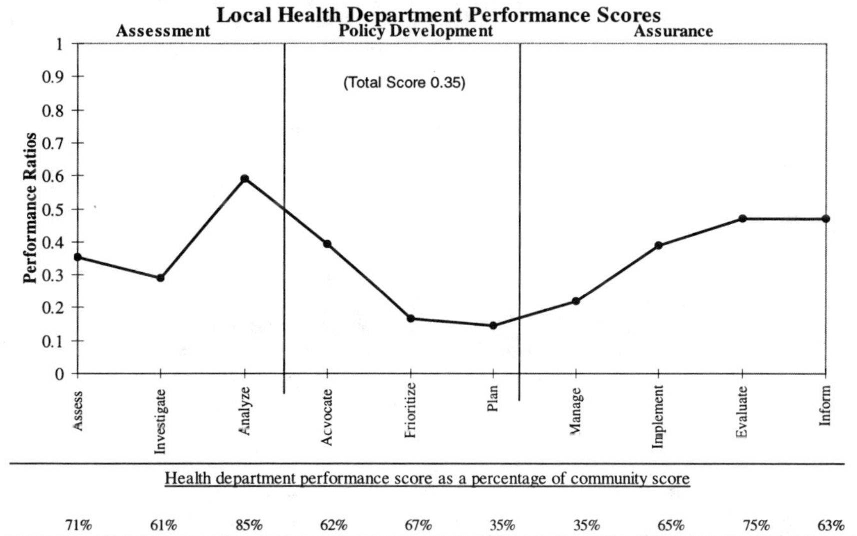

Figure 2. Health department scores for Southwest Washington.

The local health department is reported to perform core public health functions at ~35% of the maximum possible level, thereby contributing almost two-thirds of the community performance level (**Figure 2**). Like community performance, health department performance is highest for the *assurance* function and lowest for the *policy development* function. Among the ten public health practices, health department performance appears highest for the practices of *analyzing the determinants of health, evaluating health programs and services*, and *informing and educating the public*. Health department performance appears lowest for the practices of *developing plans and policies*, and *prioritizing health needs*. Organizations other than the local health department contribute the greatest share of effort to the practices of *managing health programs and resources* (65% of total effort), and *developing plans and policies* (65% of total effort).

When we examine organization-specific rates of participation in public health activities, hospitals, public agencies, and nonprofit agencies appear to participate in the largest proportion of activities (**Figure 3**). Hospitals, local government agencies, and nonprofit agencies participate more in policy development activities than in assessment and assurance activities. In contrast, state health agencies participate most frequently in assessment activities. Universities participate only in policy development and assessment activities, while federal agencies are directly involved in local public health activities only for the function of assessment.

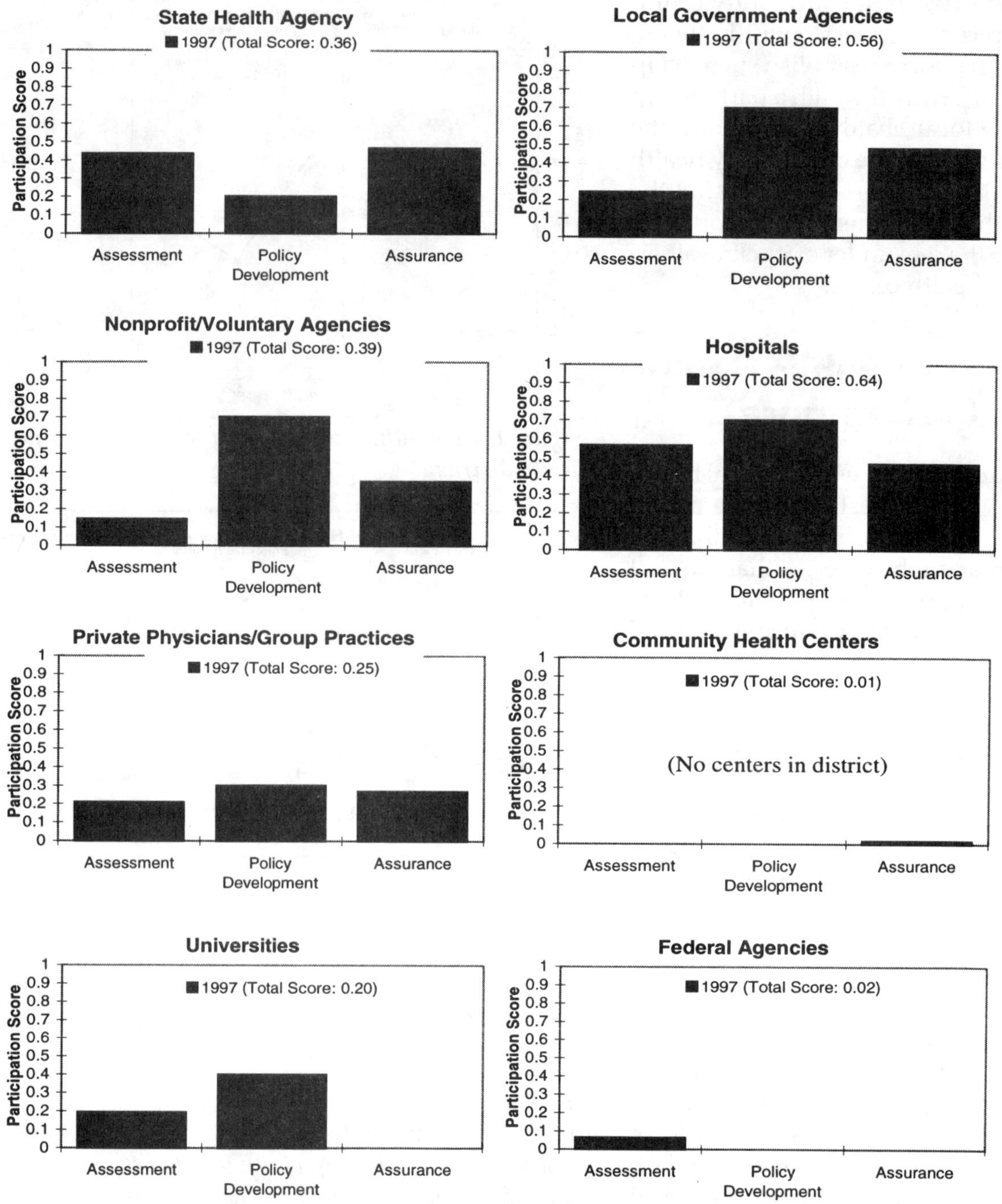

Figure 3. Participation in public health activities by other organizations, 1997 (as reported by the local health director).

Measures of public health performance for the Southwest Washington Health District suggest that the unique interorganizational arrangements for public health delivery are successfully assuring access to needed services. Community public health performance is highest for the assurance function, despite the fact that many public health services are no longer directly provided by the local health department. Indeed, organizations other than the local health department appear to contribute the majority of effort in *managing health programs and resources* within the jurisdiction. Nevertheless, the health department retains a dominant role in other assurance practices, such as *evaluating health programs and services,* and *informing and educating the public.* The health department appears to have found an effective division of labor by transferring direct responsibilities in program management to other organizations while retaining responsibilities in program evaluation and education.

The relatively low performance scores for policy developments activities is somewhat surprising given the extensive community planning activities that are underway through the jurisdiction's Community Choices effort. A detailed examination of the performance scores reveals that most of the community's policy development efforts are directed at advocacy and constituency-building activities. The community has not yet been fully effective in other policy development activities such as informing candidates for elective office about community health priorities and developing written agreements among community health organizations that define shared functions and responsibilities. The health director anticipates that as the Community Choices effort matures, these other policy development practices will be incorporated into its scope of activity.

Future Prospects and Projections

The local health department serving the Southwest Washington Health District has undergone dramatic changes in its organization and operation over the past decade. Nonetheless, the department has maintained relatively high levels of public health performance through partnerships with other community organizations. This success has motivated the department to consider additional public health responsibilities that might be effectively transferred to other community organizations. The department has begun to explore the potential for service transfers in areas such as family planning services, sexually transmitted disease services, and immunization services.

It remains to be determined whether there are practical limits to the scale and scope of public health responsibilities that can be successfully transferred to private providers. The existing service transfers appear more viable in urbanized parts of the jurisdiction (Clark County), as compared to the rural areas in Klickitat and Skamania Counties. These rural counties contain fewer private providers and therefore fewer potential partners that could share public health responsibilities with the local health department. The populations residing in these areas also face greater socioeconomic and geographic barriers to health care than the residents of more urbanized areas of the jurisdiction. As a consequence, the health department has found it necessary to maintain direct involvement in public health delivery in these rural areas, while it shares these responsibilities with other community providers in more urbanized areas.

The health department's growing reliance on other community organizations for direct provision of public health services suggests the need for more formalized mechanisms of interorganizational coordination and management. Currently, many of the health department's shared responsibilities in public health service delivery are not supported by formal contracts and performance expectations. These interorganizational arrangements are carried out largely through informal agreements and expectations among organizations. To be sure, efforts such as the Community Choices initiative create an effective forum for communication and informal collaboration among the organizations contributing to public health. However, these informal mechanisms of coordination and control may become difficult to manage as relationships among organizations grow in their complexity. As the health department continues to share more public health responsibilities with its current collaborators, and as the health department establishes collaborative relationships with more community organizations, it may require more formalized interorganizational structures to manage effectively these relationships.

The Southwest Washington Health District offers a compelling example of a successful reorganization of local public health practice through privatization approaches. The success of these approaches appears to hinge on two critical factors. First, and perhaps most importantly, the health department maintains strong, collaborative relationships with community providers that have both the capacity and the willingness to assume responsibilities in local public health delivery. The community's two dominant providers—a hospital and an HMO—share the health department's commitment to improving community health. Second, the health department is successfully developing expanded roles in assessment, evaluation, and education to balance its diminishing responsibilities in direct service provision. For these reasons, the experience of Southwest Washington in public health privatization may not be readily generalizable to other jurisdictions. A unique set of circumstances at the organization and community levels has enabled the health department to develop and sustain its interorganizational arrangements for public health delivery. Nevertheless, the experience of the Southwest Washington Health District provides yet another example of how core public health functions can be successfully carried out through broad community collaboration.

References

1. American Medical Association. *Physician Data by County*. Chicago, Ill: AMA; 1992.
2. American Hospital Association. *AHA 1997 Guide to the Health Care Field*. Chicago, Ill: AHA; 1997.
3. Group Health Association of America. *1995 Directory of HMOs*. Washington, DC: GHAA; 1995.
4. US Department of Commerce. *1995 Consolidated Federal Funds Report*. Washington, DC: Census Bureau; 1997.
5. Lasker R. 1997. *Medicine and Public Health: The Power of Collaboration*. New York: New York Academy of Medicine.
6. Gordon RL, Gerzoff RB, Richards TB. Determinants of local health department expenditures, 1992 through 1993. *Am J Public Health*. 1997; 87(1):91-95.
7. Washington Health Foundation. *Inventory of Washington Hospital Community-based Activities*. Seattle, Wash: Washington Health Foundation; 1997.

Chapter 16
Case Study of Thurston County, Washington

Key Attributes

- Transitioning personal health services responsibility from local health department to community providers.
- Limited but growing interaction between local health department and managed care plans.
- Strong collaborative relationship between community hospital and local health department.
- Active community health assessment and planning processes with broad community participation.
- Strong community-based organizations with active involvement in public health issues.

Community Characteristics

Demographic and Socioeconomic Characteristics

Thurston County borders Washington State's Puget Sound ~60 miles southeast of Seattle. The county contains almost 190 thousand residents, many of whom reside in Washington's capital city of Olympia (**Table 1**). Census data indicate that minority groups comprise a small but growing proportion of the county population, of which 92% are White, 4% are Asian, 2% are African American, and 1% are Native American. The local economy continues to expand beyond its historical dependence on the timber industry, which has substantially declined over the last decade with the increase in federal logging restrictions. State government is now the county's largest employer; health care institutions comprise six of the county's top 10 employers. The work force is well educated, but per capita income remains below the state and national averages. Census data from 1990 suggest that ~10% of individuals and 7% of families in Thurston County maintain incomes below the federal poverty threshold.

Community Health Status Indicators

Thurston County mirrors state and national trends with respect to leading causes of death. For the period 1980-1991, heart disease was responsible for one third of county deaths, while cancers caused 25% of deaths and cerebrovascular disease caused 8% of these deaths. Cancer exists as the leading cause of death among Thurston County residents age 45 and older. For all cancers combined, Thurston County's age-adjusted cancer incidence rate exceeds that of the state as a whole (427 per 100,000 in 1993). The county ranks first or second among all Washington counties for the incidence of cancers of the esophagus, stomach, oral cavity / pharynx, kidney, pancreas, and cervix. However, the county

Table 1
Demographic Characteristics: Thurston County, Washington

Population (1990)	161,238
Median age in years	35.0
Percent 65 years and older (1990)	6.8
Percent non-White (1990)	8.1
Percent speaking a language other than English at home (1990)	6.6
Percent completing high school degree (1990)	86.5
Percent of individuals below federal poverty level (1989)	10.1
Median household income (1989)	$30,976
Average percent unemployed (1991)	5.9

Data from US Department of Commerce, Bureau of the Census.

Table 2
Health Status Indicators: Thurston County, Washington, 1996

Infant mortality rate per 1000 live births	3.7
Percent of births to mothers age 10-17	3.2
Percent of infants with low birth weight	4.6
Percent of births with prenatal care later than first trimester	22.8
Deaths per 100,000 population, age-adjusted	766.7
Cancer, all types	202.8
Lung cancer	66.3
Female breast cancer	28.9
Heart disease	213.4
Cerebrovascular diseases	56.6
Chronic obstructive pulmonary diseases	50.0
Suicide	18.2
Pneumonia and Influenza	25.9
HIV / AIDS	4.2
Diabetes mellitus	24.9
Homicide	3.9

Data from Washington State Department of Health (unpublished data, 1997).

experiences cancer incidence rates below the statewide rates for several common cancers, including those of the lung (52 per 100,000), female breast (111 per 100,000) prostate (136 per 100,000), and rectum/colon (39 per 100,000).

The county's infant mortality rate stands at 3.7 per 1000 live births for the period 1993, a rate which meets the nation's Year 2000 objective of 7.0 per 1000 (**Table 2**). Approximately 4.6% of Thurston County infants born during 1996 were low birth weight (less than 2500 g), somewhat lower than the statewide low birth weight rate. Steady improvements have been made in the proportion of pregnant women who receive prenatal care during the first trimester—77% of women did so in 1996, compared with 73% in 1991 and only 63.2% in 1989. Maternal smoking has been a persistent problem among Thurston County residents, with more than 12% of pregnant women reporting smoking during 1991.

Infectious diseases remain an important cause of illness and disability in Thurston County, although incidence rates for many diseases are below state and national averages. Among reportable diseases, only the incidence rates for *Escherichia coli*, giardiasis, and salmonellosis exceeded the statewide rates during 1992. Through year-end 1993, a total of 59 cases of AIDS have been reported in Thurston County since reporting began in 1984. From this statistic, health officials have estimated that 590 to 1180 county residents are HIV positive. Although no cases of measles, mumps, or rubella were recorded during 1992, a 1993 survey indicated that only 50% of 2-year-olds are up-to-date on immunizations. The last measles outbreak in the county occurred in 1990. The proportion of county residents diagnosed with active tuberculosis has steadily decreased since 1989, although the proportion of individuals testing positive for TB infection has increased during this same period. These figures emphasize the continued need for an effective treatment program to prevent disease progression from latent infection to active TB. Deaths due to pneumonia and influenza have also increased since 1989, with these diseases accounting for 3.5% of all county deaths during the period 1989-1991.

Environmental health measures suggest that substantial proportions of the county population face health risks due to air, water, and soil pollution. Only 36% of the county population are served by municipal or community sewers, in comparison to 68% statewide. Periodic surveys of on-site sewage disposal systems have found septic tank failure rates of up to 54% in some neighborhoods. The county experienced 5.8% of the state's hazardous materials spills during 1992 (227 spills) and has 7% of the state's designated hazardous waste sites within its jurisdiction. Despite the risks posed by the county's aging housing stock, a state screening and reporting system for blood lead levels found no incidence of blood lead levels exceeding the minimum risk level (10 mg/dL) during 1993.

Table 3
Health Resources: Thurston County, Washington

Number of nonfederal physicians (Number per 100,000 population) 1992[a]	383 (217)
Family practice	58 (33)
General practice	12 (7)
Internal medicine	36 (20)
Obstetrics/gynecology	19 (11)
Pediatrics	24 (14)
Number of community hospital beds (FY1995)[b]	431
Beds per 100,000 population	244
Number of community hospitals (FY1995)[b]	2
Number of HMOs (1995)[c]	7
Number of federally qualified health centers (1994)[d]	1
Total number of clinic sites	1
Local public health expenditures (1997)	$7,216,140
Percent from direct federal sources	0%
Percent from state sources (including federal pass-throughs)	22%
Percent from local sources	17%
Percent from Medicaid	2%
Percent from Medicare	0%
Total federal funding for community health centers (1996)[e]	$109,972
Total federal funding for migrant health centers (1996)[e]	0
Total federal block grant funds for preventive health services (1996)[e]	$2,053,159
Total federal block grant funds for maternal and child health services (1996)[e]	$8,967,119
Total federal block grant funds for substance abuse services (1996)[e]	$619,356
Total federal funding for homeless health services (1996)[e]	0
Total federal funding for National Health Service Corporation (1996)[e]	0

[a]*Data from American Medical Association Physician Masterfile.*[1]
[b]*Data from American Hospital Association.*[2]
[c]*Data from American Association of Health Plans.*[3]
[d]*Data from US Bureau of Primary Health Care (unpublished data, 1994).*
[e]*Data from US Department of Commerce.*[4]

Local Health Resources and Manpower

A relatively small and stable collection of health care organizations comprise the local health system that serves Olympia, Washington (**Table 3**). Prime among these providers is the Group Health Cooperative of Puget Sound, a large, nonprofit health maintenance organization (HMO) with a 50-year history in the Pacific Northwest region. At least five other managed care plans report operations in Thurston County, but Group Health Cooperative enjoys the largest share of the roughly 25% of the population that receives care from HMOs. Under a 1915(b) Medicaid-waiver program from the US Health Care Financing Administration, Thurston County residents who receive Medicaid benefits through participation in the federal Aid to Families with Dependent Children (AFDC) program are required to receive their health care coverage through state-approved HMOs. Group Health Cooperative and two other plans have received this approval and are currently serving the ~10,000 Medicaid beneficiaries who are recipients of the AFDC program in Thurston County.

Two general acute-care hospitals serve residents of Thurston County and surrounding areas. St. Peter Hospital, part of the nonprofit Sister's of Providence multihospital system, operates a 327-bed facility in northeastern Olympia. St. Peter also operates an HMO for serving Medicaid beneficiaries, in conjunction with its family practice residency program. Six miles to the west, Capital Medical Center operates as a 110-bed facility owned by the national for-profit hospital corporation Columbia/HCA. In total, these facilities provide the county with ~230 hospital beds per 100,000 population.

Approximately 383 active nonfederal physicians practice in the county, yielding a ratio of 217 physicians per 100,000 residents. The local health director reports that some rural areas of the county remain underserved because of the clustering of providers in urban areas. Thirty-nine percent of these physicians practice in the primary care specialties of family medicine, general practice, internal medicine, obstetrics and gynecology, and pediatrics. Although no federally funded health centers operate within the county, St. Peter's Hospital operates a community clinic in collaboration with Group Health Cooperative and the county health department. This clinic serves as a major source of primary care for underserved populations in the county, including uninsured and underinsured individuals, and Medicaid beneficiaries who are not eligible for HMO enrollment. These three organizations also collaborate in operating a homeless health clinic for residents of area homeless shelters. Because for many years the community was served by only one hospital (St. Peter), local health care institutions and providers maintain a long history of cooperation rather than competition. The construction of a new hospital (Capital Medical Center) in 1985 and its conversion to for-profit status soon thereafter has introduced new competitive dynamics into the local health care market.

The Local Health Department

The Thurston County Department of Public Health and Social Services serves as an important provider of personal and population-based health services in the community. The department provides personal health services in the areas of family planning, immunizations, sexually transmitted disease prevention and treatment, maternal and child health services, and communicable disease control. In addition, the department maintains substantial population-based health activities in areas such as health education and outreach, community health assessment, and environmental protection and monitoring. As the county's "umbrella agency" for health and social services, the department also administers programs in areas such as mental health treatment, substance abuse prevention and treatment, developmental disabilities services, and child protective services.

Organizational Structure

The Department of Public Health and Social Services exists as one of 12 administrative departments within the county government system. A three-member elected board of county commissioners provides overall governance for the department, and serves as the local board of health. Acting as the board of health, this body establishes broad policy and programmatic objectives for the department and makes annual budgetary decisions. An administrative director for the department reports directly to the county commissioners.

A Thurston County native, Patrick Libby, maintains a 12-year tenure as department director. Mr. Libby began his career at the health department just as county commissioners were dismantling a multicounty public health district that had served Thurston County and neighboring Mason County for almost two decades. Disagreements over the financial responsibilities and policy-making authorities of counties and cities within the district forced the dissolution of this intergovernmental arrangement. Thurston County commissioners hired Mr. Libby to develop a county health department from the vestiges of the former multicounty organization. Much of Mr. Libby's early years with the department were therefore devoted to executing the administrative and financial reforms that moved the department from a district health department to a combined public health and social services agency operating at the county level.

A full-time, physician-trained health officer reports directly to the department director and maintains responsibility for county medical functions. These functions include providing oversight and consultation for the department's clinical staff and personal health programs, issuing public health orders authorized by state law, and maintaining linkages with the local medical community. In carrying out these responsibilities, Health Officer Dr. Diana Yu, MD, MSPH, draws upon the professional relationships she established during her years as a practicing pediatrician before joining the department in 1990.

The department comprises four divisions that collectively administer all county-operated health and social programs. A *personal health division* houses the department's clinical programs in primary and preventive care areas, including: HIV/AIDS education, testing, and case management; family planning counseling and outreach; immunization delivery; sexually transmitted disease testing and treatment; communicable disease detection, tracking, and treatment; breast and cervical cancer prevention and control services; maternity case management; nutrition services under the federal Special Supplemental Food Program for Women, Infants, and Children (WIC); and other child health services. An *environmental health division* administers assessment and enforcement programs for food safety, vector control, wastewater and drinking water safety, ground and surface water protection, solid waste and hazardous waste control, and community noise control. This division also contains an environmental health laboratory that conducts bacterial analyses of drinking water, surface water, sewage treatment plant effluent, sediments, and shellfish. A *social services division* administers county programs for mental health service delivery, chemical dependency prevention and treatment, developmental disabilities service delivery, family support services, and child protection activities. Finally, a *fiscal and administrative division* houses department-wide functions for grants management, purchasing, payroll, and epidemiology.

Service Areas

Personal Health Services

The health department's involvement in personal health services has changed over the last decade as community health needs and resources have evolved within the county. Under the state's Medicaid managed care initiative, the scope of services directly provided by the health department has diminished somewhat as managed care plans have assumed responsibility for certain services. Nevertheless, the department served over 68,000 clients through its personal health programs in 1996, up from 18,500 clients during calendar year 1989. More than 800 new clients receive care through the department's public health clinics each month.

Maternal and child health services. One health service that the health department provided before the 1994 Medicaid managed care initiative—Early Periodic Screening, Diagnosis, and Treatment services—has now been transitioned to the three managed care plans that enroll Medicaid beneficiaries in Thurston County. Under federal Medicaid regulations, all Medicaid beneficiaries under the age of 20 are eligible for these periodic examinations, which mandate the early detection and treatment of physical, dental, and mental health problems. In transferring responsibility for these services to managed care plans, the health department also transferred its de facto obligation to provide sick care services to children who presented at the department's well child exam clinics. In total, this transition has allowed the health department to eliminate ~1.5 full-time equivalent (FTE) hours of pediatric nurse practitioner services.

The local health department continues to provide many other types of maternal and child health services to Medicaid beneficiaries and other community residents who lack adequate access to care. Prime among these services is the department's maternity case management and support initiative known as the First Steps program. This program provides in-home health education and counseling services to Medicaid-eligible and other high-risk pregnant women regarding appropriate nutrition, health behaviors, and prenatal care services during their pregnancies. The program also provides tracking, follow-up, and support services to encourage women to obtain prenatal care services from their primary care providers at appropriate intervals. The health department's team of community health nurses provides these services.

Under the state's Medicaid managed care program, the local health department is allowed to directly bill the state Medicaid program on a fee-for-service basis for the prenatal support services it provides to Medicaid beneficiaries. Under this program, Medicaid beneficiaries may choose to receive these services from their managed care plans rather than from the local health department, and these plans must cover the cost of these services under the capitated contracts that they negotiate with the state Medicaid agency. The Medicaid agency adjusts the capitated reimbursement rates it pays to Medicaid managed care plans on an annual basis, based in part upon the proportion of beneficiaries who access prenatal support and other "direct billable" services from local health departments. Despite implementation of the Medicaid managed care program in 1994, the number of women served through the local health department's First Steps program has remained relatively stable over the past five years. More than 300 women received prenatal support services and almost 70 women received case management services during calendar year 1995. The local health director anticipates that, as managed care plans further develop the expertise and capacity for providing these services and as beneficiaries develop greater familiarity with these plans, the health department will transition more responsibility for these services to the local managed care plans.

The department provides a range of other services in the area of maternal and child health. A high-risk infants and children program provides case management, assessment, education, and counseling services to the families of children considered at-risk for adverse health events due to premature birth, low birth weight, or substance abuse during pregnancy. The department also administers the county's child protective services program, which assists in identifying and investigating cases of child abuse or neglect, and ensures the health and safety of children in these family environments. The department's program for children with special health care needs provides assessments, referrals, and support services for families and children with chronic or disabling health conditions. Finally, the department administers an active oral health program for children, which includes school-based health education activities and a dental sealant program for low-income children.

Immunization services. The local health department operates an active immunization program that targets infants, children, and adults through a variety of initiatives. Direct provision of vaccinations continues to be an important component of this program, although the growing role of private providers in immunization delivery is expected to reduce the need for health department activities. During 1995, the department directly administered over 2300 does of the measles, mumps, and rubella (MMR) vaccine to individuals who did not have access to immunization services through private providers. The health department continues to immunize Medicaid beneficiaries who are enrolled in managed care plans but who choose to seek care from the department's clinics. As with maternity case management services, immunization services are classified "direct billable" services under the state's Medicaid managed care initiative, allowing the health department to seek fee-for-service reimbursement from the state Medicaid agency when Medicaid beneficiaries are served.

Several of the health department's community immunization projects are administered in collaboration with other local health care providers. The department operates on-site immunization clinics at all of the county's public elementary schools each year in cooperation with Group Health Cooperative. These clinics administer the second scheduled MMR vaccine to area sixth graders. Group Health Cooperative also assists the department in operating annual influenza and pneumonia vaccine clinics for at-risk and elderly adults. The department is also actively engaged in developing a community-wide immunization tracking system in collaboration with local physician practices and hospitals. As part of this development, the department assists local physician practices in implementing a computer-based immunization record review system called CASA, which was developed by the US Centers for Disease Control and Prevention. One final component of the department's immunization program entails providing free state-supplied vaccine to area physicians and hospitals and conducting training and review sessions with these providers regarding appropriate vaccine administration and storage practices. The department supplies vaccine to 31 private health care providers within the county.

Sexually transmitted disease services. Another major component of the local health department's personal health services division, sexually transmitted disease services are delivered through the department's clinic to county residents 14 years of age and older. These services include counseling and testing for HIV / AIDS and other sexually transmitted diseases, contact tracing and follow-up for individuals exposed to sexually transmitted diseases, and referral to community providers for infected individuals to receive appropriate treatment. The department's sexually transmitted disease services are classified as "direct billable" services under the state's Medicaid managed care program, thereby allowing Medicaid beneficiaries who are enrolled in managed care plans to choose between receiving care from the their managed care plan or from the health department clinic. The local health director reports that, because of excess demand for these services in the community, implementation of Medicaid managed care in Thurston County has not resulted in a substantial decline in the number of clients served through its sexually transmitted disease clinics.

Family planning services. The department operates a family planning clinic that provides reproductive health services, family planning counseling, and sexuality health education services to area residents. The clinic served ~2100 clients during calendar year 1995, of whom 30% were under 20 years of age, and 79% reported family incomes within 150% of the federal poverty level. A special "teen clinic" operates within the larger family planning clinic and provides targeted reproductive health care and counseling services to adolescent women. Recognizing the substantial overlap between family planning and sexually transmitted disease service needs, the department is currently integrating these two functions within a single clinic. Departmental administrators hope to realize improvements in efficiency and effectiveness through the consolidated delivery of these services.

As with selected other health department services, family planning services are classified as "direct-billable" under the state Medicaid managed care program, allowing the department to continue providing these services to Medicaid beneficiaries on a fee-for-service basis despite their enrollment in private managed care plans. Departmental administrators report that implementation of Medicaid managed care in Thurston County has not substantially affected the volume or intensity of services delivered through the family planning clinic.

In addition to clinical services, the department's family planning staff administers a collection of health education interventions throughout the community in areas such as birth control, parenting skills, puberty, and the prevention of sexually transmitted diseases and

HIV / AIDS. These interventions typically take the form of presentations at area schools, community centers, neighborhood groups, and professional associations. Health department records indicate that these community presentations reached almost 8000 school-age residents, 129 families, and 273 health and human service professionals during calendar year 1995.

Other personal health services. The department administers several additional personal health services for special populations within Thurston County. The department processes over 1300 tuberculosis skin tests through its tuberculosis control program, a state-mandated initiative that endeavors to control the disease through surveillance, treatment, and prevention. The department administers periodic tests to high-risk individuals, including health workers, group facility residents and workers, substance abuse treatment clients, and contacts of known tuberculosis cases. In cooperation with community providers, clinical staff from the health department provide follow-up to all confirmed tuberculosis cases through both home and clinic visits. Directly observed therapy is maintained for all cases during their contagious phases and for noncompliant cases throughout their treatment process. The department also conducts training sessions with community health and human service providers regarding correct practices for diagnosing and treating the disease.

The health department also manages two interorganizational consortia that provide coordinated services for the prevention and treatment of HIV and AIDS. The first of these entities, the Thurston County HIV Prevention Coalition, includes participation from the local Red Cross chapter, several community youth organizations, and a local affiliate of Planned Parenthood. In cooperation with these agencies, the health department delivers over 2000 HIV antibody counseling and testing sessions annually, and conducts partner notification for individuals testing positive for HIV. The consortium also conducts HIV prevention education and training sessions for students of area schools (grades 5 through 12), health professionals, members of community groups, and special at-risk populations (including residents of correctional facilities and clients of drug dependency programs). An expanding syringe exchange program and a new peer education project round out the consortium's major activities. The health department chairs a second interorganizational consortium, the Thurston County HIV Care Consortium, which brings together major service providers to insure coordination and comprehensiveness in service delivery. The health department serves as the focal point for this coordination by providing case management for area HIV patients and their families. The department manages a caseload of more than 50 clients who reside within the county, linking these individuals and their families with appropriate clinical, social, and mental health services. Federal funding under the Ryan White Act help to sustain this project.

Finally, the health department operates a program for providing breast and cervical health screening services to low-income women who lack insurance coverage for these services. A state pass-through grant from the federal Centers for Disease Control and Prevention helps to fund this effort, which targets the estimated 4600 women in Thurston County age 40 and older who have incomes below the federal poverty level. Through this program, the department conducts public education sessions on the importance of regular breast self-exams, clinical breast exams, yearly Pap smears, and age-appropriate mammograms. Through education and outreach efforts, the department identifies women who are eligible for the federally funded screening program and makes referrals to community physicians who have agreed to serve eligible women under this program. The department also maintains a tracking system to assure that identified women receive the needed screening services.

Environmental Health Services

The health department maintains responsibility for a comprehensive range of county programs and services that aim to maintain and improve environmental quality within the community. Responsibilities in such diverse areas as land use permitting, gravel mine inspection, shellfish resources management, and noise pollution control allow the department to develop coordinated, multifaceted interventions to address environmental health issues within the county. The health department has acquired these responsibilities in part through flexible state legislation that in many cases has given municipalities the choice to participate in functions often reserved for state agencies. A creative and responsive county board of commissioners has also encouraged the health department's expansive role in environmental issues.

Water quality initiatives comprise a substantial portion of the health department's environmental health agenda. The department reviews the proposed drinking water supply of all proposed land use and building projects within the county, and inspects the location and construction of all wells and drinking water systems. Other water quality responsibilities include septic tank and sewage system inspection, certification of sewage system developers and installers, surface water and ground water quality monitoring, and surveillance of water quality in shell-fishing areas.

The department maintains responsibility for a wide range of programs and services that target human living environments. These responsibilities include solid waste disposal permitting and inspection; regulation of hazardous waste transportation and disposal; land use permitting for all construction and development projects within the county; licensing and inspection of gravel mines, swimming pools, and schools; vector control; and noise pollution monitoring and enforcement. Finally, the department maintains an active food safety program that includes periodic inspection of all permanent and temporary food establishments and the training and licensing of all food service workers within the county.

Social Services

As an "umbrella" human services agency, the Thurston County Department of Public Health and Social Services provides many types of services not traditionally administered within local health departments. These include chemical dependency prevention and treatment services, educational and support services for individuals with developmental disabilities, mental health treatment services, and counseling and support services for children, youth, and families. The department provides many of these services through contracts with community-based service providers, while assuming direct responsibility for activities such as case management, resource development, community education, evaluation, and advocacy.

The department administers county mental health services through a partnership with neighboring Mason County. Since November 1993, this two-county regional service network has operated as a prepaid health plan under the state's managed mental health care program for Medicaid beneficiaries. Under this arrangement, the regional service network has functioned much like an HMO in that it receives capitated funding from the state Medicaid agency and manages mental health service delivery through capitated subcontracting arrangements that it establishes with area mental health service providers. Through this initiative, the department has gained valuable experience in operating within managed care systems. Department administrators report that this experience in the mental health arena has aided the department in responding to the more recent challenges of public health delivery under Medicaid managed care.

Infrastructure and Resources

For calendar year 1997, the department maintains a staff of 96 FTE positions within the public health services division and 17 FTE positions within the social services division. These staffing levels represent a modest decrease of almost 4 FTE positions from 1996 levels. A total budget of more than $7,216,000 is allocated for public health services and $1,735,611 for social services during 1997. This latter amount does not include the more than $10 million in state "pass through" funding that the department administers to local social services providers. Approximately 17% of the public health division's budget is derived from local government sources, which include county general fund appropriations and contractually defined contributions from cities and towns within the county. State grants and contracts comprise ~12% of revenues, while federal pass-through funding represents another 10% of the budget. Medicaid reimbursement amounts to only 2% of the public health division's total budget, with another 5% being derived from the county's share of Medicaid federal matching funds received by the state. Fees collected by the department for permits, licenses, and personal health services generate ~40% of the public health division's annual budget. The department collects fees for environmental health activities such as food establishment permits, water system certifications and testing, sewage system permits, land use reviews and permits, solid waste disposal permits, and school facility reviews. Additionally, the department assesses patient fees for delivering certain personal health services, medications, and supplies using a sliding fee schedule based on family income and size.

Other Contributors to Local Public Health Practice

State Health Agencies

Complementing the county's thriving public health and social services agency is a range of other public and private organizations that play important roles in addressing public health issues in Thurston County. Certainly, Washington's state health agencies contribute substantially to the local public health system that serves the state's capitol city. Three separate agencies hold responsibility for state health programs and services in Washington. The Department of Health oversees traditional public health services, including programs in infectious disease control, maternal and child health, environmental health, epidemiology, health statistics, and health facilities and services licensing. The Department of Social and Health Services administers the state's Medicaid program, as well as a wide range of mental health and social services programs. Finally, the Washington State Health Care Authority administers a state-sponsored health insurance plan for individuals not eligible for other public insurance programs, as well as the state system for financing community health centers.

The Department of Health carries out many of its public health initiatives through grants, contracts, and cooperative agreements with local health departments. Thurston County and Washington's 32 other local health departments are decentralized units of local government that rely on the state agency primarily for funding and technical assistance. Thurston County's health director indicates that his interaction with the state health department began to expand when the department was carved out of a larger umbrella human services agency in 1988. This reorganization appeared to make state public health officials more visible and accessible to Thurston County staff. More recently, the development and implementation of the statewide Public Health Improvement Plan has created enhanced opportunities for interaction and collaboration between Thurston County's Public Health Agency and the state Department of Health. This initiative, created by state legislation in 1993, established an administrative framework and a funding stream for enhancing the public health system's capacity to protect and promote health within the state. The enabling legislation requires the state health department to revise and update an improvement plan every two years, in collaboration with other public and private organizations that contribute to public health within the state. During the first 4 years of this ongoing initiative, state officials have worked closely with Thurston County staff, along with officials from other local health departments, in designing new systems for financing, delivering, and evaluating local public health services under the Public Health Improvement Plan initiative. Specific areas of interaction have included the following: identifying core public health functions and capacities that should be maintained by state and local public health agencies; developing a system for measuring the adequacy of these functions and capacities in local jurisdictions; and designing new, performance-based contracting and reimbursement systems for state-financed public health services. Thurston County's health agency has actively participated in the development and implementation of these activities, and its staff has served as important advocates for the Public Health Improvement Plan initiative.

Thurston County's interaction with the Washington Department of Social and Health Services (DSHS) primarily involves financing issues for public health and mental health services under the state's Medicaid program. The local health department provides several types of public health services that are eligible for direct, fee-for-service reimbursement from DSHS under Medicaid. These services include immunizations, maternity case management, sexually transmitted disease services, and family planning services. For other personal health services, DSHS establishes contracts with approved managed care plans that assume responsibility for addressing the health service needs of Medicaid beneficiaries. Thurston County's health director reports that the local health department to date has not maintained much interaction with DSHS in monitoring and evaluating the performance of managed care plans that serve Medicaid beneficiaries within its jurisdiction. The local health director hopes to secure a future role for his department in these activities, which currently remain within the domain of DSHS. Thurston County's health department also maintains financial relationships with DSHS through the prepaid health plan program for mental health services under Medicaid, and through other social service programs that receive federal and state pass-through funds in areas such as developmental disabilities, substance abuse, child protection, and family support.

Finally, Thurston County's Health Department interacts with the Washington State Health Care Authority primarily through its Primary Health Care Services division. This division provides funding, technical assistance, and training to public and nonprofit community health centers which serve low-income and underserved populations within the state. Health centers that participate in this program include federally qualified community and migrant health centers, public hospital-affiliated clinics, and clinics operated by local public health departments. Thurston County staff interacts with this division regularly to secure funding and consultation for both the county's public health clinic and the community clinic operated collaboratively with St. Peter Hospital and Group Health Cooperative.

County health department officials maintain relatively little involvement with the health care authority's other major initiative, the Washington Basic Health Plan. This plan provides managed care coverage to more than 200,000 state residents who are not insured through other public or private health plans, in exchange for a sliding-scale premium based upon family income. By expanding health insurance coverage among the uninsured, this plan holds the potential to reduce local health departments' current responsibilities in providing personal health services to this population group. Additionally, this plan may create opportunities for local health departments to develop service agreements and other collaborative arrangements with the private health plans that contract to serve these groups. To date, Thurston County Health Department officials indicate that they continue to experience a strong demand for services among the uninsured—a trend they attribute to excess demand for the types of personal health services they provide. Furthermore, health department officials have not yet experienced much success in forging service agreements with the managed care plans that serve enrollees of the Basic Health Plan. Thurston County's health director remains optimistic that as the Basic Health Plan expands to cover larger numbers of private providers and larger numbers of the uninsured, the health department will be able to transition more of its responsibilities in direct service provision to these providers. These developments would also create an imperative for the local health department to work closely with the state health care authority to assure that sufficient contract provisions and evaluation systems are in place to serve adequately the health care needs of the uninsured in Thurston County. Unfortunately, state budgetary limits on the number of individuals who can enroll in the Basic Health Plan continue to constrain the growth of the program (a waiting list of almost 36,000 individuals existed as of July 1997).

Community Hospitals

St. Peter Hospital

For much of the last century, Thurston County was served by a single, nonprofit community hospital affiliated with the Catholic Church. St. Peter Hospital, part of the Sisters of Providence -multihospital system, maintains a long history of addressing health care needs in the community, with a particular emphasis on serving vulnerable populations such as individuals living in poverty. The hospital encompasses a 327-bed acute care facility, a community health clinic staffed in part by members of the hospital's family practice residency program, and an HMO that serves over 20,000 commercial members and several thousand Medicaid beneficiaries.

As the only nonprofit hospital in the county, St. Peter provides the majority of uncompensated care for both inpatient and ambulatory care services. The hospital's community health clinic, referred to as the Community Care Clinic, provides primary care services to a large proportion of the community's uninsured and underinsured populations, as well as to Medicaid beneficiaries. St. Peter operates the Community Care Clinic in collaboration with numerous other community organizations, including the local health department, Group Health Cooperative, and the local community action council. The clinic was originally launched during the late 1970s in response to the dismantling of a state program for providing health care services to low-income refugees. Currently, the clinic is incorporated as an independent, nonprofit organization with a governing board comprised of members from the contributing organizations. St. Peter provides the facilities for the clinic, and members of the hospital's family practice residency program staff the clinic along with volunteers from Group Health, the local health department, and private physician practices. Clinic operating expenses are covered through grants from St. Peter, Group Health, the local health department, and the state health care authority. A dental clinic is also operated through the Community Care Clinic with funding from the state authority.

Another community health initiative operated collaboratively by St. Peter Hospital, Group Health, and the local health department—the homeless health clinic—provides primary care services to residents of Olympia's downtown homeless shelters. All three organizations collaborate in funding and staffing the clinic and in securing additional grant funding from the state health care authority. St. Peter independently operates a third health clinic that provides prenatal care and support services to low-income women who are unable to access these services from private community physicians. Although Medicaid eligibility expansions and the state Medicaid managed care initiative have reduced the demand for services through this clinic, St. Peter continues to operate this vital safety-net program for community members who still face financial barriers to prenatal care. The team of obstetricians and nurse midwives who staff this program serve ~350 women annually.

St. Peter Hospital maintains a long history of involvement in managed care delivery, which it has more recently applied to the care of vulnerable populations through the state Medicaid managed care initiative. The hospital's earliest experience with managed care began soon after Group Health Cooperative opened its Olympia clinic in 1972. Through capitated contracts, St. Peter now provides ~70% of the HMO's inpatient care days. Using experience gained through its partnership with Group Health, St. Peter initiated its own HMO during the late 1980s as part of a statewide health plan developed by the Sisters of Providence. With the implementation of Medicaid managed care in 1994, St. Peter's HMO was one of three managed care plans designated to enroll Medicaid beneficiaries in Thurston County. In operating a Medicaid managed care plan, St. Peter administrators report that the hospital is able to combine its substantial experience in managed care with its long history of service to vulnerable populations. Through this plan the hospital is able to assure coordinated delivery of a comprehensive range of health services to these populations, rather than the episodic care often provided through its community clinics and hospital departments. St. Peter administrators view the move to Medicaid managed care in Thurston County as a promising strategy for improving access to care for vulnerable populations. Already, the hospital reports a 10% decline in visits to its emergency room by Medicaid beneficiaries since the implementation of managed care. This result may suggest that beneficiaries are obtaining appropriate access to primary care services in nonemergent community settings.

In addition to directly providing and managing health services, St. Peter Hospital plays an active role in community health assessment and policy development efforts within Thurston County. A corporate policy adopted during the 1980s requires all hospitals within the Sisters of Providence system to conduct an annual assessment of health needs within the communities they serve. For several years, administrators at St. Peters completed an independent assessment that entailed a review of area health and socioeconomic statistics, an analysis of hospitalization data, and interviews with community residents and community organizations regarding their perceptions of the most pressing health issues. These assessments were then used as part of the hospital's annual strategic planning process to determine how programs and services could be modified to meet outstanding community health needs. Beginning in 1994, St. Peter linked its assessment process to the community health assessment process undertaken by the local health department. In doing so, the hospital has been able to use the health department's assessment work for its own strategic planning purposes. At the same time, St. Peter has become a critical participant in the health department's assessment process. The hospital has maintained active participation on several of the community intervention task forces that were formed in response to findings from the assessment process. Hospital staff chairs the task force on indoor and outdoor air quality and participates on task forces on increasing immunization rates among preschool children and designing community surveillance systems for dental health and immunization status.

Capital Medical Center

A relative newcomer to the local hospital market, Capital Medical Center, is a 110-bed hospital established in 1985 by the for-profit hospital chain Hospital Corporation of America (HCA). Now a member of the nation's largest for-profit health care system, Columbia/HCA, the hospital includes an ambulatory care center, a diabetes wellness center, and a home health service in addition to its inpatient services divisions. The hospital's administrator reports that majority of patients served by the hospital are Medicare beneficiaries (~55%) and commercially insured individuals (~30%). Medicaid beneficiaries comprise ~10% of the hospital's patient population, with private pay and charity care patients comprising the remaining 5% of this population. Approximately 2% of the hospital's annual budget is devoted to charity care and bad debts (eg, unpaid medical bills).

As a new addition to the local health care community, the hospital continues to work at developing relationships with Thurston County's existing health organizations. Two recent developments appear to have facilitated Capital Medical Center's involvement in community health issues. First, the local health department's community health assessment process, which began in 1994, provides an opportunity for the hospital to begin collaborating with other community organizations to address health issues of common concern. As contributors to this process, staff from the hospital serves on community task forces addressing community fitness, nutrition practices, and preschool immunization rates. Administrators suggest that these activities allow the hospital to acquire new insight regarding health needs in the community and regarding the resources and capacities that other health organizations maintain within the community. In turn, the community health assessment process allows the hospital to contribute its unique perspectives and expertise as a large, investor-owned medical care facility in the community.

A second development in the community—the growth of managed care delivery, especially for Medicaid beneficiaries—has motivated the hospital's involvement in community health issues. As growing proportions of local employers move to managed health care delivery, Capital has faced an imperative to enhance its own involvement with managed care delivery in order to remain competitive with St. Peter Hospital and its exclusive alliance with Group Health Cooperative, the area's largest HMO. To this end, the hospital has expanded its involvement in providing health promotion and disease prevention services within the community. This expansion is undertaken to achieve two related purposes: (1) to improve the hospital's ability to compete for contracts with managed care organizations and their enrollees and (2) to promote health and reduce risks among the growing number of managed care enrollees served by the hospital. Expanded services include the following: a special wellness center for diabetes patients that is designed to facilitate improved management of diabetes on an outpatient basis; a community education division that conducts free seminars for patients, community members, and health professionals on high-priority health issues; an enhanced mammography program accredited by the American College of Radiology; a nutritional counseling program staffed by registered dietitians; and an occupational health program that includes employee health screenings and work place safety consultations.

As part of the hospital's move to primary and preventive care, the hospital has acquired six primary care clinics located in outlying, rural areas of the community. Two of the clinics are staffed by physicians who are employed by the hospital, and the remaining four are staffed by nurse practitioners. These clinics have expanded the hospital's involvement in providing care to vulnerable population groups such as underserved Medicaid and Medicare beneficiaries. The hospital's involvement in this area has grown markedly since the implementation of Medicaid managed care in 1994, as the hospital's clinics participate as providers in the network of Thurston County's largest Medicaid managed care provider, Kitsap Physician Services. Under this arrangement, the hospital receives capitated reimbursement from the managed care plan to provide a comprehensive range of primary care and specialty services through its medical center and network of primary care clinics. This arrangement creates an additional imperative for the hospital to develop expertise in serving vulnerable population groups and to forge working relationships with the many other community organizations that may contribute to the health of this population. Relationships with many of these organizations, such as the local health department, are still under development. At a minimum, the health department's community assessment process provides the hospital with a forum in which to explore these types of relationships.

Managed Care Plans

For many years, the local managed care market has been dominated by the large, nonprofit Group Health Cooperative of Puget Sound. Consistent with its nonprofit mission of community service, Group Health has maintained a long history of involvement in community health activities. During the 1980s, new managed care plans began operating in Thurston County as this form of health care delivery grew in popularity as a strategy for cost containment and accountability. These plans included a nonprofit HMO affiliated with St. Peter Hospital, as well as several for-profit corporations that expanded their operations from Seattle. The implementation of Medicaid managed care in Thurston County during 1994 brought in another health plan, Kitsap Physician Services, which had successfully operated under a Medicaid managed care demonstration program in several neighboring counties. Interaction between Thurston County's public health system and this diverse collection of managed care plans has continued to grow throughout these developments.

Group Health Cooperative

Group Health Cooperative is a staff-model HMO based in Seattle with a 50-year history in the northwest and more than 500,000 enrollees. The 1997 merger of this plan with the nation's largest nonprofit HMO, Kaiser Permanente, makes this organization part of a national network of prepaid health care providers. Group Health's Olympia health district serves ~50,000 enrollees, which accounts for ~20% of the area's commercially insured population and 25% of the nonmilitary insured population. The Olympia district is managed as a decentralized, local administrative unit of Group Health Cooperative, with two multispecialty ambulatory medical centers serving as the focal points of service delivery in the district. These centers employ a medical staff of almost 100 full-time equivalent staff, including board certified physicians, physician assistants, nurse practitioners, nurse midwives, optometrists, and mental health professionals. Unlike other units of Group Health Cooperative, the Olympia district does not operate any inpatient facilities, but rather it maintains an exclusive contract with St. Peter Hospital for most inpatient care services and selected outpatient services.

Group Health engages in many community health initiatives through partnerships with the local health department and St. Peter Hospital. The HMO is a vital contributor of funding, staff, and management expertise for the homeless health clinic and the community care clinic that are jointly operated by the three organizations. Additionally, Group Health collaborates with the local health department in several community-based initiatives to improve immunization rates among both children and adults. The HMO contributes teams of nursing staff to administer scheduled childhood immunization boosters in Thurston County schools. The HMO also operates community influenza vaccination clinics annually to increase senior citizen vaccination coverage rates within the county. As part of this initiative, Group Health solicits the participation of other private physicians in providing free and reduced-fee influenza vaccinations to seniors. Although the HMO continues to meet resistance from some community physicians, the organization continues to expand the number of private providers who participate in the program. These initiatives target all age-appropriate community members, rather than only those residents who are members of Group Health's HMO. As one motivation for its involvement in these initiatives, Group Health's administrator suggests that for public health issues such as infectious diseases, community-wide interventions are often more effective than HMO-specific interventions in helping to improve the health of its enrolled populations.

Group Health also administers a wide range of health promotion and disease prevention interventions within its own population of enrolled members. Given the large market share that the HMO maintains in the community, these internal activities often have substantial "spillover" effects on the health of the larger community in Thurston County. The HMO maintains an extensive, computerized childhood immunization tracking and support system that includes automatic generation of patient and provider reminders regarding scheduled immunizations. This system enables the HMO to insure that more than 70% of its enrollees under the age of 2 years are up-to-date on scheduled immunizations, in comparison to the 50% immunization rate for other community members within the county. A similar tracking system for senior influenza vaccinations enables the HMO to continually improve its vaccination rate among this group of enrollees. Other health promotion initiatives include the following: routine group counseling sessions regarding diabetes management; an active smoking cessation program; tracking and reminder systems for age-appropriate breast and cervical cancer screenings; and an expanding program for developing clinical practice guidelines in areas such as childhood immunizations, breast cancer screening, tobacco cessation, prostate specific antigen screening, and cervical cancer screening.

Group Health's involvement in community health issues includes the provision of care for vulnerable populations through the state's Medicaid managed care initiative. Group Health's Olympia district serves as a Medicaid managed care provider for Thurston County as well as the neighboring Lewis County. As of mid-year 1995, the plan served 1800 Medicaid recipients through a capitated contract with the state Medicaid agency. Group Health has experienced marked success in meeting the complex health and social service needs of Medicaid recipients. By adopting strategies such as extended clinic office hours and flexible appointment scheduling protocols, the plan has rapidly become an important source of care for vulnerable and underserved populations in Thurston County.[5]

Group Health maintains a history of collaboration with the local health department in serving vulnerable populations. Under a state-funded prenatal care program for low-income women begun in the late 1980s (known as First Steps), Group Health has provided obstetrical services for high-risk pregnant Medicaid beneficiaries who are identified and managed by the local health department. Through this program, Group Health staff gained experience in serving vulnerable population groups that face complex health, social, and economic problems. This collaborative program continues to operate successfully for Medicaid beneficiaries who are not enrolled in managed care plans; however, contracting Medicaid managed care plans such as Group Health Cooperative now may choose to provide these case management services to the Medicaid beneficiaries who are enrolled in their plans.

Several other linkages between Group Health Cooperative and Thurston County's local health department are notable. First, Group Health continues to play a vital role in the health department's ongoing community health assessment process. Staff from the HMO serves on task forces that are now addressing dental health issues, fluoridation efforts, and preschool immunization rates. Group Health staff is also collaborating with the health department in developing an earthquake emergency preparedness plan for the county. The frequency of seismic activity in the region lends added importance and urgency to this effort. Finally, Group Health and the local health department are working to resolve a quirk in the HMO's process for laboratory testing that results in delays in the reporting of communicable diseases. Because the HMO uses a centralized laboratory in Seattle, laboratory tests that reveal reportable communicable diseases for Olympia enrollees are reported to the King County health department rather than to the Thurston County agency. In conjunction with the health department, Group Health is designing a new laboratory reporting process that will enable direct reporting to the appropriate county health department. The strong working relationships between Group Health and Thurston County's health department greatly facilitate the adoption of timely and creative responses to many community health issues.

Group Health's administrator observes that most of the interaction that occurs between the HMO and the local health department are initiated by the department. Given the department's primary focus on public health issues and given the HMO's primary focus on medical care delivery for its enrolled populations, this arrangement seems entirely appropriate. In many areas, the local health department may hold a better vantage point for identifying community health issues and strategies for addressing issues through collaboration. Nevertheless, Group Health has initiated some of the collaborative efforts, such as the jointly sponsored childhood immunization effort in local schools and community centers and the jointly sponsored influenza vaccination campaign for seniors. For these issues, Group Health administrators clearly recognized the need for a community-level effort in order to impact health among its enrolled members.

Kitsap Physician Services

The dominant plan serving Medicaid beneficiaries in Thurston County is Kitsap Physician Services, a physician-sponsored health plan that serves a four-county area that includes Thurston County. Originally formed as a local Blue Shield plan, Kitsap Physician Services now operates as an independent managed care plan that primarily serves state and federal employees, Medicaid beneficiaries, and low-income enrollees in the state's Basic Health Plan. In total, ~35% of the plan's 75,000 enrollees are Medicaid beneficiaries. In Thurston County, the plan covers ~8000 of the 10,000 Medicaid beneficiaries who are enrolled in managed care plans.

Kitsap gained early experience in serving vulnerable populations through its participation in the US Health Care Financing Administration's Medicaid managed care demonstration program, which operated in a neighboring county during the late 1980s and early 1990s. When the state Medicaid managed care initiative began implementation in Thurston County during 1994, the local medical society requested Kitsap to begin operations in the county so that area physicians could participate as Medicaid managed care providers by contracting with the plan.

As a physician-sponsored plan, Kitsap contracts with individual physicians and groups on a capitated basis to provide or arrange for a comprehensive set of health services to the enrollees that select them as their primary care providers. Under the capitated reimbursement system, primary care physicians who contract with Kitsap are financially at risk for all medically necessary services covered by the state Medicaid program, including inpatient and specialty services. Because Medicaid beneficiaries enrolled in managed care plans are allowed to self-refer to local health departments for services such as childhood immunizations, maternity case management, and sexually transmitted disease services, Kitsap maintains contractual agreements with the departments in most of the counties in which it operates. These contracts allow Kitsap to reimburse health departments on a fee-for-service basis at rates that exceed the those that the departments would receive by "direct billing" the state Medicaid agency for these services. These contracts also allow Kitsap to receive timely information about the services their enrollees receive from health departments, so that they can accurately track service utilization and identify outstanding service needs (such as underimmunized children).

To date, Kitsap has not been successful in establishing service contracts with Thurston County's local health department, despite the plan's willingness to do so. The local health department's reluctance to establish such contracts stems primarily from their desire to encourage private providers to develop their own capacities and expertise to provide these services adequately to Medicaid beneficiaries. The health department continues to serve as a provider of last resort for these services and is able to directly bill the state Medicaid agency for services it provides to Medicaid beneficiaries. Nonetheless, the department's hope is that eventually private providers will be able to fully address the service needs of vulnerable populations in Thurston County, so that direct provision of these services by the health department will no longer be necessary. Health department administrators report that this goal has already been achieved for well child health examinations, allowing the health department to discontinue providing this service now that Medicaid managed care providers can fully meet the community's need. By choosing not to establish Medicaid service contracts with managed care plans such as Kitsap, the department anticipates that these plans will be motivated to develop their own internal capacities for delivering a comprehensive range of personal health services to Medicaid beneficiaries and other vulnerable populations. While this transition takes place, the health department continues to provide specified personal health services to these clients, but plans such as Kitsap are unable fully integrate health department services into their own delivery and management systems.

Despite the absence of formal, contractual relationships, Kitsap continues to build a strong working relationship with the local health department and other community service providers. Kitsap administrators meet regularly with Thurston County's medical director to insure that the plan's practices for services such as childhood immunization, maternity case management, and communicable disease control are consistent with those provided through health department programs. Similarly, Kitsap works to establish strong relationships with other community agencies who are likely to serve vulnerable populations in the area, such as public and private social service agencies, transportation and child care providers, community mental health centers, substance abuse treatment centers, and violence prevention programs. The plan works to keep its primary care providers aware of available community services, so that appropriate referrals and consultations can be made for their clients. In a related effort, Kitsap maintains a staff of five beneficiary advocates who provide Medicaid enrollees with information and counseling on how to access needed health and social services both from within the plan and from outside community service providers. Through these initiatives, Kitsap administrators hope to expand and improve their ability to serve Medicaid beneficiaries and other vulnerable populations in Thurston County. As a relative newcomer to the community, the plan appears to be achieving success in carving out an appropriate role for its organization among an established network of community health providers.

Other Health Plans

At least five other managed care plans operate in Thurston County, all of which are part of larger organizations based in Seattle. The Good Health Plan, owned by the nonprofit Sisters of Providence health system and affiliated with St. Peter Hospital, operates Thurston County's third Medicaid managed care plan. Although it currently covers only a small number of Medicaid beneficiaries, the plan appears well poised to expand its involvement in serving this population as well as beneficiaries of the state's Basic Health Plan, given the hospital's long history in serving vulnerable population groups. St. Peter's strong relationships with the local health department also make this plan a promising participant in the department's endeavors to transition some of its current service responsibilities to private managed care organizations. Other plans operating within Thurston County include the for-profit corporations of HealthFirst Partners, PacifiCare, and QualMed as well as the nonprofit HealthPlus plan. Several of these plans serve Medicaid beneficiaries in other counties or states, making them likely candidates for future involvement in this arena, especially if the state's Medicaid managed care initiative and Basic Health Plan program are expanded to create more potential enrollees in Thurston County. At this time, Thurston County's local health department maintains little if any interaction with these remaining four health plans.

Other Community Organizations

A wide range of other community organizations makes valuable contributions to the local public health system serving Thurston County. The Community Action Council, which began in the 1960s with funding from the US Office of Economic Opportunity, provides a broad array of health and social support services to community residents. These services include the following: nutritional supplementation under the federal Special Supplemental Food Program for Women, Infants, and Children (WIC); maternal case management services for low-income women through the state First Steps program; homeless services; housing assistance; food programs; substance abuse treatment services; and domestic abuse services. A community-based organization named Together conducts policy development, planning, advocacy, and community mobilization efforts around issues involving tobacco use, the abuse of alcohol and other drugs, and youth violence. This organization also collaborates with the Community Action Council and other community organizations in operating multipurpose human service centers in three low-income neighborhoods and three low-income apartment complexes. In addition to social support services, these centers provide health education and substance abuse prevention services to area residents. An active local chapter of the United Way helps to finance the community's homeless health clinic and to conduct community assessments of health issues affecting teenage youth in the community. The local medical and dental societies play valuable roles in developing policies and plans for addressing community health issues and in educating and mobilizing area health professionals around these issues. A local restaurant association participates in shaping policies and regulations regarding the prevention of food-borne diseases and the training of food handlers. Area public school administrators maintain involvement in policy development and planning activities regarding child and adolescent health issues such as violence, tobacco use, and substance abuse. Finally, public health and medical school faculty from the Seattle-based University of Washington interact frequently with the local health department for purposes such as providing technical assistance for public health assessment and surveillance efforts and implementing training programs for public health and medical professionals. These organizations and numerous others have also contributed to the local health department's ongoing community health assessment process.

Measures of Public Health System Performance

The local health director's assessments of public health performance in 1992 and 1997 reveal a steady improvement in the availability and adequacy of public health services in Thurston County during this 5-year period (**Figure 1**). The total performance score for the jurisdiction as a whole rises from 43% of the maximum possible score to 53% during this period—a 23% increase in jurisdictional performance. The largest increases in performance appear to occur within the core public health functions of *policy development* and *assessment*. Among policy development activities, we note a 100% increase in the performance of efforts to set priorities among health needs, an 11% increase in public health advocacy activities and a 20% increase in efforts to develop plans and policies to address priority health issues. Among assessment activities, we note a 60% increase in efforts to assess community health needs and a 92% percent increase in efforts to analyze the determinants of health needs. Community performance of public health activities appears to have declined during the 1992-1997 period for only two public health practices. A 22% decrease in performance is noted for the practice of investigating the occurrence of health effects and health hazards, and a 50% decrease in performance emerges for the practice of evaluating health programs and providing quality assurance.

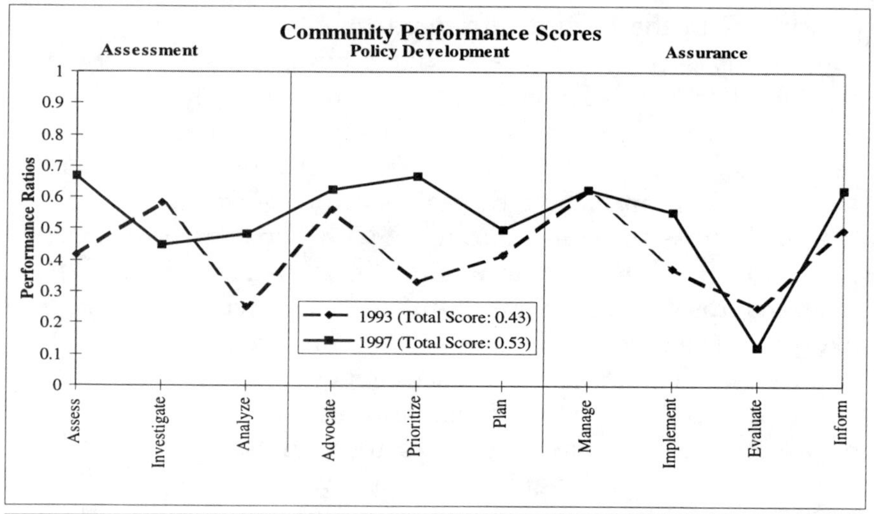

Figure 1. Community public health performance scores for Thurston County.

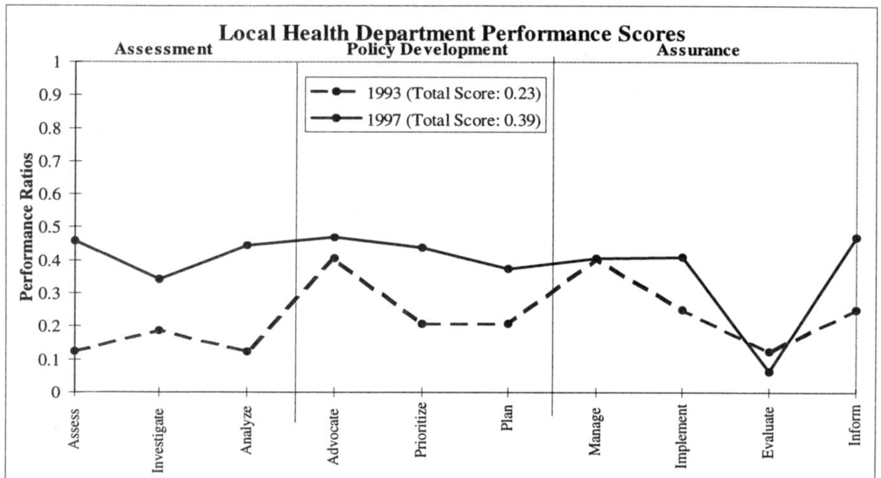

Health department performance score as a percentage of community score

	Assess	Investigate	Analyze	Advocate	Prioritize	Plan	Manage	Implement	Evaluate	Inform
1993:	30%	32%	50%	72%	62%	50%	65%	67%	50%	50%
1997:	69%	76%	92%	75%	66%	75%	65%	74%	50%	75%
Chg:	+129%	+138%	+83%	+04%	+05%	+50%	0%	+11%	0%	+50%

Figure 2. Local health department performance scores for Thurston County.

When we examine only those public health practices that are directly performed by Thurston County's local health department, it appears that the department's performance has also increased substantially during the 1992-1997 period (**Figure 2**). Overall, the department's performance score increases from 23% of the maximum possible score in 1992 to 39% in 1997, representing a 70% increase in performance. When we express the department's total performance score as a percentage of the community performance score, we find that this ratio increases from 53% in 1992 to 74% in 1997—an increase of 38% in the proportion of total community effort that is performed by the local health department. The largest increases in health department performance appear to occur within the core public health functions of *assessment* and *policy development*. Among assessment activities, the largest increases in performance are reported for the practices of assessing health needs in the community (266% increase) and analyzing the determinants of identified health needs (255% increase). Among policy development activities, the largest performance increases are reported for the practices of setting priorities among health needs (111% increase) and developing plans and policies to address

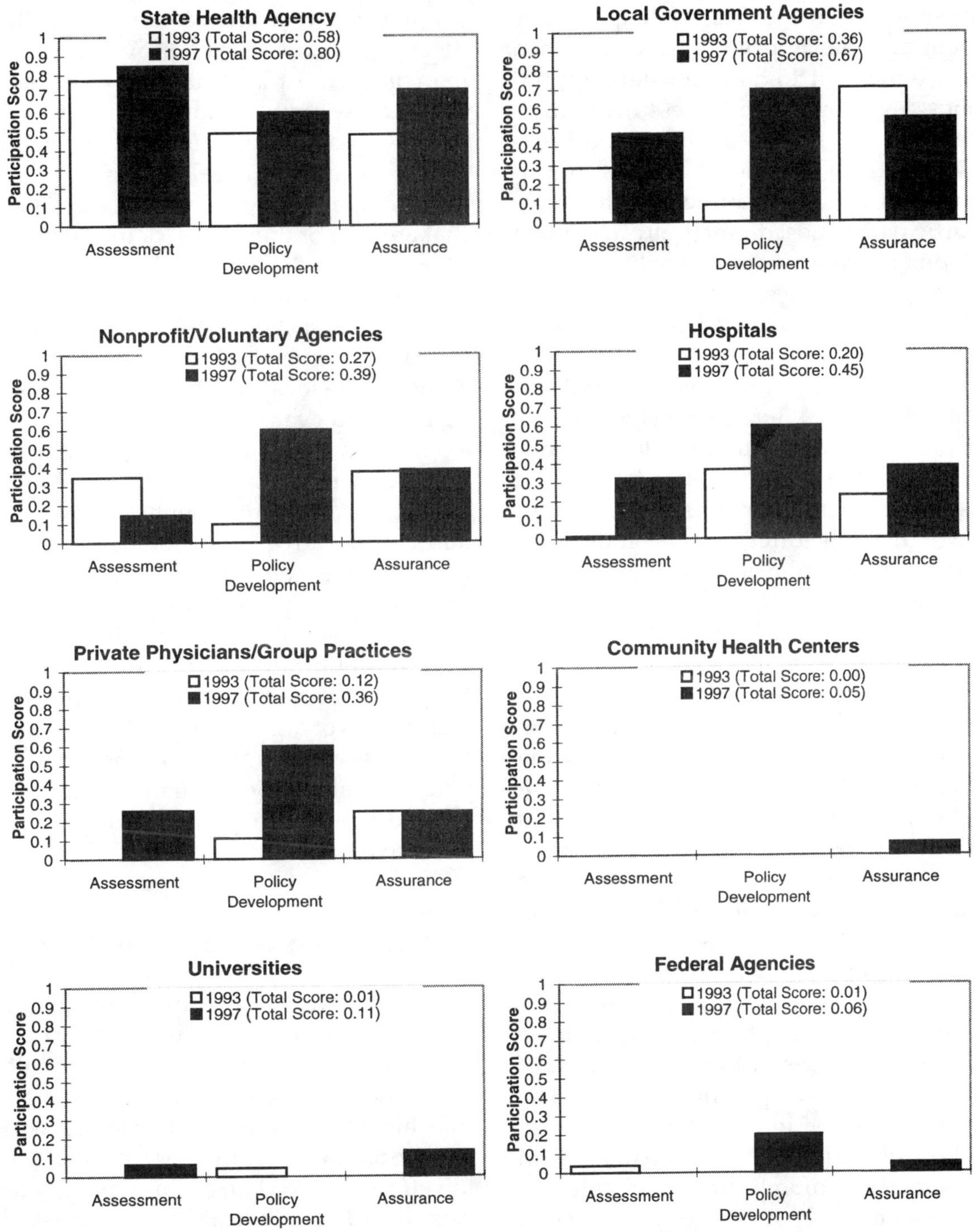

Figure 3. Participation in local public health activities by other organizations, 1993 and 1997 (as reported by the local health director).

priority health needs (80% increase). For activities involving the core public health function of *assurance,* performance increases are reported for two practices (implementing programs and informing/educating the public), while a 50% decrease in performance is reported for the practice of evaluating programs and providing quality assurance. Local health department performance for the practice of managing resources and developing organizational structure appears unchanged between 1992 and 1997.

Participation in public health activities by organizations other than the local health department appears to have increased substantially between 1992 and 1997, according to the local health director reports (**Figure 3**). Participation by state health agencies appears to have markedly increased for the functions of assurance and policy development. In contrast, participation by local government agencies appears to have declined for assurance activities but to have substantially increased for policy development and assessment activities. Many types of organizations—including local government agencies, federal agencies, hospitals, physicians, and nonprofit agencies—appear to have increased their participation most dramatically in the area of policy development activities. Additionally, community health centers, universities, and federal agencies all appear to have initiated new efforts in assurance activities during the 1992-1997 period.

Results from the performance assessments in Thurston County offer some interesting insight regarding the changes taking place within the local public health system during the 1990s. Health department administrators report that their organization is gradually moving away from the direct provision of many personal health services and transitioning these responsibilities to other organizations within the community as they develop the capacity and expertise for serving Medicaid beneficiaries and other vulnerable and underserved populations. Our performance assessments suggest that the health department's role in public health performance is nevertheless growing substantially over the time period in which this transition is taking place, especially for policy development and assessment functions. This experience seems to support the notion that local health departments can maintain and even improve public health delivery in the wake of policy initiatives that transfer service responsibilities from public to private health care organizations. In the case of Thurston County, decreases in responsibility for direct service provision appear to be more than offset by increases in the performance of assessment and policy development activities. The result is an overall increase in public health performance within the jurisdiction, as well as an increase in the proportion of total community effort performed by the health department. In responding to health system changes such as privatization and Medicaid managed care, the local health department has achieved an expanded role rather than diminished role within the local public health system.

It is somewhat disconcerting that the two areas of diminished community performance during the 1992-1997 period involve investigating health risks and evaluating health programs and services. Policy initiatives which give private organizations enhanced responsibilities in service delivery to vulnerable populations may also create barriers for public health agencies in obtaining timely information about health risks within these populations. Effective arrangements for sharing health-related data between the local health department and private providers such as Medicaid managed care plans have not yet been devised in Thurston County, although progress is underway in specific areas such as childhood immunization. At the same time, the local health department to date has had very little input and access to the evaluation strategies that are part of the state's Medicaid managed care initiative. These developments appear to be reflected in the results of our performance assessment, and they point out the need for further work at both local and state levels to insure that health care reform initiatives do not erode local capabilities for public health investigation and evaluation.

Findings regarding the participation of community organizations in public health activities seem to reflect the local health department's ongoing efforts to maintain collaborative partnerships with a wide array of organizations contributing to health within the community. The department's community health assessment process and the community task forces that grew from this effort appear to have opened new avenues for participation in policy development activities for many types of organizations. As these task forces begin to address community health issues through surveillance and intervention, many organizations may also expand their participation in the assessment and assurance functions.

Future Prospects and Projections

Thurston County exemplifies a public health system that thrives upon stable, long-term relationships between health care organizations while also capitalizing upon the ability of these organizations and relationships to adapt rapidly to changes within the health care system. To date, the system appears to be responding effectively to changes brought about by state policies regarding Medicaid beneficiaries and the uninsured. The local health department's strategy of transitioning selected responsibilities in personal health services delivery to private organizations continues to be balanced with an expanding role in assessment and policy development activities. Whether this strategy will prove effective for the full range of personal health services currently performed by the department remains far from clear. Limits on the expansion of the state's Medicaid managed care program and its parallel program for the low-income uninsured are likely to preserve a role in clinical services provision for the local health department and other safety-net providers in the community for the foreseeable future.

The health department's collaborative relationships with many of the other health and human service organizations in the community prove to be valuable assets in responding to community health issues. The quality of these relationships are in many ways a product of the careful leadership and vision provided by the local health department and its long-time partners such as St. Peter Hospital and Group Health Cooperative. The ability to maintain and expand these relationships in the wake of growing marketplace competition and policy change exists as a daunting challenge for the health department and its partners. Nevertheless, the current constellation of organizations within Thurston County's public health system appears well positioned to anticipate and respond to these emerging threats and opportunities.

References

1. American Medical Association. Physician Data by County. Chicago, Ill: AMA; 1992.
2. American Hospital Association. AHA 1997 *Guide to the Health Care Field*. Chicago, Ill: AHA; 1997.
3. Group Health Association of America. 1995 Directory of HMOs. Washington, DC: GHAA; 1995.
4. US Department of Commerce. 1995 *Consolidated Federal Funds Report*. Washington, DC: Census Bureau; 1997.
5. McLaughlin CP, Halverson PK, Mays GP. Group health cooperative and the public health system serving Olympia, Washington. In Halverson PK, Kaluzny AD, and McLaughlin CP, eds. *Managed Care and Public Health*. Gaithersburg, Md: Aspen Publishers; 1998: 222-232.

Part III: Conclusions

Chapter 17

Changing and Durable Local Health Departments

Some of the few generalizations that can be made with certainty about local public health agencies are that they differ from each other and they differ from their past. These organizations are shaped by local circumstances and by changing state and national policies affecting their financing and operation. The dynamic nature of local public health agencies is not a new phenomenon. From their very beginnings in the late nineteenth century they have embraced innovations in technology and practice to address newly emerging threats to the public's health.

The Changing Nature of Local Public Health

The first locally organized public health departments were established in order to cope with community problems of sanitation and epidemic disease. The need for maternity and infant health care quickly expanded the spectrum of public health services, especially in rapidly growing industrial cities and among immigrant populations. Nutritional programs, school health, safety in public accommodations, housing codes, and immunizations quickly joined the expanding services of local public health departments. This fascinating history is expertly described in Duffy's book on the history of the New York City Health department.[1] This history is more than the story of public health in New York, as it reflects the growth of the public health movement across the nation. Local health departments became substantially involved in personal health care after World War I when the status of women became an issue of growing national concern. High maternal mortality rates prompted the establishment of maternal and child health services among the rapidly expanding county and municipal health departments. The crisis of World War II saw another surge in publicly sponsored personal health care when communities of young families mushroomed around newly established military bases. At the height of the war, one out of seven newborns in the United States was delivered and cared for under the auspices of public health departments.[2] During those years, national indicators of maternal health outcomes improved appreciably. New entitlements to medical care were established in the 1960s with the passage of Medicaid and Medicare. Limitations of access to care among private providers stimulated the growth of comprehensive clinics in local health departments and in free-standing community health centers, organized and financed largely by governmental appropriations. Maternity and Infant Care as well as Children and Youth health care programs were similarly established in many underserved areas. Public health departments were the principle sponsors of these programs.[3] The history of health care in this century is replete with evidence of the dynamic and responsive nature of local public health. Scant evidence in this history suggests a tradition bound and unchanging establishment.

Many well-accepted innovations in community health care originated and became established by the work of public community clinics. Such practices include establishment of telephone hotlines to provide 24-hour access to counseling and services; the training of nurses and other providers for expanded roles in health care; and the incorporation of clinic users in policy development and governance of health care services. Public health departments share with community health centers the merits of these and other changes.

Change has been a hallmark of local public health throughout its history, no less so than in the past decade when token enrollments in health maintenance organizations (HMOs) escalated to involve more that half the population in managed care plans. Our surveys suggest that many local health department are now involved in working relationships with managed care plans.[4] In about half the instances, these relationships are formalized under contract. The case studies provide interesting and useful information on the variability and ingenuity represented in these contracts.

Associated with the growth of enrollments in managed care plans, there has been a decline in the offering of comprehensive ambulatory care by local health departments. Public health clinics continue to feature maternal and child health services, communicable disease control, family planning, sexually transmitted disease clinics, health education and a variety of screening programs. Exceptions to these generalizations are numerous and worthy of examination.

One of the most striking changes in characteristics of local health departments focuses on relationships to different levels of government. A study of exemplary departments in the late 1970s suggested that these relationships were in substantial ways the surrogates of federal government in the exercise of public policy.[5] This interpretation was supported by data on the extensive support departments received from federal agencies through such initiatives as the maternal and infant health programs, the children and youth programs, community and migrant health centers, and regional commissions such as those for the coastal plains and Appalachia. Exemplary health departments were entrepreneurial in their ability to secure support from such national grant programs. Many of these federal programs were phased out or substantially diminished by the Reagan administration in 1981. The most enterprising public health departments were then those that were successful in gaining support from state and local government, and increasingly from fee income.[6] No health department today could be convincingly characterized as a surrogate of federal government operational at local levels. A summary of outstanding features from each of the current case studies is presented in **Table 1**.

Partnerships with Managed Care

A wide range of accommodations between health departments and managed care plans is illustrated by the case studies. The Memphis / Shelby County health department has a distinguished history of offering full service ambulatory care in strategically located neighborhood clinics (Chapter 12). In that jurisdiction, Medicaid clients are all enrolled in managed care plans, many of which have in turn contracted with the health department to continue offering the same full range of services to the same patients as previously served. The biggest difference is that Medicaid funds, instead of being paid directly to the health department provider, now flow through the hands of managed care intermediaries. Multnomah County is rightfully proud of a health department that has offered comprehensive health care in full service clinics in each sector of the county (Chapter 14). In addition, HMOs in Portland have served for many years as models of managed care at its best. The health department has sometimes in the past served as broker to enroll Medicaid clients in the HMOs. Under a plan that commits most Medicaid clients to HMOs, the health department formed its own HMO in close collaboration with the university hospital and with a statewide network of community and migrant health centers. The publicly sponsored HMO competes with the commercial plans for Medicaid enrollees. The competition has been wholesome. When the commercial HMOs recognized that the health department's enrollees benefited from many enhancements to traditional prenatal and postnatal care, contracts were written for the health department to offer the same enhancements to Medicaid clients enrolled in the private HMOs. The private HMOs pay the health department for these enhancements. The Thurston County health department is another example where the public clinic renders enhanced maternity support services to Medicaid client enrolled in commercial plans (Chapter 16). In Thurston County, the health department bills Medicaid for many services (eg, family planning, diagnosis and treatment of sexually transmitted disease) rendered to patients who are enrolled in managed care plans. Annually, the state Medicaid agency then adjusts the capitation payments to managed care plans, taking into consideration this duplicate payment for services. When Medicaid clients in Milwaukee were enrolled in managed care, the local health department eventually retrenched many of its clinical services including its own HMO previously operated in collaboration with several community health centers (Chapter 13). Subsequently, a serious measles outbreak revealed a large unimmunized population of children creating both financial and public relations concerns for the managed care plans that served this population. Recognizing that the health department had unique skills for reaching vulnerable populations, the managed care plans developed jointly sponsored programs with the health department for

Table 1
Key Features of Local Public Health Case Studies

Denver, Colo

- Integrated organization encompassing health department, hospital, network of CHCS, and an HMO for Medicaid and county employees.
- As of January 1997, it is an independent health care authority (quasi-governmental institution) which is separate from local and state government administration. It contracts with the county to perform statutorily defined public health and indigent care services.
- Strong collaborative relationships with other public and nonprofit healthcare providers, such as the University Hospital, the local Catholic hospitals, and the local Children's' Hospital. Limited interaction with the for-profit hospitals and managed care plans which are rapidly gaining market share within the jurisdiction

Multnomah County, Ore

- Operates its own Medicaid HMO in collaboration with the University Hospital, a neighboring local health department, and a statewide network of C/MHCs.
- Operates its own network of public health clinics providing a wide range of clinical services.
- Maintains strong relationships with other HMOs and hospitals in the jurisdiction, despite also being a competitor. This includes contracting with other Medicaid HMOs for providing public health services to their enrollees.
- Considering entering the commercial HMO market for serving employed groups.

Thurston County, Wash

- Has discontinued providing well child services through its public health clinics. The department reports that Medicaid managed care plans and the state's managed care program for the uninsured have eliminated the need for these services to be provided.
- The department continues to provide many other types of public health services to Medicaid beneficiaries, even if they are enrolled in managed care plans. These services include maternity support services, immunizations, sexually transmitted disease services, and family planning services. State Medicaid regulations allow the department to directly bill the state Medicaid agency for these services, even for serving managed care enrollees.
- Maintains strong collaborative relationship with the area's dominant managed care plan, Group Health Cooperative. Collaborative activities include jointly sponsored child and adult immunization clinics, jointly supported homeless health clinic and community clinic for the uninsured, and collaboration in conducting a community health assessment process.
- Maintains strong collaborative relationship with the area's Catholic hospital, including operating a community clinic for the uninsured.
- Relatively limited interaction with other HMOs or the other, for-profit, hospital. The department has not taken steps to establish contractual agreements with those HMOs enrolling Medicaid beneficiaries or the uninsured. The health director feels that such agreements might discourage plans from developing the necessary capacity and expertise to serve these individuals.

Milwaukee, Wis

- The health department operates a network of public health clinics that have reduced their involvement in providing some types of clinical services (eg, sick care). Much of this has been achieved through collaborative arrangements with CHCs.
- The health department maintains close working relationships with area hospitals and managed care plans. During the 1980s, the health department operated its own Medicaid HMO in collaboration with several CHCs. More recently, a measles outbreak in 1989-1990 motivated the formation of closer relationships between the health department and local health plans. Currently, the health department maintains contracts with HMOs for providing immunization and lead screening services. Additionally, HMOs and hospitals participate with the health department on an array of community health initiatives.

(continued)

Table 1 *(continued)*
Key Features of Local Public Health Case Studies

Beloit, Wis

- The health department has developed several "one-stop shopping" community centers for delivering integrated health and social services. The department has been successful in securing continued funding for these services even though the demonstration grants for these projects have expired.
- The health department maintains strong relationships with the local hospital and local physician clinic. The department's medical director is a member of the clinic and serves as a vice president in the local hospital. These relationships allow the department to insure that uninsured residents receive needed health services through these providers. (The health department does not directly provide primary care services beyond categorical public health services.) These relationships also allow the department to secure the support and participation of the clinic and hospital in community health initiatives, such as a home visitation program for newborn infants, a case management program for the medically indigent, and a maternity case management program for high-risk women.
- The health department's interaction with managed care plans remains limited to contracts with its home nursing service.
- The health department's interaction with the other major hospital serving the area remains limited.

Genesee County, Mich

- Strong interaction with community-based organizations. A grant from the W. K. Kellogg Foundation helped the department to develop a formalized structure for interacting with these groups. These groups now play major roles in public health program development and implementation, planning, advocacy, and community outreach.
- Strong and growing interaction with hospitals.
- Strong interaction with the medical community.
- Strong and growing interaction with the major employer and union.
- Interaction with managed care plans remains limited to joint planning activities.

Southwest Washington Health District, Wash

- Over the past decade, responsibility for the provision of many personal health services has been transferred from the health department to the local hospital.
- Expanded efforts in population-based activities, including a community health information line and an office for public health program evaluation.
- Strong relationship with the local hospital, including joint programs and joint planning activities.
- Strong relationship with the dominant managed care plan in the jurisdiction (Kaiser), including joint programs and joint planning activities.

Memphis-Shelby County, Tenn

- Continues to provide comprehensive primary care services through its public health clinics.
- Maintains contractual relationships with multiple managed care plans for providing primary care and case management services to Medicaid enrollees.
- Relationship with the public hospital has been complicated by the move to Medicaid managed care, especially referral patterns.

---

programs such as immunization and lead screening of children.

An earlier series of case studies of exemplary local health departments attempted to identify determinants that helped development of the outstanding programs.[5] All departments benefited from well-prepared and dedicated leadership, but those assets were in each instance complemented by local political leadership—a mayor or commissioner—who made public health a high priority on the local political agenda. That synergism still seems to pertain in the new case studies with one important variation. Genesee County, Michigan, was one of the sites for a Kellogg Foundation demonstration project that sought to develop strong working relationships linking public health departments with community groups and with academic institutions. In Genesee County, the Kellogg sponsorship has terminated, but the strong linkage between the health department and community groups endures. Neighborhood associations and churches are among the groups represented on a health department advisory board. A full-time health educator, skilled at community organization, assists the work of the advisory board. In a complex atmosphere of competing managed care plans and ambitious hospitals, the leadership of the health department emerges as the preeminent force in local health policy negotiation. Strong community support is a telling asset in this dynamic. The county commissioners are not unsupportive of public health, but the driving force appears to be a strong base of informed community investment in public health. This community-based support may prove to be the most durable kind of political sponsorship.

Public Health Performance

Serial measures of public health performance were applied to the case study jurisdictions over a 2- to 3-year period, covering a time when managed care growth and public health reform were intensive. The measurement method, described in Chapters 1 and 8, was based on a conceptual framework of public health practice established by the National Academy of Sciences Institute of Medicine, and refined by working groups convened by the US Centers for Disease Control and Prevention.[7] Measures from the case study jurisdictions indicated that overall levels of public health performance changed little, usually in the direction of improvement. Performance in specific public health practices revealed some interesting changes. Policy development activities improved in most jurisdictions, and were associated with greater health department interaction with hospitals, community health centers, and managed care plans. Activities involving public health assessment tended to decline, indicative of voids and uncertainties about how health care under a variety of managed care plans would be monitored and evaluated. The practice of informing and educating the public declined in several jurisdictions. Improvements in overall public health performance were not always attributable to increased action by the health department. About 25% of the public health effort in most jurisdictions could be attributed to agencies other than the local health department.[7] Over the span of these studies, organizations other than the local health department made growing contributions to public health performance. Increased contributions by managed care plans were not apparent except as they were reflected indirectly in the expanding involvement of hospitals in public health activities

The methods used for measuring public health performance in these studies proved useful, particularly for serial measurement over time. The methods proved especially helpful for identifying the source and scope of public health practice by all contributors in a jurisdiction—including both governmental and private organizations. By linking to specific managerial strategies and public health practices, these performance measurement methods provide insight about practical applications needed to improve local public health systems.

The Status of Local Health Departments

Local health departments at the dawn of the 21st Century are different but not diminished in the wake of dramatic changes in the financing and provision of medical care. Some health departments, but not all, have scaled back their programs of comprehensive ambulatory care. Some changes have occurred in the provision of routine categorical and preventive services (eg, maternal and child health, family planning, diagnosis and treatment of sexually transmitted disease, communicable disease control), but the public health role continues to be substantial, sometimes at the insistence of local managed care providers. Some of them have recognized the special skills of public health in assuring nonmedical enhancements to health care and in reaching certain vulnerable populations.

In the communities of our study, public health departments are playing expanding roles in policy development and planning. They have developed strong working relationships with local physicians, hospitals, and social agencies. These interorganizational arrangements continue to evolve; present circumstances will not necessarily prevail into the future, and many uncertainties are unanswered. There is no suggestion, however, that local public health departments will play diminished or constricted roles in assuring community health.

One of the uncertainties requiring attention is the matter of monitoring community health status and evaluating the effects of health system change on public health. Small declines in performance of the public health assessment function are ominous signs that these important aspects of public health are not receiving the attention they deserve. Evaluating quality of care and monitoring community health outcomes against national and community objectives deserve increased attention. Local public health departments, if provided with sufficient resources, are perhaps the only entities that can assure that these important functions are carried out in the public interest and on a community-wide basis.

Conclusions and Future Prospects

Local health departments remain the focal point of public health practice, although their forms and functions have substantially changed over the years. Meanwhile, the array of public health collaborators, contributors, stakeholders, and even competitors is clearly expanding. Evidence from national trends and detailed case studies lead to the conclusion that local public health practice remains effective and responsive to the larger political, social, economic, and health environment–largely through continual evolution in its structures, processes, and outcomes. As a dynamic field of practice, public health appears largely successful in weathering the challenges posed by managed health care, privatization initiatives, health care mergers and closures, shifts in health policy and funding streams, new and resurgent health threats, demographic changes, and a host of related trends and issues. In many cases, local public health organizations do not merely react and adapt to these larger trends, but rather they often drive changes in their political, social, economic, and health care environments.

The public health organizations examined in this book achieve evolutionary changes through a variety of strategies and with varying levels of success. Some of these strategies and outcomes may be transferable to other situations, while others may be inextricably linked to specific local contexts. Rather than providing explicit guidelines for future initiatives in local public health practice, the trends and models identified here should serve as examples of the diverse structures, practices, relationships, resources, and outcomes that are possible within local communities.

Though it maintains a rich history, public health appears as a dynamic field of practice characterized by continual innovation – particularly at the local level. Public health exists as an open system in many communities, allowing the free entry of new organizations, new technologies, and new information that may contribute to the health of the population. This dynamism and openness is a reason for optimism about the continued success of local public health practice in protecting and improving the health of communities. Successful efforts in public health improvement are far from automatic in the current health environment, however. Communities are challenged by an accelerating rate of change in population health needs and risks, and in available health resources, technologies, and delivery systems. These challenges can only be addressed through informed, evidence-based, and entrepreneurial public health practice. Governmental public health organizations cannot sustain these activities alone, and neither can the private sector. The ever-present challenge lies in bringing together the broadest possible array of public and private resources in the most effective and efficient ways possible. Local health departments remain at the heart of these endeavors.

References

1. Duffy T. *A History of Public Health in New York City 1866-1966*. New York: Russell Sage Foundation; 1974.
2. Elliot MM, Freedman LR. Four years of the E.M.I.C. Program. *Yale J Biol Med J*. 1947;199(4): 621-635.
3. Kotch JB, Coulter ML, Porter CQ, Miller CA. Productivity and selected indicators of care in Maternity and Infant Care and Children and Youth Projects according to sponsorship. *J Med Syst*. 1988;12(5):285-294.
4. Halverson PK, Mays GP, Kaluzny AD, Richards TB. Not so strange bedfellows: models of interaction between managed care plans and public health agencies. *Milbank Q*. 1997;75(1):113-138.
5. Miller CA, Moos MC. *Local Health Departments: Fifteen Case Studies*. Washington, DC: American Public Health Association; 1981.
6. Miller CA, Moore KS, Richards TB, Kotelchuck M, Kaluzny AD. Longitudinal observations: a preliminary report. *J Public Health Policy*. 1993;401(1): 34-50.
7. Halverson PK, Miller CA, Kaluzny AD, Fried BJ, Schenck SE, Richards TB. Performing public health functions: the perceived contribution of public health and other community agencies. *J Health Human Serv Admin*. 1996;18(3):288-303.

Part IV: Appendices

Appendix A

Local Public Health Assessment Survey (Revised March 1994)

Portions of this survey have been taken from APEX/PH, The Core Component Survey of Local Health Departments, the National Association of County & City Health Officials (NACCHO), 1990. Certain questions pertaining to the 10 core functions were adapted from the detailed definitions provided by the Public Health Practice Program office in their September 1991 report.

Questions 6–8 under Assessment were developed using the Health Status Indicators from the Centers for Disease Control and Prevention.[1]

Questions 7 and 8 under Assurance were developed using categories for Environmental and Personal Health Services outlined in *The Profile of State and Territorial Public Health Systems: United States, 1990*.[2]

This instrument gathers information and perceptions from a local public health officer in order to:

1. Estimate the extent that the jurisdiction of the local health department (LHD) is served by the three core public health functions assessment, policy development, and assurance[2];
2. Estimate the performances of the local health department in rendering those functions as they are disaggregated into 10 separate public health practices assess, analyze, investigate; advocate/build constituencies; set priorities, develop plans; manage, implement, evaluate, inform and educate the public;
3. Indicate the nature and extent that other agencies at local, regional, and state levels contribute to the performance of the 10 public health practices on behalf of the jurisdiction.
4. Provide the potential for making comparisons among health departments on the nature and extent of their performance, and for tracking changes over time in a given health department's performance.

Indicators

The indicators are of two types: generalized descriptions of performance, and specific designations of program content. The generalized indicators are adapted from a schedule developed by Turnock and Handler, keyed to the same three public health functions and the 10 practices identified above. Modifications in the Turnock/Handler schedule were required in order to incorporate the concept of community coverage from a variety of providers.

The specific indicators are clustered within two functional areas: assessment and assurance. The assessment items were incorporated from CDC's Consensus Set of Indicators for Assessing Community Health Status and Monitoring Progress toward the Year 2000 Objectives.[1] The specific indicators for the assurance function were adapted from the environmental and personal health services items identified in *The Profile of State and Territorial Public Health Systems: United States, 1990*.[2]

Results

Your responses to this survey will be aggregated into a profile intended to display the extent that the population served by your health department is covered by generally accepted public health practices and the extent that the coverage is supplied by your health department. Recognizing that agencies other than the health department make important contributions to public health practice in patterns that vary widely from one community to another our display will also attempt to illustrate the pattern that prevails in your community. Those findings will be shared with you in the hope that you will provide us with guidance on the accuracy and utility of our findings.

C. Arden Miller, MD	*Karen Strazza Moore, MPH*
Principal Investigator	*Project Director*

References

1. Centers for Disease Control and Prevention. Consensus set of indicators for Assessing Community Health Status and Monitoring Progress toward the Year 2000 Objectives. *MMWR Morb Mortal Wkly Rep.* 1991; 40(27); 450-451.
2. Centers for Disease Control and Prevention. *The Profile of State and Territorial Public Health Systems: United States, 1990.* Atlanta, Ga: Centers for Disease Control, US Department of Health and Human Services; October 1991.
3. Institute of Medicine. *The Future of Public Health.* Washington, DC: National Academy Press 1988.
4. Centers for Disease Control. *Steering Committee for Measuring Public Health Capacity.* Atlanta, Ga: Public Health Practice Program Office; 1991. Processed report.

Instructions

The following questionnaire is mailed to health department directors who are asked to respond. They should confer with colleagues sufficiently to enable a response to every query. Responses will be recorded by an interviewer during a scheduled and taped telephone call.

The format follows a consistent rationale:

- Is the jurisdiction of the health department covered by a given public health practice?
- How completely does the coverage respond to need? Answer on a five-point scale from:

0	1	2	3	4
Not at all	Some	Half	Most	The need is met

- What agencies help perform the service/practice for the jurisdiction?
- Examples: Local health department
  District health department
  State health department
  Community or migrant health center
  Etc.
- What portion of the current performance of the service/practice in question is contributed by the local health department? Answer on a five-point scale:

None				All
0	1	2	3	4

In addition to general queries about public health practices, there are a series of questions gathering similar information on some specific services. The format is a little different, enabling response by a check mark. For example:

	Provided by Health Dept	Provided by Other Agencies	Names of Other Agencies	The Need Is Fully Met
Family Planning	✓	✓	Planned Parenthood Hospital clinics Migrant health center Private MDs	

We realize that many local health departments will not have all of the activities and programs mentioned in the survey; however, we would like to get some idea of the relationship of local health departments to these activities and programs and the extent that the community is served. If services to the local jurisdiction are rendered by the state, district, or regional health department, these should be designated as an "other agency."

Date ______________________ Time ______________________

Interviewer ______________________

Respondent ______________________

Title ______________________

Health Department ______________________

State ______________________

I. Assessment Activities

The first set of questions in this section concerns the collection of data and the conduct of epidemiological studies.

1. In the jurisdiction served by your health department is there a regular process of needs assessment to describe the prevailing health status and needs of the community, incorporating locally specific morbidity, mortality, and vital statistics data? (assess)

   _____ Yes   _____ No

   1.1 If Yes ASK: In your judgment, how adequate and timely are the data developed by this process?

0	1	2	3	4
I	I	I	I	I
Not at all	**Some**	**Half**	**Most**	**The need is met**

   1.2 What agencies are involved in performing the needs assessment for your jurisdiction? (Please circle all appropriate responses.)

   A) State Government Agencies
   B) City/County Government Agencies
   C) Nonprofit/Community Agencies
   D) Hospitals
   E) MDs/Private Clinics
   F) Community/Migrant Health Centers (Section 329/330 Agencies)
   G) Universities
   H) Federal Agencies
   I) Others (specify) ____

   1.3 On the scale below, representing the total effort for this assessment, please indicate the share contributed by the local health department:

0	1	2	3	4
I	I	I	I	I
Not at all	**Some**	**Half**	**Most**	**The need is met**

2. In the past three years has there been a survey for your jurisdiction to assess participation in appropriate age-specific preventive and screening services? (assess)

   _____ Yes   _____ No

   2.1 If Yes ASK: In your judgment, how adequate are these surveys?

0	1	2	3	4
I	I	I	I	I
Not at all	**Some**	**Half**	**Most**	**The need is met**

   2.2 What agencies are involved in performing such surveys for your jurisdiction? (Please circle all appropriate responses.)

   A) State Government Agencies
   B) City/County Government Agencies
   C) Nonprofit/Community Agencies
   D) Hospitals
   E) MDs/Private Clinics
   F) Community/Migrant Health Centers (Section 329/330 Agencies)

G) Universities
H) Federal Agencies
I) Others (specify)

2.3 On the scale below, representing the total effort for these surveys, please indicate the share contributed by the local health department:

None				All
I	I	I	I	I
0	1	2	3	4

3. Within the past three years has the population in your jurisdiction been surveyed for behavioral risk factors? (assess)

_____ Yes   _____ No

3.1 If Yes ASK: In your judgment, how adequate are these surveys?

0	1	2	3	4
I	I	I	I	I
Not at all	**Some**	**Half**	**Most**	**The need is met**

3.2 What agencies were involved in conducting the surveys? (Please circle all appropriate responses.)

A) State Government Agencies
B) City/County Government Agencies
C) Nonprofit/Community Agencies
D) Hospitals
E) MDs/Private Clinics
F) Community/Migrant Health Centers (Section 329/330 Agencies)
G) Universities
H) Federal Agencies
I) Others (specify) ____________________

3.3 On the scale below, representing the total effort for these surveys, please indicate the share contributed by the local health department:

None				All
I	I	I	I	I
0	1	2	3	4

4. In the past three years in your jurisdiction, has there been timely investigation of any unusual adverse health events? (investigate)

_____ Yes   _____ No

4.1 If Yes ASK: In your judgment, how adequate were the investigations?

0	1	2	3	4
I	I	I	I	I
Not at all	**Some**	**Half**	**Most**	**The need is met**

4.2 What agencies conduct such investigations for your jurisdiction?
(Please circle all appropriate responses.)

A) State Government Agencies
B) City/County Government Agencies
C) Nonprofit/Community Agencies
D) Hospitals
E) MDs/Private Clinics
F) Community/Migrant Health Centers (Section 329/330 Agencies)
G) Universities
H) Federal Agencies
I) Others (specify) ____________________

4.3 On the scale below, representing the total effort for these investigations, please indicate the share contributed by the local health department:

None				All
|	|	|	|	|
0	**1**	**2**	**3**	**4**

5. In the past three years in your jurisdiction, has there been a review of hospital discharge data to determine age-specific leading causes of hospitalization? (investigate)

_____ Yes _____ No

5.1 If Yes ASK: How adequate was the review?

0	**1**	**2**	**3**	**4**
|	|	|	|	|
Not at all	**Some**	**Half**	**Most**	**The need is met**

5.2 What agencies perform this review for your jurisdiction?
(Please circle all appropriate responses.)

A) State Government Agencies
B) City/County Government Agencies
C) Nonprofit/Community Agencies
D) Hospitals
E) MDs/Private Clinics
F) Community/Migrant Health Centers (Section 329/330 Agencies)
G) Universities
H) Federal Agencies
I) Others (specify) ____________________

5.3 On the scale below, representing the total effort for this review, please indicate the share contributed by the local health department:

None				All
|	|	|	|	|
0	**1**	**2**	**3**	**4**

6. In the past three years in your jurisdiction, has there been a review of work-related morbidity and mortality? (investigate)

_____ Yes _____ No

6.1 If Yes ASK: In your judgment, how adequate was the review?

0	1	2	3	4
Not at all	Some	Half	Most	The need is met

6.2 What agencies are involved in such a review?
(Please circle all appropriate responses.)

A) State Government Agencies
B) City/County Government Agencies
C) Nonprofit/Community Agencies
D) Hospitals
E) MDs/Private Clinics
F) Community/Migrant Health Centers (Section 329/330 Agencies)
G) Universities
H) Federal Agencies
I) Others (specify) ____________________

6.3 On the scale below, representing the total effort for this review, please indicate the share contributed by the local health department:

None				All
0	1	2	3	4

7. In the past three years in your jurisdiction, has there been an analysis of data on children two years of age who have been immunized with the basic series? (analyze)

_____ Yes _____ No

7.1 If Yes ASK: In your judgment, how adequate was this analysis?

0	1	2	3	4
Not at all	Some	Half	Most	The need is met

7.2 What agencies perform these analyses for your jurisdiction?
(Please circle all appropriate responses.)

A) State Government Agencies
B) City/County Government Agencies
C) Nonprofit/Community Agencies
D) Hospitals
E) MDs/Private Clinics
F) Community/Migrant Health Centers (Section 329/330 Agencies)
G) Universities
H) Federal Agencies
I) Others (specify) ____________________

7.3 On the scale below, representing the total effort for this review, please indicate the share contributed by the local health department:

None				All
0	1	2	3	4

8. In the past three years in your jurisdiction, has there been an analysis of health services needed by high-risk population groups? (analyze)

_____ Yes _____ No

8.1 If Yes ASK: In your judgment, how adequate was this analysis?

0	1	2	3	4
Not at all	Some	Half	Most	The need was fully met

8.2 What agencies perform these analyses for your jurisdiction?
(Please circle all appropriate responses.)

A) State Government Agencies
B) City/County Government Agencies
C) Nonprofit/Community Agencies
D) Hospitals
E) MDs/Private Clinics
F) Community/Migrant Health Centers (Section 329/330 Agencies)
G) Universities
H) Federal Agencies
I) Others (specify) ________________________________

8.3 On the scale below, representing the total effort for these analyses, please indicate the share contributed by the local health department:

None				All
0	1	2	3	4

The following are sets of indicators for assessing health status outcomes in your jurisdiction. Please indicate with a ✓ in the appropriate column if these data are: 1) available for your jurisdiction; 2) collected by your health department; and/or 3) collected by other agencies serving your jurisdiction. In column IV, indicate with a ✓ if the need for these data is fully met and timely. If any of these data are collected by other agencies, please fill in the corresponding letters for those agencies in column V, using the key located at the bottom of the page.

9. For the items listed below please provide the most appropriate response to describe the availability of timely data on process indicators for your jurisdiction. (investigate)

	I Indicator Available for Entire Jurisdiction ✓	II Available from LHD ✓	III Available from Other Agencies ✓	IV The Need for Data Is Met ✓	V Other Agency(ies) (Use Key)
a. Basic series immunization rate for children age 2 years and under (proportion of children under 2 who have been immunized with basic series)	____	____	____	____	____________ ____________
b. Pneumococcal pneumonia/influenza immunization rate for adults (proportion of adults aged > 65 who have been immunized)	____	____	____	____	____________ ____________
c. Proportion of assessed rivers, lakes, estuaries that support beneficial uses (fishing and swimming approved)	____	____	____	____	____________ ____________
d. Proportion of women receiving a Pap smear (at interval appropriate for age)	____	____	____	____	____________ ____________
e. Proportion of women receiving a mammogram (at interval appropriate for age)	____	____	____	____	____________ ____________
f. Proportion of population uninsured for medical care	____	____	____	____	____________ ____________
g. Proportion of population without regular source of primary care services (including dental service)	____	____	____	____	____________ ____________

Key: Other Agencies

A) State Government
B) City/County Government Agencies
C) Nonprofit/Community Agencies
D) Hospitals
E) MDs/Private Clinics
F) Community/Migrant Health Centers (Section 329/330 Agencies)
G) Universities
H) Federal Agencies
I) Other (specify)

10. Does your jurisdiction have available timely data on the following specific indicators for analyzing health status outcomes for your jurisdiction? (analyze)

	I Indicator Available for Entire Jurisdiction ✓	II Available from LHD ✓	III Available from Other Agencies ✓	IV The Need for Data Is Met ✓	V Other Agency(ies) (Use Key)
a. Race/ethnicity specific infant mortality rate	____	____	____	____	____
b. Death rates (per 100,000 population) for:					
1. Motor vehicle crashes	____	____	____	____	____
2. Work-related injury	____	____	____	____	____
3. Lung cancer	____	____	____	____	____
4. Breast cancer	____	____	____	____	____
5. Cardiovascular disease	____	____	____	____	____
c. Incidence rates (per 100,000 population) for:					
1. Acquired Immunodeficiency Syndrome	____	____	____	____	____
2. Measles	____	____	____	____	____
3. Tuberculosis	____	____	____	____	____
4. Primary and secondary syphilis	____	____	____	____	____
d. Percentage of children < 5 with blood-lead levels exceeding 10 µg/dL	____	____	____	____	____
e. Incidence of hepatitis (all types) (per 100,000 population)	____	____	____	____	____
f. Proportion of children aged between 6–8 and 15 years with one or more decayed primary/permanent teeth	____	____	____	____	____

11. Does your jurisdiction have available timely data on the following risk factor indicators for the jurisdiction being served? (analyze)

	I Indicator Available for Entire Jurisdiction ✓	II Available from LHD ✓	III Available from Other Agencies ✓	IV The Need for Data Is Met ✓	V Other Agency(ies) (Use Key)
a. Incidence of low birthweight (< 2500 grams)	____	____	____	____	____________ ____________
b. Adolescent birth rate (females age 10–17 years)	____	____	____	____	____________ ____________
c. Level of prenatal care (% of mothers with no prenatal care during 1st trimester of pregnancy)	____	____	____	____	____________ ____________
d. Childhood poverty (proportion of children living in families below the poverty level)	____	____	____	____	____________ ____________
e. Air quality (proportion of persons living in jurisdiction exceeding US EPA standards for air quality during previous year)	____	____	____	____	____________ ____________
f. Age-specific cigarette smoking rates	____	____	____	____	____________ ____________
g. Age-specific obesity rates	____	____	____	____	____________ ____________
h. Hypertension	____	____	____	____	____________ ____________
i. Hypercholesterolemia	____	____	____	____	____________ ____________
j. Confirmed abuse and neglect of children	____	____	____	____	____________ ____________

Key: Other Agencies (use for questions 10 and 11)

A) State Government
B) City/County Government Agencies
C) Nonprofit/Community Agencies
D) Hospitals
E) MDs/Private Clinics
F) Community/Migrant Health Centers (Section 329/330 Agencies)
G) Universities
H) Federal Agencies
I) Other (specify)

II. Policy Development

In the next set of questions we are concerned with activities thought to be part of the development and implementation of health policy.

1. Has there been within the past three years a public review of the public health mission and role for your agency's jurisdiction? (advocacy / constituency)

    _____ Yes   _____ No

    1.1 If Yes ASK: On the scale provided below please indicate your judgment of the adequacy of this public review.

0	1	2	3	4
|	|	|	|	|
Not at all adequate	**Some**	**Half**	**Most**	**Fully adequate**

    1.2 What agencies were involved in the conduct of the review?
    (Please circle all appropriate responses.)

    A) State Government Agencies
    B) City / County Government Agencies
    C) Nonprofit / Community Agencies
    D) Hospitals
    E) MDs / Private Clinics
    F) Community / Migrant Health Centers (Section 329 / 330 Agencies)
    G) Universities
    H) Federal Agencies
    I) Others (specify) ____________________

    1.3 On the scale below, representing the total effort for this review, if any, please indicate the contribution of your local health department:

None				**All**
|	|	|	|	|
0	1	2	3	4

2. Do you and your senior staff members regularly participate in meetings with other community health organizations? (advocacy / constituency)

    _____ Yes   _____ No

    2.1 If Yes ASK: How effective are these meetings for coordinating efforts responsive to community needs?

0	1	2	3	4
|	|	|	|	|
Not at all	**Some**	**Half**	**Most**	**The need for coordination is met**

    2.2 What agencies initiate these meetings?
    (Please circle all appropriate responses.)

    A) State Government Agencies
    B) City / County Government Agencies
    C) Nonprofit / Community Agencies
    D) Hospitals

E) MDs / Private Clinics
F) Community / Migrant Health Centers (Section 329 / 330 Agencies)
G) Universities
H) Federal Agencies
I) Others (specify) ______________________________

2.3 On the scale below, indicate the extent that the local health department serves as convener for such meetings:

Never				Always
0	1	2	3	4

3. Is your jurisdiction served by a process which regularly informs elected officials about the potential public health impact of actions under their consideration? (advocacy / constituency)

_____ Yes _____ No

3.1 If Yes ASK: In your judgment, how adequate is this process?

0	1	2	3	4
Not at all adequate	Some	Half	Most	Fully adequate

3.2 What government agencies are involved in this informational process for your jurisdiction? (Please circle all appropriate responses.)

A) State Government Agencies
B) City / County Government Agencies
C) Nonprofit / Community Agencies
D) Hospitals
E) MDs / Private Clinics
F) Community / Migrant Health Centers (Section 329 / 330 Agencies)
G) Universities
H) Federal Agencies
I) Others (specify) ______________________________

3.3 On the scale below, representing the total performance of this informational process, please indicate the share contributed by the local health department:

None				All
0	1	2	3	4

4. Do elected or other government officials in your jurisdiction strongly advocate for public health? (advocacy / constituency)

_____ Yes _____ No

4.1 If Yes ASK: In your judgment, how vigorous is this advocacy?

0	1	2	3	4
Absent	Some	Half	Most	Very strong

4.2 List the title of officials who conduct such advocacy for your jurisdiction.
(Please circle all appropriate titles.)

A) County Supervisor/Commissioner
B) City/County Council Member
C) County Executive/Manager
D) Mayor
E) State Representative/Senator
F) Public Health Officials
G) Board of Health
H) Others (specify) ______________________________

4.3 On the scale below, please indicate the extent that your local health department can promote such advocacy:

No				**No Limitation**
I	I	I	I	I
0	**1**	**2**	**3**	**4**

5. Within the past three years has a priority list of proposed or expanded community health initiatives been developed for your jurisdiction responsive to assessed problems and resources? (prioritize)

_____ Yes _____ No

5.1 If Yes ASK: In your judgment, how complete is this list?

0	**1**	**2**	**3**	**4**
I	I	I	I	I
Not at all	**Some**	**Half**	**Most**	**The need is met**

5.2 What agencies participated in the development of such a list for your jurisdiction?
(Please circle all appropriate responses.)

A) State Government Agencies
B) City/County Government Agencies
C) Nonprofit/Community Agencies
D) Hospitals
E) MDs/Private Clinics
F) Community/Migrant Health Centers (Section 329/330 Agencies)
G) Universities
H) Federal Agencies
I) Others (specify) ______________________________

5.3 On the scale below, please indicate the contribution to this effort by the local health department:

None				**All**
I	I	I	I	I
0	**1**	**2**	**3**	**4**

6. Does your health department have an explicit annual policy agenda? (prioritize)

_____ Yes _____ No

6.1 If Yes ASK: In your judgment, how adequate is this agenda?

0	**1**	**2**	**3**	**4**
I	I	I	I	I
Not at all adequate	**Some**	**Half**	**Most**	**Fully adequate**

6.2 What agencies participated in the development of your heath department's policy agenda? (Please circle all appropriate responses.)

A) State Government Agencies
B) City/County Government Agencies
C) Nonprofit/Community Agencies
D) Hospitals
E) MDs/Private Clinics
F) Community/Migrant Health Centers (Section 329/330 Agencies)
G) Universities
H) Federal Agencies
I) Others (specify) ______________________________

6.3 On a scale of 0–4, representing the total performance for preparing this agenda, please indicate the share contributed by the local health department:

No contribution				**Provides all the effort**
0	**1**	**2**	**3**	**4**

7. Within the past year have candidates for elective office been advised about your jurisdiction's health status and priorities? (prioritize)

_____ Yes _____ No

7.1 If Yes ASK: How extensive are these advisements?

0	**1**	**2**	**3**	**4**
Not at all	**Some**	**Half**	**Most**	**The need is met**

7.2 What agencies have given such advisements for your jurisdiction? (Please circle all appropriate responses.)

A) State Government Agencies
B) City/County Government Agencies
C) Nonprofit/Community Agencies
D) Hospitals
E) MDs/Private Clinics
F) Community/Migrant Health Centers (Section 329/330 Agencies)
G) Universities
H) Federal Agencies
I) Others (specify) ______________________________

7.3 On the scale below, representing the total performance for initiating these advisements, please indicate the share contributed by the local health department:

None				**All**
0	**1**	**2**	**3**	**4**

8. Does your jurisdiction have available a timely community health action plan that was developed with public and constituency participation? (plan)

_____ Yes _____ No

8.1 If Yes ASK: How adequate is this plan?

0	1	2	3	4
Not at all adequate	**Some**	**Half**	**Most**	**Fully adequate**

8.2 What agencies have developed such a plan for your jurisdiction? (Please circle all appropriate responses.)

A) State Government Agencies
B) City / County Government Agencies
C) Nonprofit / Community Agencies
D) Hospitals
E) MDs / Private Clinics
F) Community / Migrant Health Centers (Section 329 / 330 Agencies)
G) Universities
H) Federal Agencies
I) Others (specify) ______________________________

8.3 On the scale below, representing the total performance in developing this plan, please indicate the share contributed by the local health department:

None				**All**
0	1	2	3	4

9. Are reports on local health needs, resources, and priorities regularly shared among state, regional, and local health boards and administrators? (plan)

_____ Yes _____ No

9.1 If Yes ASK: How complete is the sharing of these reports?

0	1	2	3	4
Not at all	**Some**	**Half**	**Most**	**The need is met**

9.2 What agencies initiate the sharing of these reports for your jurisdiction? (Please circle all appropriate responses.)

A) State Government Agencies
B) City / County Government Agencies
C) Nonprofit / Community Agencies
D) Hospitals
E) MDs / Private Clinics
F) Community / Migrant Health Centers (Section 329 / 330 Agencies)
G) Universities
H) Federal Agencies
I) Others (specify) ______________________________

9.3 On a scale of 0–4, representing the total initiative for sharing these reports, please indicate the contribution by the local health department:

None				**All**
0	1	2	3	4

10. Within your jurisdiction are there agreements in writing among financing and provider agencies in order to define shared power and function? (plan)

_____ Yes _____ No

10.1 If Yes ASK: How functional are these agreements?

0	1	2	3	4
Not at all	**Some**	**Half**	**Most**	**Fully operative**

10.2 What agencies are involved in such agreements for your jurisdiction? (Please circle all appropriate responses.)

A) State Government Agencies
B) City/County Government Agencies
C) Nonprofit/Community Agencies
D) Hospitals
E) MDs/Private Clinics
F) Community/Migrant Health Centers (Section 329/330 Agencies)
G) Universities
H) Federal Agencies
I) Others (specify) ______________________________

10.3 On the scale below, please indicate the extent the local health department promotes such agreements:

Not at all				**Prime mover**
0	1	2	3	4

III. Assurance

1. In the past three years, have health codes which apply to your jurisdiction been reviewed to assure they were up to date? (manage)

_____ Yes _____ No

1.1 If Yes ASK: How rigorous is this program?

0	1	2	3	4
Not at all	**Some**	**Half**	**Most**	**The need is met**

1.2 What agencies perform this function for your jurisdiction? (Please circle all appropriate responses.)

A) State Government Agencies
B) City/County Government Agencies
C) Nonprofit/Community Agencies
D) Hospitals
E) MDs/Private Clinics
F) Community/Migrant Health Centers (Section 329/330 Agencies)
G) Universities
H) Federal Agencies
I) Others (specify) ______________________________

1.3 On the scale below, representing total performance for maintaining local health codes, please indicate the share contributed by the local health department:

None				**All**
0	1	2	3	4

2. In the past three years in your jurisdiction, have public health services been reviewed to assure they comply with applicable professional and regulatory standards? (manage)

_____ Yes _____ No

2.1 If Yes ASK: In your judgment, how thorough are these monitoring activities?

0	1	2	3	4
Not at all	Some	Half	Most	The need is met

2.2 What agencies conduct such reviews in your jurisdiction?
(Please circle all appropriate responses.)

A) State Government Agencies
B) City/County Government Agencies
C) Nonprofit/Community Agencies
D) Hospitals
E) MDs/Private Clinics
F) Community/Migrant Health Centers (Section 329/330 Agencies)
G) Universities
H) Federal Agencies
I) Others (specify) ____________________

2.3 On the scale below, representing the total performance of these reviews, please indicate the contribution by the local health department:

None				All
0	1	2	3	4

3. In the past year in your jurisdiction, has there been a program to assure environmental safety? (implement)

_____ Yes _____ No

3.1 If Yes ASK: In your judgment, how adequate are these programs?

0	1	2	3	4
Not at all	Some	Half	Most	The need is met

3.2 What agencies perform these functions in your jurisdiction?
(Please circle all appropriate responses.)

A) State Government Agencies
B) City/County Government Agencies
C) Nonprofit/Community Agencies
D) Hospitals
E) MDs/Private Clinics
F) Community/Migrant Health Centers (Section 329/330 Agencies)
G) Universities
H) Federal Agencies
I) Others (specify)

3.3 On the scale below, please indicate the relative contribution by the local health department to environmental safety:

None				All
0	1	2	3	4

For the following survey items in the appropriate column, please indicate with a ✓ if this system or service is: 1) available for your jurisdiction; 2) provided by your health department, and/or 3) other agencies serving your jurisdiction; and 4) if the need for this system/service is fully met. If any of these services are provided by other agencies, please fill in the corresponding letter for these agencies in column V, using the key located at the bottom of the page.

4. Is your community served by a system for inspection and licensure of: (implement)

System/Service	I Available for Entire Jurisdiction ✓	II Available Available from LHD ✓	III from Other Agencies ✓	IV The Need Is Met ✓	V Other Agency(ies) (Use Key) ✓
a. Food and milk control	____	____	____	____	____________
b. Health facility safety/quality	____	____	____	____	____________
c. Recreational facility safety/quality	____	____	____	____	____________
d. Compliance with restaurant standards	____	____	____	____	____________

5. Is your community served by any of the following forms of health education? (implement)

System/Service	I	II	III	IV	V
a. HIV Prevention program	____	____	____	____	____________
b. Family Life Education in schools	____	____	____	____	____________

Key: Other Agencies

A) State Government
B) City/County Government Agencies
C) Nonprofit/Community Agencies
D) Hospitals
E) MDs/Private Clinics
F) Community/Migrant Health Centers (Section 329/330 Agencies)
G) Universities
H) Federal Agencies
I) Other (specify)

6. In the past year in your jurisdiction, has there been a program to assure access to basic personal health services for those unable to afford them? (implement)

_____ Yes   _____ No

6.1 If Yes ASK: In your judgment, how adequate are these services?

0	1	2	3	4
Not at all	**Some**	**Half**	**Most**	**The need is met**

6.2 What agencies perform these services in your jurisdiction?
(Please circle all appropriate responses.)

A) State Government Agencies
B) City/County Government Agencies
C) Nonprofit/Community Agencies
D) Hospitals
E) MDs/Private Clinics
F) Community/Migrant Health Centers (Section 329/330 Agencies)
G) Universities
H) Federal Agencies
I) Others (specify)

6.3 On the scale below, representing the total performance of this function, please indicate the contribution by the local health department:

None				**All**
0	1	2	3	4

The following is a list of possible programs which may exist in your jurisdiction. For each program, please indicate with a ✓ whether this service is currently provided by your local health department and/or other agencies. If the service is provided for your jurisdiction by another agency or agencies, please fill in the corresponding letters for those agencies, using the key located at the bottom of the page.

Indicate with a ✓ if the need for this service is fully met.

7. Is the jurisdiction served by programs to provide environmental protection in the following areas? (implement)

Service	Provided by or through Health Dept ✓	Provided by Other Agency(ies) ✓	Other Agency(ies) (Use Key)	The Need Is Met ✓
a. Air quality control	___	___	___	___
b. Hazardous waste management	___	___	___	___
c. Individual water supply management	___	___	___	___
d. Occupational health and safety	___	___	___	___
e. Water supply safety	___	___	___	___
f. Radiation control	___	___	___	___
g. Sewage disposal systems	___	___	___	___
h. Solid waste management	___	___	___	___
i. Vector and animal control	___	___	___	___
j. Water pollution control	___	___	___	___

Key: Other Agencies
A) State Government
B) City/County Government Agencies
C) Nonprofit/Community Agencies
D) Hospitals
E) MDs/Private Clinics
F) Community/Migrant Health Centers (Section 329/330 Agencies)
G) Universities
H) Federal Agencies
I) Other (specify)

8. Is the jurisdiction served by programs to provide personal health services in the following areas? (implement)

Service	Provided by or through Health Dept ✓	Provided by Other Agency(ies) ✓	Other Agency(ies) (Use Key)	The Need Is Met ✓
a. AIDS testing and counseling	____	____	____________	____
b. Well-child preventive care	____	____	____________	____
c. Dental health prophylaxis screening and treatment or referral	____	____	____________	____
d. Drug abuse treatment	____	____	____________	____
e. Emergency medical services	____	____	____________	____
f. Family planning	____	____	____________	____
g. Home health care	____	____	____________	____
h. Immunizations	____	____	____________	____
i. Mental health services	____	____	____________	____
j. Prenatal care	____	____	____________	____
k. Sexually transmitted diseases diagnosis and treatment	____	____	____________	____
l. Tuberculosis diagnosis and treatment	____	____	____________	____

Key: Other Agencies

A) State Government
B) City/County Government Agencies
C) Nonprofit/Community Agencies
D) Hospitals
E) MDs/Private Clinics
F) Community/Migrant Health Centers (Section 329/330 Agencies)
G) Universities
H) Federal Agencies
I) Other (specify)

9. In the past year in your jurisdiction, has there been any evaluation of the effect that public health services have on community health? (evaluate)

_____ Yes _____ No

9.1 If Yes ASK: In your judgment, how adequate are these assessments?

0	1	2	3	4
Not at all	Some	Half	Most	The need is met

9.2 What agencies conduct such assessments for your jurisdiction? (Please circle all appropriate responses.)

A) State Government Agencies
B) City/County Government Agencies
C) Nonprofit/Community Agencies
D) Hospitals
E) MDs/Private Clinics
F) Community/Migrant Health Centers (Section 329/330 Agencies)
G) Universities
H) Federal Agencies
I) Others (specify)

9.3 On the scale below, representing the total performance of these assessments, please indicate the contribution by the local health department:

None				All
0	1	2	3	4

10. In the past year in your jurisdiction, has there been any evaluation of the effect that budget changes for your health department would have on public health problems? (evaluate)

_____ Yes _____ No

10.1 If Yes ASK: In your judgment, how adequate is this assessment?

0	1	2	3	4
Not at all	Some	Half	Most	The need is met

10.2 What agencies conduct such assessments for your jurisdiction? (Please circle all appropriate responses.)

A) State Government Agencies
B) City/County Government Agencies
C) Nonprofit/Community Agencies
D) Hospitals
E) MDs/Private Clinics
F) Community/Migrant Health Centers (Section 329/330 Agencies)
G) Universities
H) Federal Agencies
I) Others (specify)

10.3 On the scale below, representing the total performance of these assessments, please indicate the contribution by the local health department:

None				All
|	|	|	|	|
0	1	2	3	4

11. Is a process in place to inform the public about the current health status of the community? (inform and educate)

_____ Yes _____ No

11.1 If Yes ASK: In your judgment, how adequate is this process?

0	1	2	3	4
|	|	|	|	|
Not at all	**Some**	**Half**	**Most**	**The need is met**

11.2 What agencies have implemented such a process in your jurisdiction? (Please circle all appropriate responses.)

A) State Government Agencies
B) City/County Government Agencies
C) Nonprofit/Community Agencies
D) Hospitals
E) MDs/Private Clinics
F) Community/Migrant Health Centers (Section 329/330 Agencies)
G) Universities
H) Federal Agencies
I) Others (specify)

11.3 On the scale below, representing the total performance of this process, please indicate the contribution by the local health department:

None				All
|	|	|	|	|
0	1	2	3	4

12. Are reports on health status and programs regularly prepared and disseminated to the local media? (inform and educate)

_____ Yes _____ No

12.1 If Yes ASK: Are these reports published?

0	1	2	3	4
|	|	|	|	|
Not at all	**Some**	**Half**	**Most**	**The need is met**

12.2 What agencies regularly provide such reports to the media for your jurisdiction? (Please circle all appropriate responses.)

A) State Government Agencies
B) City/County Government Agencies
C) Nonprofit/Community Agencies
D) Hospitals
E) MDs/Private Clinics
F) Community/Migrant Health Centers (Section 329/330 Agencies)

G) Universities
H) Federal Agencies
I) Others (specify)

12.3 On a scale of 0–4, representing the total performance of this function, please indicate the contribution by the local health department:

None				All
0	1	2	3	4

That is all of the questions we have. Thank you for your time and the important responses you have given. These data will be very helpful in our attempts to characterize the public health system at the local level.

Appendix B

Scoring for Local Public Health Assessment Survey

The following are instructions intended to assist in scoring the Local Public Health Assessment Survey (Revised March, 1994). Along with definitions of terms and directions for scoring are examples of scoring of indicators, as well as scoring sheets and a graphic profile of a hypothetical jurisdiction and local health department (LHD). Finally, blank scoring sheets and a blank graph are included to facilitate scoring.

There are two types of indicators used in the survey: general and specific. General indicators are those that are in the four-part format and refer to broad descriptions of performance. Specific indicators are those which are in the checklist format and refer to particular designations of program content. Each of these indicators are scored differently and will be discussed separately below.

We appreciate your interest in the survey. If you make use of it we would be pleased to learn of your experience. If you require clarification on the administration or scoring of the survey please call (919) 966-3807.

Definitions for Core Public Health Functions and Practices[1,2]

Assessment: The regular systematic collection, assembly, analysis and dissemination of information on the health of the community. Assessment practices are specifically:

Assess the health needs of the community.
Investigate the occurrence of health effects and health hazards in the community.
Analyze the determinants of identified health needs.

Policy development: The exercise of the responsibility to serve the public interest in the development of comprehensive public health policies by promoting the use of scientific knowledge base in decision making. Policy development practices are specifically:

Advocate for public health, build constituencies and identify resources in the community.
Set priorities among health needs.
Develop plans and policies to address priority health needs.

Assurance: The assurance to constituents that services necessary to achieve agreed-upon goals are provided by encouraging actions of others (private or public), requiring action through regulation, or providing service directly. Assurance practices are specifically:

Manage resources and develop organizational structure.
Implement programs.
Evaluate programs and provide quality assurance.
Inform and educate the public.

References

1. Dyal WW. *Public Health Infrastructure and Organizational Practice Definitions.* Atlanta, Ga: Division of Public Health Systems, Public Health Practice Program Office, Centers for Disease Control and Prevention; August 22, 1991.
2. Turnock B, Handler A. *Surveillance of Effective Public Health Practice. Preliminary and Draft Set of Performance Standards and Performance Indicators.* Chicago, Ill: School of Public Health, University of Illinois at Chicago; June 1992.

Instructions for Scoring

The indicators are distributed among the three public health functions and ten practices as follows:

	Indicators:	
	General	Specific
I. Assessment Function		
Assess (Nos. 1, 2, 3)	3	–
Investigate (Nos. 4, 5, 6 ,9)	3	7
Analyze (Nos. 7, 8, 10, 11)	2	23
II. Policy Development		
Advocate/Constituency Building (Nos. 1, 2, 3, 4)	4	–
Set Priorities (Nos. 5, 6, 7)	3	–
Plan (Nos. 8, 9, 10)	3	–
III. Assurance		
Manage (Nos. 1, 2)	2	–
Implement (Nos. 3, 4, 5, 6, 7, 8)	2	28
Evaluate (Nos. 9, 10)	2	–
Inform and Educate (Nos. 11, 12)	2	–

Scores can be calculated for each function and practice, as well as for public health performance overall. Responses to the survey result in two separate sets of scores, those for the jurisdiction as a whole, and those indicating the extent to which efforts were provided by the local health department. Because some practices are linked with more indicators than others, scores are never reported in raw numbers but as proportions of a possible perfect score, calculated separately for each practice. Practice scores are aggregated into function and overall scores.

Both general and specific indicators allow for the identification of other agencies involved in the given activity to be identified, using the key provided.

General Indicators:

Jurisdictional performance. A maximum possible jurisdictional score for each general indicator is 40 points. Jurisdictional scores for each general indicator are determined by responses to the adequacy scale attached to each indicator:

	Not at All	Some	Half	Most	Fully Adequate
	|	|	|	|	|
Jurisdictional points:	0	10	20	30	40

Health department performance. The local health department's performance is estimated for general indicators from the scale which assigns a proportion to the LHDs contribution to the total adequacy of the jurisdiction's performance for that indicator. For each general indicator:

	None				All
	|	|	|	|	|
LHD contribution:	0	25%	50%	75%	100%

To calculate the LHD score for general indicators, multiply the jurisdictional score by the percent of LHD contribution. The LHD score is an indication of the portion of jurisdictional effort which is contributed by the LHD.

Example of General Indicator Scoring:

The two general indicators associated with the Inform/Educate practice (found on pages 37-38 of the Survey) will be used to demonstrate indicator scoring and deriving a practice score. Arbitrary responses will be shown to serve as examples.

11. Is a process in place to inform the public about the current health status of the community? (inform and educate)
_____ Yes _____ No

11.1 If Yes ASK: In your judgment, how adequate is this process?

0	1	2	3	4
Not at all	**Some**	**Half**	**Most**	**The need is met**

11.2 What agencies have implemented such a process in your jurisdiction? (Please circle all appropriate responses.)
A) State Government Agencies
B) City/County Government Agencies
C) Nonprofit/Community Agencies
D) Hospitals
E) MDs/Private Clinics
F) Community/Migrant Health Centers (Section 329/330 Agencies)
G) Universities
H) Federal Agencies
I) Others (specify)

11.3 On the scale below, representing the total performance of this process, please indicate the contribution by the local health department:

None				**All**
0	1	2	3	4

12. Are reports on health status and programs regularly prepared and disseminated to the local media? (inform and educate)
_____ Yes _____ No

12.1 If Yes ASK: Are these reports published?

0	1	2	3	4
Not at all	**Some**	**Half**	**Most**	**The need is met**

12.2 What agencies regularly provide such reports to the media for your jurisdiction? (Please circle all appropriate responses.)
A) State Government Agencies
B) City/County Government Agencies
C) Nonprofit/Community Agencies
D) Hospitals
E) MDs/Private Clinics
F) Community/Migrant Health Centers (Section 329/330 Agencies)
G) Universities
H) Federal Agencies
I) Others (specify)

12.3 On a scale of 0–4, representing the total performance of this function, please indicate the contribution by the local health department:

None				**All**
0	1	2	3	4

In this example, the response to question 11 was "yes," a process is in place to inform the public about the current health status of the community. As is indicated by the response to 11.1, this process is considered to be adequate most of the time. The #3 is assigned 30 jurisdictional points - this is the jurisdictional score for this indicator. Finally, as is indicated by the response to 11.3, the LHD is considered to contribute half of this effort. The #2 is assigned the value of 50%. To calculate the LHD score for this indicator, multiply the jurisdictional points time 50%: 30 + .50 = 15. The agencies outside of the LHD which are also involved in implementing the informing process are indicated in 11.2, in this case B and C (City/County Government Agencies, and Non-profit/Community Agencies).

The response to question 12 was also "yes," reports on health status and programs are regularly prepared and disseminated to the local media. (NOTE—if the answer to a general indicator is "no," both jurisdictional and LHD scores = 0.) This process is considered adequate half of the time, so the jurisdictional score is 20. All of the effort is contributed by the LHD, so the LHD score is 20 + 100% = 20. Since all of the effort was contributed by the LHD, no other agencies were involved, and there is no response to 12.2.

To calculate the inform/educate jurisdictional practice score, add the jurisdictional scores for the corresponding indicators and divide by the total possible points for those indicators. The jurisdictional scores for questions 11 and 12 equal 50, and the total possible points is 80 (the maximum possible score for a general indicator is 40), so the jurisdictional inform/educate practice score is 50/80 = 0.63.

Follow the same process to calculate the LHD practice score. The LHD scores totaled 35, and there were again 80 possible points, so the LHD inform/educate practice score is 35/80 = 0.44.

Specific Indicators:

Jurisdictional performance. A maximum possible jurisdictional score for each specific indicator is 10 points. Jurisdictional performance is scored based on the extent to which community need is met, regardless of provider. Full points are given if the column "the need is met" is checked. Partial points are given if "the need is met" is not checked, but the service is available from either the LHD, other agencies, or both. No points are awarded if none of columns II, III, or IV are checked. Column I is not considered when scoring.

The specific indicators for jurisdictional performance are scored on the following three-point scale:

Need met (regardless of provider) = 10 points
Need not met but service available somewhere = 5 points
Need not met and no agency providing service = 0 points

Health department performance. A maximum possible LHD score for each specific indicator is also 10 points. LHD scoring is similar to jurisdictional scoring, with the exception that partial points are only awarded if community need is not met and the service that is available is provided by the LHD, and no points are awarded if community need is not met and the LHD offers no service.

Specific indicators for LHD performance are scored on the following three-point scale:

Need met (regardless of provider) = 10 points
Need not met and LHD offers service = 5 points
Need not met and LHD offers no service = 0 points

As a rule of thumb, if "the need is met" is checked, then both the jurisdictional and LHD scores will be 10. If it is not checked, neither will be 10.

This scoring practice is consistent with the assurance concept of public health practice.

Example of Specific Indicator Scoring:

4. Is your community served by a system for inspection and licensure of: (implement)

	I Indicator Available for Entire Jurisdiction ✓	II Available from LHD ✓	III Available from Other Agencies ✓	IV The Need for Data Is Met ✓	V Other Agency(ies) (Use Key)
a. Food and milk control	____	____	____	____	____________ ____________
b. Health facility safety / quality	____	____	____	____	____________ ____________
c. Recreational facility safety / quality	____	____	____	____	____________ ____________
d. Compliance with restaurant standards	____	____	____	____	____________ ____________

Key: Other Agencies

A) State Government
B) City / County Government Agencies
C) Nonprofit / Community Agencies
D) Hospitals
E) MDs / Private Clinics
F) Community / Migrant Health Centers (Section 329 / 330 Agencies)
G) Universities
H) Federal Agencies
I) Other (specify)

In this example, "the need is met" is checked for both a and b, so both jurisdictional and LHD scores for these indicators 10. "The need is met" is not checked for either c or d, so neither scores for these indicators will be 10. The only column checked for c is "available from LHD." In this case both scores are 5, the LHD score because it provides the inspection and licensing in question, and the jurisdictional score because that service is provided within the jurisdiction by some agency. "Available form other agencies" is checked for d. In this case, the jurisdictional score is 5 because the service is provided within the jurisdiction, and the LHD score is 0 because the LHD does not provide the service. Again, the check in column I does not affect the scoring.

The other agencies involved in providing the service addressed in the indicators were identified in column V for a, b, and d, those indicators for which the service was checked as being "available from other agencies." As with the general indicators, a key was used to identify these other providers.

A practice score cannot be calculated in this example because the question provided is only part one of the indicators used to assess performance with regard to the implement practice. The scores for this indicator would be added to the those for the other implement indicators (nos. 3, 5, 6, 7, and 8), and divided by the total possible points for all indicators combined (40 for each general indicator, 10 for each specific indicator, totaling 360 for the implement practice).

Final Score:

Two aggregate scores are calculated, one for the jurisdiction / community (x) and the other for the health department (y). Both scores are calculated as means of the respective proportional scores or performance ratios for the separate practices:

x = jurisdiction / community coverage
y = health department performance

Caution should be exercised not to report the y score (health department performance) independent of the x score (jurisdiction/community coverage). A community might be well protected by public health activity derived, for example, from regional or state levels, even with low levels of performance by the local health department. Important regional differences will pertain.

If scores are accumulated from a national sample of LHDs, or from a given department over time, useful comparisons and trends may be revealed.

Example—Practice, Function and Overall Scores for a Hypothetical Jurisdiction/LHD

The following pages provide examples of scoring and the resulting graphic profile for a hypothetical jurisdiction and local health department. The total possible points for each practice as well as the raw scores given per practice are provided, and the performance ratio is calculated. These are aggregated into function scores, as well as overall scores. These steps are illustrated separately for the jurisdiction as a whole, and the LHD. Blank scoring sheets and graph are provided, to be copied for use. The scoring sheets used in the hypothetical example are for totaling practice and function scores (referred to as ratios on the scoring sheets). There are additional blank scoring sheets provided that were not used with the hypothetical example to facilitate the scoring of each practice and function.

Score Sheet for Hypothetical Jurisdiction/Local Health Department

For Jurisdiction:

	Possible Points	Actual Raw Score	Performance Ratio
I. Assessment			
Assess	120	110	.92
Investigate	190	150	.79
Analyze	310	270	.87
	620	530	.85
II. Policy Development			
Advocate/build constituency	160	80	.50
Prioritize	120	90	.75
Plan	120	90	.75
	400	260	.67
III. Assurance			
Manage	80	70	.88
Implement	360	320	.89
Evaluate	80	60	.75
Inform and educate	80	70	.88
	600	520	.87

Overall Jurisdictional Score = total actual raw jurisdictional scores 1310 / 1620 = 0.81

Score Sheet for Hypothetical Jurisdiction/Local Health Department (cont.)

For Local Health Department:

	Possible Points	Actual Raw Score	Performance Ratio
I. Assessment			
Assess	120	60	.50
Investigate	190	100	.53
Analyze	310	220	.71
	620	380	.61
II. Policy Development			
Advocate/build constituency	160	80	.50
Prioritize	120	90	.75
Plan	120	80	.67
	400	250	.63
III. Assurance			
Manage	80	70	.88
Implement	360	180	.50
Evaluate	80	30	.38
Inform and educate	80	20	.25
	600	300	.50

Overall LHD Score = total actual raw LHD scores 930 / 1620 = 0.57

Overall scores for public health performance (calculated as the means of all practice performance ratios) are as follows for the hypothetical jurisdiction/local health department:

Community/Jurisdiction (x)	.81
Local Health Department (y)	.57

Interpretation:

The jurisdiction is well served by public health functions (81% of maximum performance) and most of this is rendered by the local public health department (57% of maximum performance). Policy Development is less well implemented than Assessment and Assurance. Of all public health practices performed in this hypothetical community, 70% (.57/.81) is rendered by the official public health agency. Assessment functions are contributed substantially by the work of the state health department; assurance performance is facilitated by the work of community health centers and volunteer community groups.

A profile of the survey's findings might be represented graphically as follows. Note that for the practices of advocate, prioritize and manage, the health department is reported to provide 100 percent of effort, and thus no other agencies are reported on the graphic profile to be involved.

Score Sheet for Local Health Department Assessment Survey (Rev. 3/94)

I. Assessment Function

	Possible	Raw Scores:		Ratios:	
	Points	Jurisdiction	LHD	Jurisdiction	LHD
Assess:					
Q1	40				
Q2	40				
Q3	<u>40</u>	____	____	____	____
	120				
Investigate:					
Q4	40				
Q5	40				
Q6	40				
Q9	<u>40</u>	____	____	____	____
	160				
Analyze:					
Q7	40				
Q8	40				
Q10	130				
Q11	<u>100</u>	____	____	____	____
	160				
Assessment Total:	620				

II. Policy Development Function

	Possible	Raw Scores:		Ratios:	
	Points	Jurisdiction	LHD	Jurisdiction	LHD
Advocate:					
Q1	40				
Q2	40				
Q3	40				
Q4	<u>40</u>	____	____	____	____
	160				
Prioritize:					
Q5	40				
Q6	40				
Q7	<u>40</u>	____	____	____	____
	120				
Plan:					
Q8	40				
Q9	40				
Q10	<u>40</u>	____	____	____	____
	120				
Policy Development Total:		400			

Score Sheet for Local Health Department Assessment Survey (con't)

III. Assurance Function

	Possible Points	Raw Scores: Jurisdiction	Raw Scores: LHD	Ratios: Jurisdiction	Ratios: LHD
Manage:					
Q1	40				
Q2	40	_____	_____	_____	_____
	80				
Implement:					
Q3	40				
Q4	40				
Q5	20				
Q6	40				
Q7	100				
Q8	120	_____	_____	_____	_____
	360				
Evaluate:					
Q9	40				
Q10	40	_____	_____	_____	_____
	80				
Inform/Educate:					
Q11	40				
Q12	40	_____	_____	_____	_____
	80				
Assurance Total:	600				

For Jurisdiction:

	Possible Points	Actual Raw Score	Performance Ratio
I. Assessment			
Assess	120		
Investigate	190		
Analyze	310	_____	_____
	620		
II. Policy Development			
Advocate/build constituency	160		
Prioritize	120		
Plan	120	_____	_____
	400		

Score Sheet for Local Health Department Assessment Survey (con't)

	Possible Points	Actual Raw Score	Performance Ratio
III. Assurance			
Manage	80		
Implement	360		
Evaluate	80		
Inform and educate	80	_____	_____
	600		

Overall Jurisdictional Score = total actual raw jurisdictional scores / 1620 = 0._______

For Local Health Department:

	Possible Points	Actual Raw Score	Performance Ratio
I. Assessment			
Assess	120		
Investigate	190		
Analyze	310	_____	_____
	620		
II. Policy Development			
Advocate/build constituency	160		
Prioritize	120		
Plan	120	_____	_____
	400		
III. Assurance			
Manage	80		
Implement	360		
Evaluate	80		
Inform and educate	80	_____	_____
	600		

Overall LHD Score = total actual raw LHD score / 1620 = 0._______

Appendix C

Twenty Merged Indicators of Local Public Health Performance

Assessment

1. For the jurisdiction served by your local health department, is there a community needs assessment process that systematically describes the prevailing health status in your community?
2. In the past three years in your jurisdiction, has the local public health agency surveyed the population for behavioral risk factors?
3. For the jurisdiction served by your local health agency, are timely investigations of adverse health events, including communicable disease outbreaks and environment health hazards, conducted on a ongoing basis?
4. Are the necessary laboratory services available to the local public health agency to support investigations of adverse health events and meet routine diagnostic and surveillance needs?
5. For the jurisdiction served by your local public health agency, has an analysis been completed of the determinants and contributing factors of priority health needs, adequacy of existing health resources, and the population groups most impacted?
6. In the past three years in your jurisdiction, has the local public health agency conducted an analysis of age-specific participation in preventive and screening services?

Policy Development

7. For the jurisdiction served by your local public health agency, is there a network of support and communication relationships which includes health-related organizations, the media, and the general public?
8. In the past year in your jurisdiction, has there been a formal attempt by the local public health agency at informing elected officials about the potential public health impact of decisions under their consideration?
9. For the jurisdiction served by you local public health agency, has there been a prioritization of the community health needs which have been identified from a community needs assessment?
10. In the past three years in your jurisdiction, has the local public health agency implemented community health initiatives consistent with established priorities?
11. For the jurisdiction served by your local public health agency, has a community health action plan been developed with community participation to address priority community health needs?
12. During the past three years in your jurisdiction, has the local public health agency developed plans to allocate resources in a manner consistent with the community health action plan?

Assurance

13. For the jurisdiction served by your local public health agency, have resources been deployed as necessary to address the priority health needs identified in the community health assessments?
14. In the past three years in your jurisdiction, has the local public health agency conducted an organizational self-assessment?
15. For the jurisdiction served by your local public health agency, are age-specific priority health needs effectively addressed through the provision of linkage or appropriate services?
16. In the past three years in your jurisdiction, has there been an instance in which the local public health agency has failed to implement a mandated program or service?
17. For the jurisdiction served by your local public health agency, have there been regular evaluations of the effect that public health services have on community health status?
18. In the past three years in your jurisdiction, has the local public health agency used professionally recognized process and outcome measures to monitor programs and to redirect resources as possible?
19. For the jurisdiction served by your local public health agency, is the public regularly provided with information about current health status, health care needs, positive heal behaviors, and health care policy issues?
20. In the past year in your jurisdiction, has the local public health agency provided reports to the media on a regular basis?

Source: Turnock BJ, Handler AS, Miller CA, 1995 (unpublished).

Appendix D

List of Organizations Contributing Material for Case Studies

Access...MedPlus Health Plan. Memphis, TN
Appalachia II Health District. Greenville, DC
Baptist Memorial Health System. Memphis, TN
Beloit Health Department. Beloit, WI
Beloit Memorial Hospital. Beloit, WI
Blue Care Network of East Michigan. Flint, MI
Capital Medical Center. Olympia, WA
Children's Hospital of Wisconsin. Milwaukee, WI
Children's Hospital. Denver, CO
CIGNA Healthcare of Colorado. Denver, CO
Cincinnati Health Department. Cincinnati, OH
CompCare Health Plan. Milwaukee, WI
Complete Health Plan. Memphis, TN
Contra Costa County Health Department. Martinez, CA
Cortland County Health Department. New Bern, NC
DeanCare Health Plan. Madison, WI
Denver Health and Hospitals. Denver, CO
Flint and Vicinity Action for Economic Development. Flint, MI
Flint Odyssey Health Awareness Center. Flint, MI
Froedtert Memorial Lutheran Hospital. Milwaukee, WI
General Motors, Health Care Initiatives. Flint, MI
Genesee County Bard of Commissioners. Flint, MI
Genesee County Community Action Agency. Flint, MI
Genesee County Health Department. Flint, MI
Genesee County Medical Society. Flint, MI
Genesis Health Pan. Milwaukee, WI
Genesys Health System. Flint, MI
Good Health Plan. Portland, OR
Greater Flint Area Hospital Assembly
Group Health Cooperative of Puget Sound, Olympia District. Olympia, WA
HealthOne System (Columbia/HCA). Denver, CO
HealthPlus of Michigan, Flint, MI
HMO-Colorado (Blue Cross and Blue Shield of Colorado). Denver, CO

HMO-Oregon (Blue Cross and Blue Shield of Oregon). Portland, OR
Hurlay Medical Center. Flint, MI
Kaiser Health Plan of Colorado. Denver, CO
Kaiser Health Plan, Vancouver Medical Center. Vancouver, OR
Kaiser Health Plan, Northwest Division. Portland, OR
Kitsap Physician Services. Olympia WA.
Lane County Health Department. Eugene, OR
LeBonheur Children's Health System. Memphis, TN
Legacy Health Systems. Portland, OR
Managed Health Services. Milwaukee, WI.
Maricopa County Department of Health Services, Division of Public Health. Phoenix, AZ
McLarent Health Care Corporation. Flint, MI
Memphis and Shelby County Community Health Agency. Memphis, TN
Memphis and Shelby County Health Department. Memphis, TN
Mercy Health System. Janesville, WI
MercyCare Health Plan. Janesville, WI
Methodist Health System. Memphis, TN
MetraHealth of Colorado. Denver, CO
Milwaukee Health Department, Milwaukee, WI
Multnomah County Health Department, Portland, OR
Newark Department of Health and Human Services, Health Division, Newark, NJ
National Association of County and City Health Officials. Washington, DC
Oregon Health Sciences University. Portland, OR
PACC Health Plan. Portland, OR
Pacificare Health Plan of Colorado (formerly FHP). Denver, CO
Phoenix Healthcare. Memphis, TN.
Porter Adventist Healthcare. Denver, CO
Portland Adventists Medical Center. Portland, OR
PrimeCare Health Plan. Milwaukee, WI
Provident Saint Anthony Hospital. Denver, CO
Providence Medical Center. Portland, OR
PruCare of Memphis health Plan. Memphis, TN
Qual-Med Plans for Health of Portland. Portland, OR
Qual-Med Plans for Health. Denver, CO
Regional Medical Center at Memphis. Memphis, TN
Restaurant Association of Washington. Olympia, WA
Rock County Health Department. Janesville, WI
Saint Francis Hospital. Memphis, TN
Saint Francis Hospital. Milwaukee, WI
Saint Joseph's Hospital. Denver, CO
Saint Joseph's Hospital. Memphis, TN
Saint Joseph's Hospital. Milwaukee, WI
Saint Mary's Hospital. Milwaukee, WI
Saint Michael Hospital. Milwaukee, WI
Saint Peter's Hospital (Providence Health System). Olympia, WA
Seattle-King County Health Department. Seattle, WA
Sinai Samaritan Hospital. Milwaukee, WI
Southern Health Plan. Memphis, TN
Southwest Washington Health District. Vancouver, WA
Thurston County Community Action Council. Olympia, WA
Thurston County Department of Health and Social Services. Olympia, WA
TLC Family Health Plan. Memphis, TN

Together. Olympia, WA
U-Care Health Plan. Madison, WI
United Auto Workers, Health Care Initiatives. Flint, MI
United States Centers for Disease Control and Prevention, Public Health Practice Program Office. Atlanta, GA
United Way of Thurston County. Olympia, WA
University Hospital. Denver, CO
University of Michigan at Flint. Flint, MI
Wellness Plan. Flint, MI
WHO Health Plan (Humana). Milwaukee, WI
Wisconsin Department of health and Family Services, Division of Health, Bureau of Public Health. Madison, WI.
Wisconsin Independent Physicians' Group. Milwaukee, WI
Yolo County Health Department. Woodland, CA

Index

Note: Page numbers followed by letters *f* and *t* indicate material presented in figures and tables, respectively.

H

I

J

K

L

M

N

O

P

R

S

T

U

W